The Duke Manual of

Pediatric Ophthalmology and Strabismus Surgery

The Duke Manual of Pediatric Ophthalmology and Strabismus Surgery

Laura B. Enyedi, MD
Professor of Ophthalmology and Pediatrics
Duke University
Durham, North Carolina

Nandini Gandhi, MD
Associate Professor of Ophthalmology
University of California Davis
Sacramento, California

Tammy L. Yanovitch, MD, MHSc
Clinical Associate Professor of Ophthalmology
Dean McGee Eye Institute
University of Oklahoma
Oklahoma City, Oklahoma

Wolters Kluwer

Philadelphia • Baltimore • New York • London
Buenos Aires • Hong Kong • Sydney • Tokyo

DukeHealth

Acquisitions Editor: Chris Teja
Development Editor: Eric McDermott
Editorial Coordinator: John Larkin
Marketing Manager: Phyllis Hitner
Production Project Manager: Sadie Buckallew
Design Coordinator: Stephen Druding
Manufacturing Coordinator: Beth Welsh
Prepress Vendor: SPi Global

9 8 7 6 5 4 3 2 1

Printed in China

Cataloging-in-Publication Data available on request from the Publisher

ISBN: 978-1-9751-5806-4

shop.lww.com

CCS1220

This book is dedicated to the many mentors and colleagues who have influenced me throughout my career, the residents who keep things "interesting" in the operating room, and especially to the Duke Pediatric Ophthalmology & Strabismus fellows I have had the honor of training. Their ideas, questions, and example have made me a better clinician, surgeon, teacher, and person, and I feel fortunate to call so many of them dear friends.

—Laura B. Enyedi, MD

Contributors

Natalie A. Afshari, MD
Stuart I. Brown M.D. Chair in Ophthalmology in Memory of Donald P. Shiley
Chief, Division of Cornea and Refractive Surgery
Vice Chair of Education
Shiley Eye Institute
University of California San Diego
La Jolla, CA

Bradley P. Barnett, MD, PhD
Assistant Professor of Ophthalmology
Duke University
Durham, NC

Paramjit K. Bhullar, MD
Resident in Ophthalmology
Duke University
Durham, NC

Derek Bitner, MD
Pediatric Ophthalmologist and Strabismus Specialist
Wolfe Eye Clinic
West Des Moines, IA

Charles J. Bock Jr, MD
Comprehensive and Pediatric Ophthalmologist and Strabismus Specialist
Randall Children's Hospital
Portland, OR

Brenda L. Bohnsack, MD, PhD
Lillian Sherman Cowen Rieger and Harold L.S. Cowen Research Professor in Pediatric Ophthalmology
Division Head, Ophthalmology
Ann & Robert H. Lurie Children's Hospital of Chicago
Northwestern University Feinberg School of Medicine
Chicago, IL

Lucas Bonafede, MD
Pediatric and Comprehensive Ophthalmologist and Strabismus Specialist
Fraser Eye Care Center
Fraser, MI

Michelle T. Cabrera, MD
Associate Professor of Ophthalmology
Chief, Division of Pediatric Ophthalmology
University of Washington
Seattle Children's Hospital
Seattle, WA

Arthika Chandramohan, MD, MPH
Clinical Fellow in Ophthalmology
University of Washington
Seattle, WA

Dinah Chen, MD
Resident in Ophthalmology
NYU Langone Medical Center
New York, NY

Xi Chen, MD, PhD
Assistant Professor of Ophthalmology
Duke University
Durham, NC

Melissa B. Daluvoy, MD
Assistant Professor of Ophthalmology
Duke University
Durham, NC

Ryan E. Davis, MD
Assistant Professor of Surgery
Uniformed Services University of the Health Sciences
Chief of Pediatric Ophthalmology
Wilford Hall Eye Center
San Antonio, TX

Derek W. DelMonte, MD
Assistant Professor of Ophthalmology
University of Colorado School of Medicine
Aurora, CO

Eniolami O. Dosunmu, MD
Assistant Professor of Ophthalmology
University of Cincinnati
Assistant Professor of Pediatric Ophthalmology and Strabismus
Cincinnati Children's Hospital Medical Center
Cincinnati, OH

Jared E. Duncan, MD
Pediatric Ophthalmologist and Strabismus Specialist
Ophthalmology Associates of Greater Annapolis
Arnold, MD
Department of Ophthalmology
Anne Arundel Medical Center
Annapolis, MD

Mays A. El-Dairi, MD
Associate Professor of Ophthalmology
Duke University
Durham, NC

Amanda L. Ely, MD
Assistant Professor of Ophthalmology
Penn State Eye Center
Hershey, PA

Laura B. Enyedi, MD
Professor of Ophthalmology and Pediatrics
Duke University
Durham, NC

Meghan S. Flemmons, MD
Assistant Professor of Ophthalmology
Vanderbilt University Medical Center
Nashville, TN

Sharon F. Freedman, MD
Professor of Ophthalmology and Pediatrics
Chief, Division of Pediatric Ophthalmology and Strabismus
Duke University
Durham, NC

Tamiesha Frempong, MD, MPH
Assistant Director of Ophthalmology
New York Eye & Ear Infirmary of Mt. Sinai
Vice Chair of Diversity and Inclusion
Mount Sinai Hospital
New York, NY

Matthew D. Gearinger, MD
Professor of Ophthalmology and Pediatrics
Flaum Eye Institute
Rochester, NY

Fatema Ghasia, MD
Associate Professor of Ophthalmology
Director of Vision Neurosciences and Ocular Motility Lab
Cleveland Clinic Lerner College of Medicine of Case Western Reserve University
Cleveland, OH

Tanya Glaser, MD
Clinical Associate Ophthalmology
Duke University
Durham, NC

Michelle S. Go, MD
Assistant Professor of Ophthalmology
University of North Carolina
Chapel Hill, NC

Maria Gomez-Caraballo, BA
Medical Student
Duke University School of Medicine
Durham, NC

Sara Fransen Grace, MD
Pediatric Ophthalmologist and Strabismus Specialist
North Carolina Eye Ear Nose & Throat and Duke Health
Durham, NC

Dilraj S. Grewal, MD
Associate Professor of Ophthalmology
Duke University
Durham, NC

Martha A. Howard, MD
Assistant Professor of Visual Science and Ophthalmology
Interim Director, Pediatric Ophthalmology and Strabismus
Yale School of Medicine
New Haven, CT

Jeffrey S. Hunter, MD
Clinical Professor of Ophthalmology
University of Texas Health Science Center -Tyler
Tyler, TX

Jing Jin, MD, PhD
Assistant Professor of Ophthalmology
Sidney Kimmel Medical College at Thomas Jefferson University
Philadelphia, PA
Pediatric Ophthalmologist
Nemours Alfred I. duPont Hospital for Children
Wilmington, DE

Kim Jiramongkolchai, MD
Assistant Professor of Ophthalmology
Wilmer Eye Institute
Johns Hopkins University
Baltimore, MD

Namita Kashyap, CO
Orthoptist
Duke University
Durham, NC

Jagger C. Koerner, MD, MBA
Assistant Professor of Ophthalmology and Pediatrics
Wake Forest Baptist Health
Winston-Salem, NC

Daniel J. Lattin, MD, MS
Courtesy Assistant Professor of Ophthalmology
University of Florida College of Medicine Jacksonville
Nemours Children's Specialty Care
Jacksonville, FL

Megan X. Law, MD
Pediatric Ophthalmologist and Strabismus Specialist
Houston Eye Associates
Houston, TX

HongVan Le, MD
Assistant Professor of Ophthalmology
University of Mississippi Medical Center
Jackson, MS

Andrew R. Lee, MD
Assistant Professor of Ophthalmology and Visual Sciences
Washington University School of Medicine
St. Louis, MO

Maria E. Lim, MD
Clinical Assistant Professor of Ophthalmology
Dean McGee Eye Institute
University of Oklahoma
Oklahoma City, OK

Alice A. Lin, MD
Comprehensive and Pediatric Ophthalmologist and Strabismus Specialist
Raleigh Eye Center
Raleigh, NC

Jason A. Liss, MD
Assistant Professor of Ophthalmology
Duke University
Durham, NC

Yasmin Poustchi Mali, MD
Assistant Professor of Ophthalmology
Lake Erie College of Osteopathic Medicine
Bradenton, FL

Miguel A. Materin, MD
Professor of Ophthalmology and Radiation Oncology
Director Ocular Oncology
Duke University
Durham, NC

Elliot C. McKee, MD
Pediatric Ophthalmologist and Strabismus Specialist
Charlotte Eye Ear Nose and Throat Associates, PA
Charlotte, NC

Prithvi Mruthyunjaya, MD, MHS
Associate Professor of Ophthalmology
Director Ocular Oncology
Byers Eye Institute
Stanford University
Stanford, CA

Mae Millicent W. Peterseim, MD
Professor of Ophthalmology
Bruce Pratt Endowed Chair for International Ophthalmology
Storm Eye Institute
Medical University of South Carolina
Charleston, SC

S. Grace Prakalapakorn, MD, MPH
Associate Professor of Ophthalmology and Pediatrics
Affiliate Faculty Duke Global Health Institute
Duke University
Durham, NC

Roshni Ranjit-Reeves, MD
Assistant Consulting Professor of Ophthalmology
Duke University
Winston-Salem, NC

Michael J. Richard, MD
Assistant Clinical Professor of Ophthalmology
Duke University
Durham, NC

Ricardo E. Rodríguez-Rosa, MD
Assistant Professor of Ophthalmology
University of Puerto Rico
San Juan, PR

Marina Roizenblatt, MD
Vitreoretinal Specialist
Federal University of São Paulo
São Paulo, Brazil

Jill C. Rotruck, MD
Assistant Professor of Ophthalmology and Visual Science
Yale Eye Center
New Haven, CT

Erin O. Schotthoefer, MD
Pediatric Ophthalmologist and Strabismus Specialist
Charlotte Eye Ear Nose and Throat Associates, PA
Charlotte, NC

Ann Shue, MD
Clinical Assistant Professor of Ophthalmology
Byers Eye Institute and Lucile Packard Children's Hospital
Stanford University
Palo Alto, CA

Evan Silverstein, MD
Assistant Professor of Ophthalmology
Virginia Commonwealth University
Richmond, VA

Sonali Talsania, MD
Assistant Professor of Ophthalmology
Columbia University Medical Center
New York, NY

Cynthia A. Toth, MD
Professor of Ophthalmology and Biomedical Engineering
Duke University
Durham, NC

Rupal H. Trivedi, MD, MSCR
Associate Professor of Ophthalmology
Storm Eye Institute
Medical University of South Carolina
Charleston, SC

Irene T. Tung, MD
Assistant Professor of Ophthalmology
Texas Children's Hospital
Baylor College of Medicine
Houston, TX

Lejla Vajzovic, MD
Associate Professor of Ophthalmology
Duke University
Durham, NC

Federico G. Velez, MD
Associate Professor of Ophthalmology and Pediatrics
Duke University
Durham, NC

Matthew S. Ward, MD
Cornea and External Disease Specialist
Riverwoods Eye Center
Provo, UT

James W. Weightman, MD
Assistant Professor of Surgery
Uniformed Services University of the Health Sciences
Bethesda, MD
Pediatric Ophthalmologist and Strabismus Specialist
Fort Belvoir Community Hospital
Fort Belvoir, VA

R. Kevin Winkle, MD
Pediatric Ophthalmology and Strabismus Specialist
Alaska Children's Eye and Strabismus
Anchorage, AK

Xinxin Zhang, MD
Resident in Ophthalmology
Duke University
Durham, NC

Video Contributors

Cody C. Blanchard, BS
Medical Student
Mercer School of Medicine
Macon, GA

Brenda L. Bohnsack, MD, PhD
Lillian Sherman Cowen Rieger and Harold L.S. Cowen
Research Professor in Pediatric Ophthalmology
Division Head, Ophthalmology
Ann & Robert H. Lurie Children's Hospital of Chicago
Northwestern University Feinberg School of Medicine
Chicago, IL

Michelle T. Cabrera, MD
Associate Professor of Ophthalmology
Chief, Division of Pediatric Ophthalmology
University of Washington
Seattle Children's Hospital
Seattle, WA

Sophie Cai, MD
Clinical Associate Ophthalmology
Duke University
Durham, NC

Melissa Daluvoy, MD
Assistant Professor of Ophthalmology
Duke University
Durham, NC

Laura B. Enyedi, MD
Professor of Ophthalmology and Pediatrics
Duke University
Durham, NC

Meghan S. Flemmons, MD
Assistant Professor of Ophthalmology
Vanderbilt University Medical Center
Nashville, TN

Sharon F. Freedman, MD
Professor of Ophthalmology and Pediatrics
Chief, Division of Pediatric Ophthalmology and Strabismus
Duke University
Durham, NC

Nandini Gandhi, MD
Associate Professor of Ophthalmology
University of California Davis
Sacramento, CA

Tanya Glaser, MD
Clinical Associate Ophthalmology
Duke University
Durham, NC

Michelle S. Go, MD
Assistant Professor of Ophthalmology
University of North Carolina
Chapel Hill, NC

Jeffrey S. Hunter, MD
Clinical Professor of Ophthalmology
University of Texas Health Science Center-Tyler
Tyler, TX

Jagger C. Koerner, MD, MBA
Assistant Professor of Ophthalmology and Pediatrics
Wake Forest Baptist Health
Winston-Salem, NC

Regina de Luna, MD
Resident in Ophthalmology
Duke University
Durham, NC

Prithvi Mruthyunjaya, MD, MHS
Associate Professor of Ophthalmology
Director Ocular Oncology
Byers Eye Institute
Stanford University
Stanford, CA

Pimpiroon Ploysangam, MD
Clinical Associate Ophthalmology
Duke University
Durham, NC

S. Grace Prakalapakorn, MD, MPH
Associate Professor of Ophthalmology and Pediatrics
Affiliate Faculty Duke Global Health Institute
Duke University
Durham, NC

Connie M. Sears, MD
Resident in Ophthalmology
Byers Eye Institute
Stanford University
Palo Alto, CA

Ann Shue, MD
Clinical Assistant Professor of Ophthalmology
Byers Eye Institute and Lucile Packard Children's Hospital
Stanford University
Palo Alto, CA

Allison C. Umfress, MD
Clinical Associate Ophthalmology
Duke University
Durham, NC

Lejla Vajzovic, MD
Associate Professor of Ophthalmology
Duke University
Durham, NC

Matthew S. Ward, MD
Cornea and External Disease Specialist
Riverwoods Eye Center
Provo, UT

Xinxin Zhang, MD
Resident in Ophthalmology
Duke University
Durham, NC

Foreword

Laura Enyedi and her contributing authors have "knocked it out of the park" with the *Duke Surgery Manual of Pediatric Ophthalmology and Strabismus Surgery*. Here you can find practical, up-to-date advice on surgical treatment of pediatric eye disease. Details of surgery for strabismus, cataract, glaucoma, nasolacrimal and oculoplastic disorders, retinopathy of prematurity, and other pediatric eye diseases are all in a single, easy-to-read volume.

Each chapter contains pearls of practical advice to keep in mind when approaching these problems. The bulleted format is easy to follow, keeps the reader engaged, and makes it easy to locate particular sections. The text provides no-nonsense, straightforward details on surgical procedures, and figures are interspersed to illustrate important points. Many chapters are augmented by videos which put you "under the microscope" with the expert performing the procedure.

Although entitled a surgical procedures manual, this book goes well beyond the technical aspects of ophthalmic procedures. Successful surgical treatment involves careful planning and meticulous postoperative care, and this book appropriately emphasizes these aspects of treatment, such as tips for successful contact lens fitting for the aphakic infant.

The next time I need to review details of a particular surgical procedure, I will reach for this volume. If I were a resident or fellow in training, it would be a "go to" resource for me when preparing for pediatric cases. Dr. Enyedi and colleagues have made a timely contribution that will serve as a valuable resource for pediatric eye surgeons worldwide.

David K. Wallace, MD, MPH
Chair
Department of Ophthalmology
Marilyn K. Glick Professor of Ophthalmology
Indiana University School of Medicine
Indianapolis, Indiana

Series Foreword

When you need to know how to approach a case that you may not commonly take care of or want to review how to approach adjustable sutures or even what to do next in the operating room when tackling a particularly challenging case, look no further. The answer lies in the pages of *The Duke Manual of Pediatric Ophthalmology and Strabismus Surgery edited by Dr. Laura Enyedi along with Drs. Nandini Gandhi and Tammy Yanovitch*. In one handy reference book such as this, you are able to explore reliable methods and techniques outlined by some of the most accomplished and competent ophthalmic surgeons, the majority of whom specialize in pediatric ophthalmology, in the United States in order to achieve your surgical goals.

At the Duke Eye Center, we decided that not only should we share pediatric ophthalmology and strabismus surgical pearls in *The Duke Manual* but also put in print some of the tips and tricks relied on in the operating room by some of the many other Duke Eye faculty in the various ophthalmic subspecialties through *The Duke Manuals of Ophthalmic Surgery* series. The intent of *The Duke Manuals* is not to circumvent traditional ophthalmic surgical training or create a substitute for the tried-and-true path to becoming a competent and skilled ophthalmic surgeon but instead to provide the student, resident, fellow, or practicing physician a review of the important factual and practical aspects of performing the different ophthalmic surgical procedures, step by step. *The Duke Manuals* series is also an invaluable resource for the surgical assistant as well as the operating room nurse as they prepare for the surgical case and anticipate the surgeon's next move.

As Series Editor of *The Duke Manuals*, it has been especially rewarding to collaborate with many outstanding individuals in the profession of ophthalmology across the country who contributed to the series. All editors and authors have either trained at Duke or trained others as faculty at Duke. This series represents countless hours of involvement and work by so many busy surgeons; it could not have come together without their dedication to sharing their knowledge with all of you.

It is our hope that *The Duke Manuals* series will serve as an excellent resource and valuable reference for students, residents, fellows, and practicing surgeons alike.

Sharon Fekrat, MD, FACS
Series Editor

Contents

Abbreviations

AC—anterior chamber
AC/A—accommodative convergence to accommodation
ACIOL—anterior chamber intraocular lens
AHP—abnormal (anomalous) head position (posture)
AMD—age-related macular degeneration
AL—axial length
APD—afferent pupillary defect
ARC—anomalous retinal correspondence
ASI—anterior segment ischemia
BI—base in
BO—base out
Botox—botulinum toxin A
BP—blood pressure
BPX—bupivacaine
BSS—balanced salt solution
BTX—botulinum toxin A
CBB—ciliary body band
CBC—complete blood count
cc—cubic centimeter
CCC—continuous curvilinear capsulorrhexis
CCT—central corneal thickness
CDI—color Doppler imaging
CGRN—Childhood Glaucoma Research Network
CHED—congenital hereditary endothelial dystrophy
CMV—Cytomegalovirus
CN—cranial nerve
CNS—central nervous system
CRAO—central retinal artery occlusion
CT—corneal transplant
CTL—contact lens
CXL—collagen cross-linking
D—diopter
DM—Descemet membrane
DMEK—Descemet membrane endothelial keratoplasty
DMR—double Maddox rod
DSEK—Descemet stripping endothelial keratoplasty
DRS—Duane retraction syndrome
DVD—dissociated vertical deviation
ECP—endoscopic diode cyclophotocoagulation
EDTA—ethylenediaminetetraacetic acid
EK—endothelial keratoplasty
EMG—electromyography
EOM—extraocular muscle
ERG—electroretinogram
ERM—epiretinal membrane
ESR—erythrocyte sedimentation rate
ET—esotropia
EUA—examination under anesthesia
FDA—Food and Drug Administration
FDT—forced duction test
FTA-ABS—Fluorescent treponemal antibody-absorption
5-FU—5-fluorouracil
G—gauge
GA—general anesthesia
GALT—Galactose-1-phosphate uridyltrans-ferase
GCA—giant cell arteritis
GDD—glaucoma drainage device
GFCS—glaucoma following cataract surgery
HES—heavy eye syndrome
HI—Harada-Ito
HSV—herpes simplex virus
HT—hypertropia
ICP—intracranial pressure
IgG—immunoglobulin G

IgM—immunoglobulin M
INR—international normalized ratio
IO—inferior oblique
IOAT—inferior oblique anterior transposition
IOFB—intraocular foreign body
IOL—intraocular lens
IOOA—inferior oblique overaction
IOP—intraocular pressure
IR—inferior rectus
IV—intravenous
J—joules
JOAG—juvenile open angle glaucoma
K-max—steepest keratometry
K-mean—mean keratometry
K-min—flattest keratometry
kg—kilogram
LF—levator function
LMA—laryngeal mask airway
LPI—laser peripheral iridotomy
LR—lateral rectus
MG—Myasthenia gravis
mg—milligram
µm—micrometer
MIOCT—microscope-integrated OCT
MISS—minimally invasive strabismus surgery
mL—milliliter
mm—millimeter
MMC—mitomycin C
MR—medial rectus
MRA—magnetic resonance angiogram
MRD—margin reflex distance
MRI—magnetic resonance imaging
MVR—microvitreoretinal
mW—milliwatt
NLDO—nasolacrimal duct obstruction
nm—nanometer
NPO—nothing by mouth
OCT—optical coherence tomography
OD—right eye
ONH—optic nerve head
OR—operating room
OS—left eye
OTC—over the counter
OU—both eyes
OVD—ophthalmic viscosurgical device
PCG—primary congenital glaucoma
PCIOL—posterior chamber intraocular lens
PD—prism diopter
PFA—platelet function assay
PFV—persistent fetal vasculature
PITS—pulled-in-two syndrome
PKP—penetrating keratoplasty
post-op—post-operative
pre-op—pre-operative
PSC—posterior subcapsular cataract
PT—prothrombin time
PTT—partial thromboplastin time
PVR—proliferative vitreoretinopathy
RB—retrobulbar
RD—retinal detachment
Rec—recession
Res—resection
RGP—rigid gas permeable
RK—radial keratotomy
ROP—retinopathy of prematurity
RPR—rapid plasma reagin
SB—scleral buckle
SES—sagging eye syndrome
SO—superior oblique
SOOA—superior oblique overaction
SR—superior rectus
SS—scleral spur
SW—Sturge Weber
TDC—transscleral diode cyclophotocoagulation
TED—thyroid eye disease
TM—trabecular meshwork
TW—tendon width
U—unit
UBM—ultrasound biomicroscopy
UGH—uveitis-glaucoma-hyphema
UVA—ultraviolet A
VA—visual acuity
VAO—visual axis opacity
VEGF—vascular endothelial growth factor
VF—visual field
VR—vitreoretinal
XT—exotropia

Section I

Anesthesia and Perioperative Considerations

CHAPTER 1

Anesthesia and Perioperative Considerations in Pediatric Ophthalmology and Adult Strabismus

Tamiesha Frempong, MD, MPH

INTRODUCTION

Anesthesia care plays a significant role in pediatric ophthalmic and adult strabismus cases. Perioperative planning has a major impact on the workflow efficiency, patient comfort and safety, and postoperative care and recovery.

Order of Surgical Cases

- Typically, patients are scheduled from youngest to oldest. Ordering by age minimizes the amount of time young children must fast prior to their procedure.
- In addition, cases are often grouped by type of procedure (ie, intraocular cases are scheduled first followed by strabismus cases, etc.). Grouping cases facilitates room set up and equipment planning.

A variety of reasons may require a patient to jump the queue. For example, an older, nervous adult patient with anxiety or one with a need to resume anticoagulation in a time-controlled fashion if a blood thinner was stopped for the purpose of surgery may need to be one of the first cases, despite an older age.

Impact of General Anesthesia on Pediatric Patients

- Distress/anxiety behaviors often exhibited at the time of anesthesia induction[1]:
  - Verbal protestations.
  - Crying, screaming, or verbally communicating fear or sadness.
  - Attempts to delay surgery or run away.
  - Nonverbal resistance such as pushing away the face mask.

- Potential sequelae of surgery and general anesthesia:
  - Postoperative pain.
  - Emergence delirium.
  - Behavioral changes:
    - General anxiety.
    - Appetite changes.
    - Sleep disturbances and nightmares.
    - Enuresis.
    - Temper tantrums.
  - Cognitive risks (see below).

Management of Pediatric Patient Stress and Anxiety Associated With General Anesthesia

- Nonpharmacologic interventions: The behavior of health care providers and parents/caregivers impact children's coping strategies and distress behaviors at anesthesia induction.[2]
  - Parents' emotion-focused behavior such as empathy, empathetic touch, and reassurance may inadvertently *increase* distress and negative coping behavior.
  - Anesthesiologist/ophthalmologist/operating room staff—humor and distracting talk such as asking about school or hobbies, in addition to medical reinterpretation (ie, anesthesia mask as part of "the astronaut game"), *lessens* a child's distress and improves coping behavior.
- Pharmacologic interventions (premedications).

> **In the United States, 50% of young children undergoing surgery receive premedication, most commonly with midazolam.[3]**

  - Midazolam—oral or rectal; used in combination with atropine for premedication, followed by ketamine and midazolam for induction of anesthesia.
    - Reliable.
    - Well tolerated.
    - Provides good postoperative analgesia.
  - Dexmedetomidine—intranasal.
    - Lowers overall anesthetic requirements by reducing sympathetic outflow in response to painful surgical stimuli.[3]
    - Has sedative, analgesic, and anxiolytic properties.[3]
  - Clonidine—oral, rectal, or caudal.
    - Does not affect respirations (in contrast to benzodiazepines).[4]
    - Effectively reduces postoperative vomiting and pain in pediatric patients undergoing ophthalmic surgery compared to placebo or benzodiazepines.[5]

Induction Methods

The factors to be considered in choosing the mask or needle for induction include preexisting respiratory disease, level of anxiety, previous experience of the patient and parents, and vein quality.[6]

- Intravenous:
  - Advantages—reduced respiratory events and postoperative behavioral issues.
  - Disadvantages—more anxiety at the time of induction.
- Mask:
  - Advantages—a better option in patients with poor vein quality.
  - Disadvantages—higher risk of respiratory events and postoperative behavioral issues.

Risk of General Anesthesia in Early Childhood

Evidence in the literature supports that *multiple exposures (not one single exposure)* to general anesthetics in children under the age of 3 years results in decreased fine motor coordination and processing speed, as well as reported behavior and reading difficulties. However, no difference in general intelligence has been found.[7] These data may serve to guide the timing of surgery and second surgeries in young children. Whenever possible, consider combining procedures with other specialties in order to minimize the risk of anesthetic exposure (ie, examination under anesthesia with a tympanostomy). However, it is important to avoid combining procedures that might increase risk of postoperative infection.

ANESTHESIA IN ADULT STRABISMUS SURGERY

Local anesthesia in conjunction with monitored anesthesia care is an option for unilateral adult strabismus cases. In some instances, it is a more desirable choice as the risk of myocardial ischemia has been shown to be lower in patients undergoing cataract surgery who receive peribulbar block compared to those cases performed under general anesthesia.[8]

- Characteristics of adult strabismus candidates for local anesthesia[9]:
  - No dementia or significant developmental delay.
  - No uncontrolled cough or tremor.
  - No excessive anxiety or claustrophobia.
  - No language barrier between the patient and surgeon.
  - No deafness.
  - No bleeding dyscrasias or coagulopathies.
  - No perforated globe.
  - Generally, medically uncompromised (ie, medically optimized from a cardiorespiratory and psychiatric standpoint).

To be clear, local anesthesia is not a replacement for general anesthesia as the patient's medical condition must be able to tolerate conversion to general anesthesia if for any reason that should become necessary. Therefore, those meeting the requirements for local anesthesia must also be eligible for general anesthesia.

Commonly Used Agents for Local Anesthesia

- Lidocaine (Xylocaine) 2%.
- Bupivacaine (Marcaine) 0.5%-0.75%.
- Hyaluronidase can be added to the anesthetic solution as the enzyme accelerates the dispersal of the agent.

Lidocaine compared to bupivacaine has a faster rate of onset (2.5 vs 5-10 minutes) and a shorter duration (2 vs 4-8 hours). Often a 50/50 mixture of these anesthetics is used particularly if a longer duration of action is desired. Same day adjustment is possible if adjustable sutures are used in strabismus cases, and the timing of the adjustment will inform whether or not the longer-acting agent is added (see Chapter 48).

Administration of Local Anesthetic

- Retrobulbar injection—typically described as within the muscle cone.
  - Advantages—excellent akinesia and sensory anesthesia of the conjunctiva, cornea, and uvea.

  - Disadvantages—risks of retrobulbar hemorrhage +/− central retinal artery occlusion, chemosis, central spread of local anesthetic causing respiratory depression and cardiac arrest, optic atrophy/vision loss, globe perforation, postoperative strabismus via intramuscular injection of anesthetic.
- Peribulbar injection—involves injection above and below the orbit and within the orbicularis oculi muscle.
  - Advantages—excellent akinesia and anesthesia, less potential for intraocular or intradural injection, easier to place, less risk of globe or optic nerve injury.
  - Disadvantages—periorbital ecchymoses, transient blindness.
- Sub-Tenon block—involves a conjunctival/Tenon cut down often in the inferonasal quadrant and the use of a curved cannula to deliver 3-5 mL of anesthetic to the episcleral space.[10]
  - Advantages—good akinesia and anesthesia.
  - Disadvantages—subconjunctival hemorrhage, chemosis, brain stem anesthesia, globe perforation, retrobulbar hemorrhage, rectus muscle dysfunction.

Risk of Retrobulbar Hemorrhage and Blood Thinner Management in Adult Strabismus Surgery

Given the aging population, more and more older adults are electing to undergo eye surgery. Strabismus surgery in older adults has increased by 24% in the last 15 years.[11,12] In the United States, the use of anticoagulation therapy has increased 38% between 2009 and 2014.[13]

- Retrobulbar hemorrhage:
  - Related to regional anesthesia.[14]
    - Peribulbar.
    - Retrobulbar.
    - Sub-Tenon.
  - Unrelated to regional anesthesia (rare).[15]
- Blood thinner management—in deciding whether to continue or discontinue anticoagulants prior to ophthalmic surgery, the surgeon and patient must weigh the risk of hemorrhage against the risk of thrombosis. Often, it is helpful to consult the patient's primary care physician to discuss appropriate blood thinner management prior to strabismus surgery.[16]

Postoperative Pain Control Following Strabismus Surgery

- Injection of sub-Tenon bupivacaine 0.75% at the end of the procedure has been shown to reduce postoperative pain in children.[17]
- Ice packs can be applied in the recovery room.
- Pain medications at discharge include acetaminophen or ibuprofen.
- Patients rarely require anything stronger for pain (eg, oxycodone) or medication for nausea (eg, ondansetron).

References

1. Chorney JM, Kain ZN. Behavioral analysis of children's response to induction of anesthesia. *Anesth Analg*. 2009;109(5):1434-1440.
2. Chorney JM, Torrey C, Blount R, et al. Healthcare provider and parent behavior and children's coping and distress at anesthesia induction. *Anesthesiology*. 2009;111(6):1290-1296.
3. FitzSimons J, Bonanno LS, Pierce S, et al. Effectiveness of preoperative intranasal dexmedetomidine, compared with oral midazolam, for the prevention of emergence delirium in the pediatric patient undergoing general anesthesia: a systematic review. *JBI Database System Rev Implement Rep*. 2017;15(7):1934-1951.
4. Bergendahl H, Lönngvist PA, Eksborg S. Clonidine in paediatric anaesthesia: review of the literature and comparison with benzodiazepines for premedication. *Acta Anaesthesiol Scand*. 2006;50(2):135-143.

5. Hsu YP, Chia-Wen Chu W, et al. Safety and efficacy of clonidine on postoperative vomiting and pain in pediatric ophthalmic surgery: a systematic review and meta-analysis. *Paediatr Anaesth*. 2019;29(10):1011-1023.
6. Sommerfield D, Von Ungern-Sternberg BS. The mask or the needle? Which induction should we go for? *Curr Opin Anaesthesiol*. 2019;32(3):377-383.
7. Warner DO, Zaccariello MJ, Katusic SK, et al. Neuropsychological and behavioral outcomes after exposure of young children to procedure requiring general anesthesia: the MASK study. *Anesthesiology*. 2018;129(1):89-105.
8. Glantz L, Drenger B, Gozal Y. Perioperative myocardial ischemia in cataract surgery patients: general versus local anesthesia. *Anesth Analg*. 2000;91:1415-1419.
9. https://www.openanesthesia.org/retrobulbar_vs-_peribulbar_block/
10. Kumar CM, Eid H, Dodds C. Sub-Tenon's anaesthesia: complications and their prevention. *Eye (Lond)*. 2011;25(6):694-703.
11. Astle AT, Foulsham T, Foss AJ, et al. Is the frequency of adult strabismus surgery increasing? *Ophthalmic Physiol Opt*. 2016;36:487-493.
12. Martinez-Thompson JM, Diehl NN, Holmes JM, et al. Incidence, types, and lifetime risk of adult-onset strabismus. *Ophthalmology*. 2014;121:877-882.
13. Barnes GD, Lucas E, Alexander GC, et al. National trends in ambulatory oral anticoagulant use. *Am J Med*. 2015;128:1300-1305.
14. Subbiah S, McGimpsey S, Best RM. Retrobulbar hemorrhage after sub-Tenon's anesthesia. *J Cataract Refract Surg*. 2007;33:1651-1652.
15. Carden SM, Good WV, Carden PA, et al. Garlic and the strabismus surgeon. *Clin Exp Ophthalmol*. 2002;30:303-304.
16. Robbins SL, Wang JW, Frazer JR, et al. Anticoagulation: a practical guide for strabismus. *J AAPOS*. 2019;23:193-199.
17. Enyedi LB, Wallace DK, Guy de LD. A double-masked randomized trial of postoperative local anesthetic pain control in pediatric strabismus surgery. *J Am Assoc Pediatr Ophthalmol*. 2017;21(2):107-111.

Suggested Readings

Davidson A, Shrivastava P, Jamson K, et al. Risk factors for anxiety at induction anesthesia in children: a prospective cohort study. *Paediatr Anaesth*. 2006;16:919-927.

Kain AN, Mayes LC, Cicchetti DV, et al. The Yale preoperative anxiety scale. How does it compare with a "gold standard"? *Anesth Analg*. 1997;85:783-788.

Kain ZN, Wang SM, Mayes LC, et al. Distress during the induction of anesthesia and postoperative behavioral outcomes. *Anesth Analg*. 1999;88:1042-1047.

Hosey MT, Macpherson LM, Adair P, et al. Dental anxiety, distress at induction and postoperative morbidity in children undergoing tooth extraction using general anesthesia. *Br Dent J*. 2006;200:39-43.

Ahmed MI, Farrell MA, Parrish K, et al. Preoperative anxiety in children risk factors and non-pharmacological management. *Middle East J Anaesthesiol*. 2011;21:153-164.

Hilly J, Hörlin AL, Kinderf J, et al. Preoperative preparation workshop reduces postoperative maladaptive behavior in children. *Paediatr Anaesth*. 2015;25:990-998.

Stargatt R, Davidson AJ, Huang GH, et al. A cohort study of the incidence and risk factors for negative behavior changes in children after general anesthesia. *Paediatr Anaesth*. 2006;16:846-859.

Holm-Knudsen R, Sjøgren P, Laub M. Midazolam and ketamine for rectal premedication and induction of anesthesia in children. *Anaesthesist*. 1990;39(5):255-257.

Ramachandran R, Rewari V, Chandralekha C, et al. Sub-Tenon block does not provide superior postoperative analgesia vs intravenous fentanyl in pediatric squint surgery. *Eur J Ophthalmol*. 2014;24(5):643-649.

Seijas O, Gomez de Liaño P, Merino P, et al. Topical anesthesia in strabismus surgery: a review of 101 cases. *J Pediatr Ophthalmol*. 2009;46(4):218-222.

Vallés-Torres J, Garcia-Martin E, Fernández-Tirado FJ, et al. Contact topical anesthesia versus general anaesthesia in strabismus surgery. *Arch Soc Esp Oftalmol*. 2016;91(3):108-113.

Section II

Pediatric Cataract Surgery

CHAPTER 2

Preoperative Considerations

Derek Bitner, MD

PREOPERATIVE EVALUATION OF PEDIATRIC CATARACT

- Perform a complete examination of both eyes to assess ocular health, vision, and cataract etiology.

All Cataracts

- Obtain vision in most reliable and age-appropriate way as possible (optotype > preferential looking > fixation).
- Assess pupils for presence of an afferent pupillary defect suggesting a more significant ocular abnormality.
- Assess ocular alignment and motility.
  - Strabismus can be evidence that the opacity is visually significant, and strabismus and amblyopia may need further treatment after cataract extraction.
  - Nystagmus is frequently seen in neonates with bilateral cataracts.
- Anterior segment evaluation should be performed undilated and dilated.
  - Cataracts may be more visually significant in the undilated state, depending on their size and location.
  - Central cataracts $\geq$ 3 mm in diameter and posterior opacities are more likely to be visually significant than anterior opacities.
  - Evaluation of the retinoscopic reflex (ie size of opacity, clarity around opacity in undilated state, any distortion of the retinoscopic streak) and assessment of the view to the posterior pole may help to determine if a cataract is visually significant in a preverbal child.
- Determine the type of cataract.
  - Anterior polar: Small isolated plaque on anterior surface of lens. Can be genetic and associated with refractive error. Often not visually significant and usually not progressive.
  - Pyramidal: Usually larger than anterior polar with extension into the anterior cortex. Usually fibrotic, may progress, and can be difficult to remove (Fig. 2.1).
  - Anterior lenticonus: Thinning of anterior capsule with lens protrusion and risk of spontaneous rupture. Associated with Alport syndrome.
  - Lamellar: Perinuclear opacity that is often hereditary and can progress (Fig. 2.2).

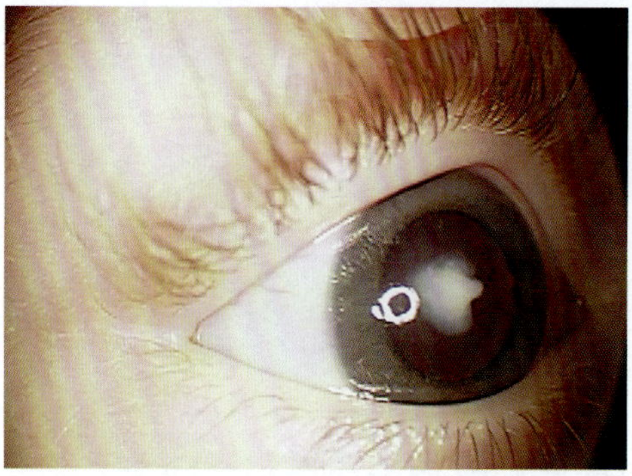

FIGURE 2.1. Anterior pyramidal cataract. This was bilateral, progressive, fibrotic, and very difficult to cut with vitrector. (Courtesy of Laura B. Enyedi, MD.)

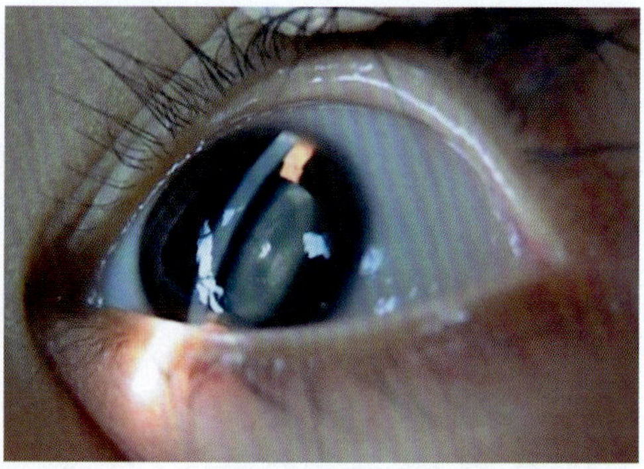

FIGURE 2.2. Lamellar cataract. Cataracts were bilateral, asymmetric, and progressive. (Courtesy of Laura B. Enyedi, MD.)

- Nuclear: Usually dense central opacity that is present at birth and can be associated with microphthalmia.
- Posterior polar: Small central capsular opacity. Usually hereditary.
- Posterior lenticonus: Weakness of posterior capsule with central protrusion. Although these lenses may rupture and lead to total cataracts, they are most frequently associated with irregular refraction that may not respond to spectacle or contact lens correction. The posterior capsule is prone to rupture with surgery.
- Posterior subcapsular: Can be congenital, traumatic, related to diabetes or chronic corticosteroid use.
- Persistent fetal vasculature (PFV): Usually unilateral, often with associated retrolental plaques. The eye is often smaller, and the plaque may be vascularized (Fig. 2.3). There may be a persistent vascular or non-vascular stalk between the optic nerve and posterior capsule (Fig. 2.4). Ciliary processes may be dragged forward and centrally, and the anterior chamber may be shallow.
- Total cataract: Nonspecific, can be associated with rupture of lens or with other forms of cataract.

- Assess anterior segment for signs of other ocular abnormalities that can affect the treatment options and prognosis including anterior segment dysgenesis (corectopia, iris atrophy, posterior embryotoxon), uveitis (posterior synechiae, keratic precipitates, cell/flare), trauma (corneal scarring, iridodonesis, phacodonesis), glaucoma (corneal enlargement, Haab's striae, elevated IOP), or PFV (small corneal diameter, elongated ciliary processes, fibrovascular stalk, atypical vessels around the lens/iris).

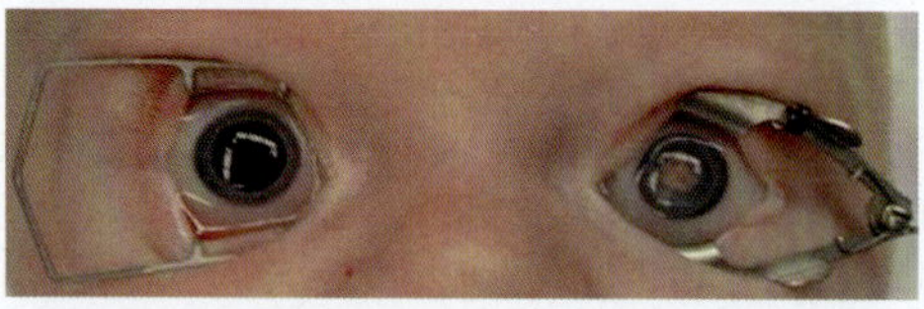

FIGURE 2.3. PFV cataract. Note the vascularity of the lens opacity and the microphthalmia. (Courtesy of Laura B. Enyedi, MD.)

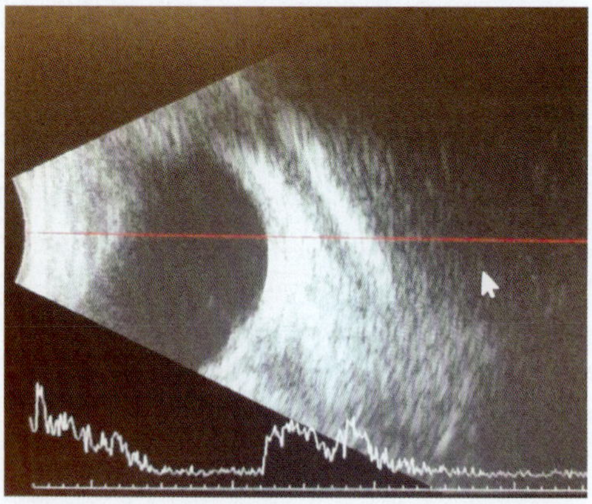

FIGURE 2.4. PFV cataract stalk. The stalk extends from the optic nerve to the posterior lens capsule. (Courtesy of Laura B. Enyedi, MD.)

- Perform complete dilated examination to assess optic nerve and retina as well as the extent of the cataract.
  - If unable to assess the posterior pole, B-scan ultrasonography should be performed to look for obvious retinal abnormalities (PFV stalk (Fig. 2.4), retinal detachment, vitritis, tumors, optic nerve abnormalities).
  - If B-scan ultrasonography is the only assessment of the posterior pole, the family should be informed that full visual potential cannot be determined until the retina and optic nerve are visualized.
- Perform cycloplegic retinoscopy.
  - Determine the presence of possible refractive or anisometropic amblyopia.
  - Assess retinoscopy streak clarity and regularity to assess how visually significant the cataract may be.
- Obtain IOL calculations via optical biometry if possible. If not able to be obtained in the clinic, ultrasonographic measurements (a-scan) can be done under anesthesia at the time of the surgery.

Unilateral Cataracts

- Assess for visual significance by obtaining visual acuity and looking at the type, location, size, and density of the cataract.
- Evaluate for reversible causes of vision loss such as significant refractive error and amblyopia (anisometropia and strabismus).
- Carefully assess for signs of PFV.

Unilateral cataracts are rarely associated with systemic conditions so further work-up is generally not needed.

Bilateral Cataracts

- Assess the parents for presence of nonvisually significant cataracts if there is not a family history.
- In the absence of family history, evaluate for systemic diseases that can present with cataracts. Blood tests may be performed as an outpatient or under anesthesia at the time of cataract surgery.
  - TORCH infections:
    - *Toxoplasmosis*: Toxoplasma IgG.
    - *Syphilis*: Fluorescent treponemal antibody-absorption (FTA-ABS), rapid plasma reagin (RPR).
    - *Cytomegalovirus*: CMV antibody IgG.
    - *Herpes simplex virus*: HSV antibody IgG.
    - *Rubella*: Rubella antibody IgG.
  - Metabolic conditions:
    - *Hypocalcemia/hypoparathyroidism*: Basic metabolic panel, calcium, phosphorous.
    - *Galactokinase deficiency*: Galactokinase, urine reducing substance.
    - *Galactosemia*: Galactose-1-phosphate uridyltransferase (GALT), urine reducing substances.
    - *Oculocerebrorenal (Lowe) syndrome*: Urine aminoacids.
    - *Cerebrotendinous xanthomatosis*: Cholestanol.
      - These are usually acquired cataracts that develop after age 4. Treatment can prevent neurologic deterioration.
  - Genetic conditions:
    - Usually autosomal dominant.
    - Numerous associated mutations make testing difficult.

- Increased frequency seen in some syndromic conditions such as Trisomy 21.
- Consider genetic evaluation.

Nonsurgical Management

- When there is a question of visual significance, conservative management should be attempted to see if surgery can be delayed.
  - Refractive error: Glasses may be prescribed for full-time wear to see if best corrected visual acuity can improve and for protection for monocular status.
  - Amblyopia: Unilateral or asymmetric bilateral cataracts may cause deprivational and/or refractive amblyopia. Polar cataracts are frequently associated with anisometropia. Occlusion therapy with spectacle correction can be utilized to attempt to improve visual acuity.
  - Strabismus: Some borderline cataracts can contribute to strabismus and strabismic amblyopia. Occlusion therapy and refractive correction may improve vision.
  - Mydriatics: Some small anterior central opacities (< 3 mm) may be treated with pharmacologic dilation to allow light to pass around the opacity. Since most mydriatics that could be used (cyclopentolate, atropine, homatropine, tropicamide) also have cycloplegic properties, appropriate spectacle correction with bifocal should be prescribed. Phenylephrine can also be used to avoid cycloplegia but may not be as effective or long-lasting.

SURGICAL PLANNING

- Exam findings can be helpful for planning surgical intervention. Age, cooperation, and anatomy will guide the surgeon to the best options regarding wound size, wound placement, optical correction choice, lens placement, capsular management, and postoperative care.
- Congenital cataract surgery should ideally be performed in the first 4-8 weeks of life. Earlier surgery is associated with better visual prognosis, but higher risk of glaucoma, and these pros and cons must be considered when deciding optimal timing. Older children whose vision is worse than 20/40 or children with significant symptoms as a result of the cataract may be considered for surgery.
- The decision to proceed with cataract surgery in a child should be made in conjunction with the child's parents or guardians.
  - The discussion should include documentation of the appropriate risks, benefits, and any potential alternatives that may arise including, but not limited to, vision loss, loss of the eye, infection, retinal detachment, uveitis, need for further surgery, risk of other ocular conditions such as glaucoma.
  - The need for refractive correction with spectacles including bifocal and/or contact lenses and the commitment to long-term follow-up for amblyopia management should be thoroughly discussed.
  - In cases of severe deprivation amblyopia, nystagmus, other significant ocular abnormalities, or when the retinal/nerve status cannot be accurately assessed preoperatively, the family should be informed that the visual potential may be guarded even with successful surgery.

Suggested Readings

Medsinge A, Nischal KK. Pediatric cataract: challenges and future directions. *Clin Ophthalmol.* 2015;9:77-90. doi: 10.2147/OPTH.S59009.

Nelson L, Olitsky S. *Harley's Pediatric Ophthalmology*. Philadelphia, PA: Wolters Kluwer; 2015.

Wilson M. Pediatric Cataracts: Overview [online]. American Academy of Ophthalmology. 2019. https://www.aao.org/disease-review/pediatric-cataracts-overview. Accessed 23 Sep. 2019.

CHAPTER 3

Medications in Pediatric Cataract Surgery

Daniel J. Lattin, MD, MS

PREOPERATIVE DILATING DROPS

- The primary goal is to achieve adequate dilation, which can be difficult in some congenital cataract patients. The secondary goal is to limit possible systemic side effects.
- Typically, a combination of cyclopentolate 1% or 2%, phenylephrine 2.5% or 5%, and/or tropicamide 0.5% or 1%, depending on the age of the patient.
  - Younger children (<2-3 years old): Duke Peds mix = Cyclopentolate 1% and phenylephrine 2.5%.
  - Older children (>2-3 years old): Duke Adult mix = Tropicamide 0.5% and phenylephrine 5%.
- If a patient is not dilating after normal drop administration, soak a cotton-tipped applicator or cellulose eye spear with the dilating drop, then place the cotton-tip into the fornix and "rough up" the conjunctiva in the fornix to aid with absorption. Leave the applicator/spearin the fornix until adequate dilation is achieved.
  - Make sure to warn the anesthesiologist to monitor the blood pressure and heart rate as the phenylephrine can cause the blood pressure to elevate and heart rate to drop quite significantly. If there are significant cardiovascular changes, remove the applicator/spear.

EPINEPHRINE 1:1000 SOLUTION

- Add to the irrigating solution (0.5 mL of epinephrine 1:1000 per 500 mL bottle) to aid with intraoperative pupillary dilation.

TRYPAN BLUE

- Can be used to help visualize the anterior capsule, especially if performing a manual capsulotomy or in dense or white cataracts (Fig. 3.1).
  - Trypan can cause the anterior capsule to be more friable and thus may increase the risk of a radial tear, although pediatric capsules tend to be more elastic than adult capsules in general.

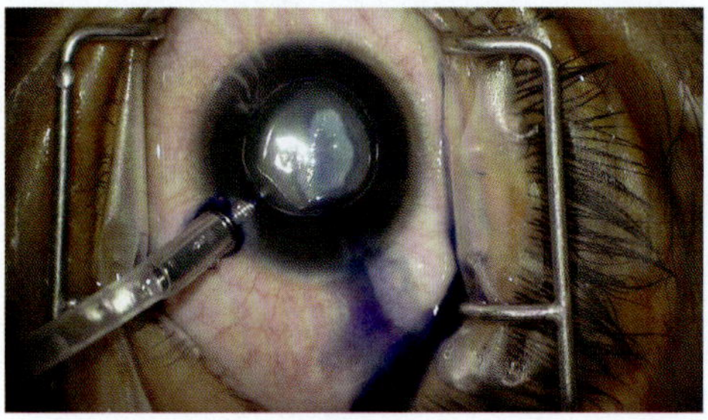

FIGURE 3.1. Trypan blue to stain dense white anterior capsule in a 11-year-old girl with count fingers (CF) vision due to traumatic cataract. (Courtesy of Jolene Rudell, MD PhD and Laura Huang, MD.)

- Prior to injecting viscoelastic, fill the anterior chamber with trypan blue and wait for ~30 seconds. Use BSS to wash out the trypan.
  - Trypan Blue can temporarily stain the corneal endothelium, so some surgeons prefer to place a filtered air bubble into the anterior chamber prior to introduction of the Trypan to minimize this effect.

OPHTHALMIC VISCOELASTIC DEVICES

- Types of ophthalmic viscoelastic devices (OVDs) and common uses:
  - High viscosity (cohesive) OVDs, for example, Provisc, Healon:
    - Better for creating space (expanding the capsular bag for IOL injection, dissecting adhesions, expanding the pupil, etc.).
    - Easier to remove at the end of a case.
    - Can rapidly leave the anterior chamber during surgery.
  - Superviscous (high molecular weight) OVDs, for example, Healon GV:
    - Useful for flattening the anterior lens when performing a manual anterior capsulotomy.
    - Will cause very high postoperative IOPs if left in the anterior chamber.
  - Low viscosity (dispersive) OVDs, for example, Viscoat, Ocucoat:
    - Can be used to help protect the corneal endothelium, or to "plug" a defect in the posterior capsule to prevent vitreous loss.
    - Often combined with a cohesive OVD in a "soft shell" technique.
      - Use a dispersive OVD to fill the anterior chamber, then inject a cohesive or high molecular weight OVD directly on to the anterior capsular surface.
      - Useful for performing a manual rhexis to combine the benefits of dispersive and cohesive OVDs.
    - Harder to remove completely at the end of surgery—take extra care to adequately remove to prevent a postoperative IOP spike.
- Effect on IOP:
  - Both cohesive and dispersive viscoelastics can cause a postoperative IOP spike in the first 24-48 hours after surgery if not removed completely at the end of the case. Consider using acetazolamide to prevent an IOP spike (see below), especially since you may not always get an ideal examination or IOP on postoperative day 1 in children.
  - If leaving a child aphakic, use of viscoelastic can be minimized; this has the additional benefit of minimizing the risk of a postoperative IOP spike.

TRIAMCINOLONE

- Two formulations:
  - Triesence is preservative-free and useful for intraocular applications (Fig. 3.2).
  - Kenalog contains a preservative (benzyl alcohol) and is best used for subconjunctival or periocular applications due to concern for retinal toxicity from the preservative.

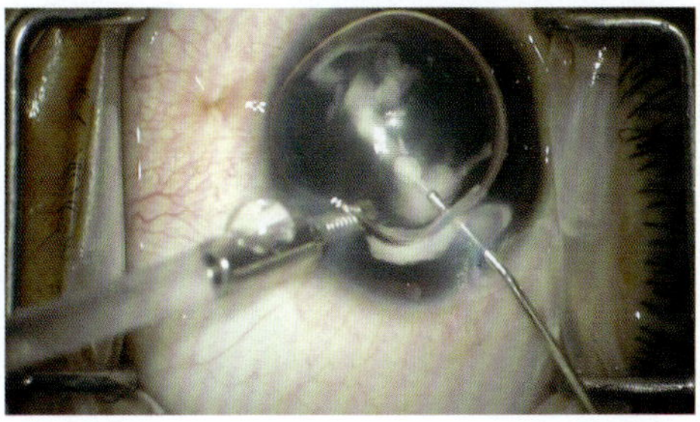

FIGURE 3.2. Triesence at the end of the case for same patient as in Figure 3.1. (Courtesy of Jolene Rudell, MD PhD and Laura Huang, MD.)

    - Because preservative-free Triesence is readily available, it is the preferred formulation for intraocular use. However, Kenalog can be used intraocularly if necessary, provided the benzyl alcohol concentration is sufficiently diluted. This can be done by diluting the Kenalog 40 mg/mL 1:10 with BSS, which will result in ~0.01% benzyl alcohol. Alternatively, one can allow the suspension of Kenalog 40 mg/mL to completely settle, remove the supernatant and then reconstitute the Kenalog with BSS 1:10. This will result in an approximate benzyl alcohol concentration of 0.001%.[1]
- Triamcinolone will "stick" to vitreous, and is useful if trying to determine if vitreous is in the anterior chamber.
    - There is a risk of elevated IOP due to a steroid response, especially if triamcinolone is placed in the vitreous.
- Triamcinolone is also useful to minimize postoperative inflammation, especially in uveitic or post-traumatic cataracts.
    - Some studies have found intracameral triamcinolone to be equivalent to oral prednisone in controlling intraocular inflammation without a significant IOP rise.[2,3]
- Triamcinolone can get trapped in the formed vitreous of children, which can lead to prolonged vitreous opacities. To avoid this:
    - If possible, only use if an IOL is placed to prevent the triamcinolone from falling into the vitreous cavity.
    - Follow injection of triamcinolone into the anterior chamber with injection of BSS or intracameral antibiotics to minimize clumping of the triamcinolone.

MIOTICS

- Miochol (acetylcholine chloride 1%) is short acting, Miostat (carbachol 0.01%) is longer acting.
- Either can be useful to produce pupil constriction at the end of a case.
    - Recommended if a three-piece IOL was placed in the sulcus.
    - May also help visualize any vitreous into the AC by highlighting "peaking" of the iris.
- Miostat also helps with IOP control in the perioperative period.[4]

INTRACAMERAL ANTIBIOTICS

- Moxifloxacin (Vigamox) is commonly used. It is preservative free and can be administered directly into the anterior chamber: 250 μg (0.05 mL of undiluted Vigamox directly from the bottle, or 0.10 mL if diluted 1:1 with BSS).
- Vancomycin (1 mg in 0.1 mL of BSS) and cefuroxime (1 mg in 0.1 mL saline 0.9%) are also used but must be compounded by a pharmacist.
- Intracameral antibiotics may be a more effective endophthalmitis prophylaxis than subconjunctival antibiotics.[5]

INTRACAMERAL FILTERED AIR

- Injecting an an air bubble can be helpful at the end of the case.
- May help mitigate IOP rises.
- Can indicate a formed anterior chamber on the first postoperative visit in an uncooperative patient.
- Useful for maintaining the anterior chamber while suturing wounds.
- Can highlight retained viscoelastic or vitreous in the anterior chamber if air bubble appears misshapen.
- If the bubble is too large it can cause pupillary block glaucoma.

SUBCONJUNCTIVAL INJECTIONS

- Subconjunctival steroids (most commonly dexamethasone) are useful to help prevent postoperative inflammation.
  - Inject ~0.2-0.5 mL of dexamethasone 4 mg/1 mL in the subconjunctival space at the end of the case, typically away from wound.
- Subconjunctival antibiotics (most commonly cefazolin) can also be administered in combination with steroids to minimize endophthalmitis risk.
  - May not be necessary if intracameral antibiotics were also given.
  - Inject ~0.2-0.5 mL of cefazolin 1 g/5 mL in the subconjunctival space at the end of the case.

SYSTEMIC STEROIDS

- Intravenous:
  - May be helpful to mitigate postoperative inflammation, administer at the end of the case.
    - Consider when placing an IOL, especially in a younger child (<10 years).
    - Consider in the setting of uveitis, trauma, previous ROP surgery, or persistent fetal vasculature (PFV). All of these may have greater than normal postoperative inflammation.
  - Methylprednisolone 1 mg/kg is a reasonable dose.
  - Anesthesia often administers IV steroids intraoperatively to prevent postoperative nausea.
- Oral:
  - If placing an IOL in a younger child (<10 years), can give 1mg/kg/day prednisolone liquid (Orapred), dosed once daily for 3-7 days, then 0.5 mg/kg/d for 3-7 additional days.
  - If performing a uveitic cataract extraction, consider using topical and/or oral steroids 2-7 days preoperatively with a prolonged taper of oral steroid postoperatively.

SYSTEMIC ACETAZOLAMIDE (DIAMOX)

- Intravenous:
  - Order 5-10 mg/kg at end of case if viscoelastics were used or if there is concern for IOP rise (eg, history of glaucoma).
- Oral:
  - Give 5 mg/kg at bedtime and again in the morning after surgery if viscoelastics were used or if there is concern for IOP rise.
  - Can crush a portion of a tablet and place in yogurt, applesauce, etc. for younger children.

TOPICAL POSTOPERATIVE MEDICATIONS

- Antibiotics
  - Moxifloxacin, Polytrim, or Maxitrol most often used.
  - Typically dosed qid for the first 1-2 weeks.
- Steroids: Minimize inflammatory response to surgery (can be quite robust in children).
  - Maxitrol or prednisolone most often used.
  - Typically dosed 4-6 times per day for the first week, often tapered over the first 4-6 weeks.
- Cycloplegics/mydriatics: Decrease ciliary spasm, reduce pain and inflammation, reduce pupillary block caused by synechiae or fibrinous membranes.
  - Cyclopentolate or atropine most commonly used, typically dosed daily to bid over the first 1-2 weeks.
- Topical nonsteroidal anti-inflammatory medications: Decrease inflammation, minimize cystoid macular edema.
  - Not used routinely, more likely to use in diabetic cataract. Consider use in uveitic cataract cases.
  - Typically dosed tid—qid for 4-6 weeks following surgery, often tapered over that time period.

References

1. Wilson ME, Trivedi RH, eds. *Pediatric Cataract Surgery: Techniques, Complications and Management*. Philadelphia, PA: Lippincott Williams & Wilkins; 2014.
2. Mohamed TA, Soliman W, Fathalla AM. Effect of intracameral triamcinolone acetonide on postoperative intraocular inflammation in pediatric traumatic cataract. *Eur J Ophthalmol.* 2016;26:114-117.
3. Ventura MC, Ventura BV, Ventura CV, et al. Outcomes of congenital cataract surgery: intraoperative intracameral triamcinolone injection versus postoperative oral prednisolone. *J Cataract Refract Surg.* 2014;40:601-608.
4. Solomon KD, Stewart WC, Hunt HH, et al. Intraoperative intracameral carbachol in phacoemulsification and posterior chamber lens implantation. *Am J Ophthalmol.* 1998;125:36-43.
5. Jabbarvand M, Hashemian H, Khodaparast M, et al. Endophthalmitis occurring after cataract surgery: outcomes of more than 480 000 cataract surgeries, epidemiologic features, and risk factors. *Ophthalmology*. 2016;123:295-301.

Suggested Reading

Wilson ME, Trivedi RH. Pediatric cataract surgery: operative and postoperative issues. In: Wilson ME, Saunders RA, Trivedi RH, eds. *Pediatric Ophthalmology: Current Thought and Practical Guide*. Berlin: Springer; 2009:325-343.

CHAPTER 4

Optical Considerations in Aphakia and Pseudophakia

Mae Millicent W. Peterseim, MD • Rupal H. Trivedi, MD, MSCR

Aphakia following cataract extraction in children may be corrected with spectacles, contact lenses (CTL), IOLs, and combinations of each. The initial surgical decision includes consideration of methods to best obtain optical correction both immediately postoperatively and as refractive needs change with growth. The extreme hyperopia of uncorrected aphakia or pseudophakia is devastatingly amblyogenic, making optical correction and amblyopia treatment imperative for the development of useful vision.

IOL implantation in children has the benefit of reducing dependency on compliance with other external optical devices (aphakic glasses and CTL) while providing at least a partial optical correction. These are important advantages to the visual development in amblyopia-prone eyes. However, concerns about primary IOL implantation in very young children include the technical difficulties of IOL implantation in small eyes, selection of the appropriate IOL power, and a higher risk of postoperative complications. While IOL use is becoming more widespread, relative contraindications to IOL implantation may include <6 months of age, severe microphthalmia, ectopia lentis, uveitis, and surgeon or parental preference.

The optical needs of the pediatric eye are expected to change with growth. Frequent follow-up and refraction update are essential, regardless of the choice for aphakic correction. This chapter provides considerations in optical correction in pediatric aphakia and pseudophakia.

APHAKIC SPECTACLES

- Option for infants with bilateral cataracts.
- Not desirable for monocular correction due to retinal size disparity.
- Create distortion—up to 30% magnification.
- Safe and easily adjusted.
- Require patient compliance.
- Heavy with poor cosmetic appearance.
- Experienced optician should determine the smallest lens and optic size that can reduce the central thickness and weight of the lens.
- Follow-up: Measure for change in refraction over glasses considering vertex distance.

- In infants and toddlers, it is satisfactory to use single vision lenses overplussed to focus at near (see below for details).
- As children age 2-3 years old become more interested in distance tasks, they should be prescribed their full cycloplegic refraction for distance with a +3 bifocal.

CONTACT LENS

- Recommended for unilateral aphakia, especially in young children.
- Creates 5%-9% magnification.
- Decreases aniseikonia in monocular cases compared with spectacles.
- Cost can be a limiting factor due to frequent replacement.
- Requires caretaker care.
- Risks include infection and corneal vascularity.
- May be a temporary solution until secondary IOL implantation.
- Types of CTL:
  - Hard lenses—rigid gas permeable (RGP):
    - Good choice for the smallest eyes.
    - Correct astigmatism and maintain shape.
    - Allow precise correction.
    - Require daily care.
  - Hydrogel:
    - For older children.
    - May be daily wear, disposable.
  - Scleral lenses:
    - For surface abnormalities unable to be fitted with conventional lenses (eg, corneal laceration with secondary scarring).
  - Silicone (Silsoft):
    - Most widely used and well tolerated in infants.
    - Mask 2 D astigmatism.
    - Resist absorption of topical ophthalmic drugs.
    - Extended wear is possible, however, increased risk of severe complications (infection and corneal vascularization). Recommendation is for weekly removal and cleaning.
    - Relative ease of insertion and removal.
    - Options:
      - Super Plus series: diameter 11.3 mm; BC 7.5, 7.7, and 7.9; power +23 D to +32 D in 3-D steps. Most aphakic infants are initially fitted with lenses that have a base curve of 7.5 mm.
        - Bausch & Lomb Patient Assistance Program SilSoft SuperPlus.
      - Aphakic series: diameter 11.3 or 12.5 mm; BC 7.5, 7.7, 7.9, 8.1, or 8.3; power +12 D to +20 D in 1-D steps.
- Initial CTL fit:
  - Fit for small and steep corneas in children relative to adults.
    - Fit immediately after cataract surgery.
    - Preoperative biometry and keratometry may help to select estimated power of CTL using following formula: CTL power = 84.4 – (3.2 × Axial Length).
    - CTL power can also be estimated using A-constant of 112.176 substituted into IOL power calculation formula.
    - For RGP lens fit, use fluorescein evaluation. Good fit should have uniform layer of stain.
    - Retinoscopy over CTL to evaluate movement and centering of the lens.
    - To provide near focus, 4 D can be added at birth, 3 D at 1 year, 2 D at 2 year, and 1 D at 3 years.

- CTL care:
  - Compliance is important.
  - Gradually increase wear by a few hours a day.
  - Teach wear schedule, insertion, removal, storage, and disinsertion.
  - Teach signs of irritation, infection, and discomfort.
  - Provide written instructions to caregivers.
  - Need to stock spare lens at home.
  - Keep backup spectacles (decrease power considering vertex distance).
- Follow-up:
  - Plan replacement of CTL 1 day to 1 week after initial insertion.
  - Examine every 3 months with refraction and fit assessment.
  - Perform retinoscopy with and without CTL.
  - Expect power decrease 0.32-0.35 D/mo.
  - Expect increased corneal diameter and flattening of cornea.
  - Cornea steepens (–0.40 D/mo) in the first 6 months.
  - Expect to replace 5-6 lenses per year.

INTRAOCULAR LENS

- Primary IOL implantation is usually not recommended for children under 7 months of age. Between age 7 months and 2 years, IOL implantation may be considered. Most children older than 2 years of age undergo primary IOL implantation.
- Hydrophobic acrylic material is most commonly used.
- IOL power calculation:
  - Axial length: Immersion.
  - Keratometry.
  - IOL power calculation formula: The Delphi expert group did not arrive at any consensus regarding which formula to use while calculating IOL power. Holladay 1 formula has been commonly used in the USA; however, gradually, Barrett's Universal II formula is becoming more popular.
  - Less accurate than in adults.
- IOL power selection: Choose initial postoperative refractive goal. Consider:
  - Myopic shift into adulthood—may initially target hyperopia with IOL, to decrease expected eventual myopia.
  - Management of changing residual refraction in childhood—expected compliance with glasses.
  - Management of amblyopia—density of amblyopia and estimated compliance to amblyopia therapy.
- Consideration for target refraction:
  - Age: Residual refraction chosen to minimize late myopia is typically based on age at surgery—the younger the age, the more myopic shift expected with growth necessitating more initial hyperopia. Delphi group suggested target ranges by age: <6 months, +6 to +10 D; 6-12 months: +4 to +6 D; 1-3 years: +4 D; 3-4 years: +3 D; 4-6 years: +2 to +3 D; 6-8 years: +1 to +2 D; >8 years: plano to +1 D. These targets should be further customized based on variables listed below.
  - Visual acuity: Known dense amblyopia is expected to improve more with less initial hyperopia.
  - Expected compliance: If compliance is estimated to be poor, target less initial hyperopia.
  - Fellow eye:
    - Bilateral cataracts: May target symmetric higher hyperopia.
    - Unilateral cataract: Target relatively less initial hyperopia to minimize anisometropia and aniseikonia.

- Family history: Child's eventual refractive error may resemble that of the family. If there is a family history of significant myopia, consider targeting more hyperopia.
- Microphthalmic eye: The highest available power may not be enough.
- Sulcus IOL placement:
  - Three-piece acrylic lenses or single-piece PMMA lenses can be placed in the sulcus. One-piece acrylic lenses are NOT suitable for sulcus placement.
  - Decrease the power by 1-2 D from the calculated power for the capsular bag. The higher the power for emmetropia, the more adjustment needed.

The "rule of 9's" can be used to adjust the calculated IOL power for sulcus placement: for IOL's 0-9 D, no adjustment; for >9-18 D, subtract 0.5 D; for >18-27 D, subtract 1.0 D; for >27 D, subtract 1.5 D.

- Managing residual refractive error:
  - Retinoscopy 2-4 weeks after surgery, then every 3 months until age 3 years, then less frequently as the refractive error stabilizes.
  - Goal to minimize blur and decrease anisometropia.
  - May be accomplished with spectacles or CTL.
  - Consider vertex distance.
  - While prescribing glasses or CTL, consider bifocal or undercorrection (–1 or –2) for near in pseudophakic eye.
  - If anisometropia over 4 D, adjust to decrease anisometropia to provide for development of binocularity.
  - For older children, when the pseudophakia is bilateral, bifocals (usually lineless progressive) are prescribed. With unilateral pseudophakia, the bifocal can be placed unilaterally, bilaterally, or not at all. This is left up to the preference of the surgeon and the patient.
- High myopia after primary IOL implantation, options:
  - Spectacles or CTL.
  - IOL exchange.
  - Piggyback secondary IOL implantation.
  - Corneal refractive surgery: LASIK or PRK.

Suggested Readings

https://www.aao.org/eyenet/article/contact-lenses-in-children-getting-it-right-lens. Accessed September 7, 2019.

Capozzi P, Morini C, Piga S, Cuttini M, Vadalà P. Corneal curvature and axial length values in children with congenital/infantile cataract in the first 42 months of life. *Invest Ophthalmol Vis Sci.* 2008;49:4774-4778.

de Brabander J, Kok JH, Nuijts RM, Wenniger-Prick LJ. A practical approach to and long-term results of fitting silicone contact lenses in aphakic children after congenital cataract. *CLAO J.* 2002;28:31-35.

Enyedi LB, Peterseim MW, Freedman SF, Buckley EG. Refractive changes after pediatric intraocular lens implantation. *Am J Ophthalmol.* 1998;126:772-781.

Lightman JM, Marshall D Jr. Clinical evaluation of back optic radius and power determination by age in pediatric aphakia due to congenital cataract fitted with a Silicone Elaster contact lens. *Optom Vis Sci.* 1996;73:22-27.

Mezer E, Rootman DS, Abdolell M, Levin AV. Early postoperative refractive outcomes of pediatric intraocular lens implantation. *J Cataract Refract Surg.* 2004;30(3):603-610.

Moore DB, Ben Zion I, Neely DE, Roberts GJ, Sprunger DT, Plager DA. Refractive outcomes with secondary intraocular lens implantation in children. *J AAPOS.* 2009;13:551-554.

Plager DA, Kipfer H, Sprunger DT, Sondhi N, Neely DE. Refractive change in pediatric pseudophakia: 6-year follow-up. *J Cataract Refract Surg.* 2002;28:810-815.

Serafino M, Trivedi RH, Levin AV, et al. Use of the Delphi process in paediatric cataract management. *Br J Ophthalmol.* 2016;100(5):611-615.

Trivedi RH, Wilson ME. Selection of an initial contact lens power for infantile cataract surgery without primary intraocular lens implantation. *Ophthalmology.* 2013;120(10):1973-1976.

CHAPTER 5

Cataract Surgery Without Intraocular Lens Implantation

Ricardo E. Rodríguez-Rosa, MD

Cataract extraction without IOL implantation may be considered for a subset of pediatric patients based on age, ocular parameters, and associated clinical diagnoses. A discussion about the surgical plan and the options for management of aphakia is advised during the preoperative evaluation.

PREOPERATIVE CONSIDERATIONS (SEE CHAPTER 2)

- Age:
  - In the Infant Aphakia Treatment Study (IATS), infants younger than 7 months of age who underwent unilateral cataract surgery with IOL implantation were more likely to have adverse events requiring secondary surgeries than those left aphakic.
  - Consider leaving infants <7 months aphakic after cataract extraction.
  - Consider IOL placement in infants younger than 7 months of age if they are likely to experience a prolonged period of uncorrected aphakia postoperatively. (see Chapters 4 and 6)
- Ocular parameters—Consider leaving infant aphakic if:
  - Corneal diameter <10 mm.
  - Axial length <17 mm.
  - History of poorly controlled uveitis: (see Chapter 7)
    - It is recommended that children with uveitis be quiet for at least 3 months prior to cataract surgery to avoid complications secondary to inflammation.
    - If good postoperative control is not anticipated, consider leaving the child aphakic to prevent fibrosis of the IOL.
  - History of trauma: (see Chapters 7 and 26)
    - If the trauma results in significant zonular dehiscence or capsular violation, there may not be adequate support for an IOL. Consider leaving these children aphakic with the option to possibly place an IOL at a later time.

SURGICAL PROCEDURE (VIDEO 5.1)

Incisions

- After completion of examination under anesthesia (if indicated), prep and drape the operative eye in sterile ophthalmic fashion.
- Place a 6-0 Silk traction suture at 3 and 9 o'clock, or a bridle suture underneath the superior rectus.
- Make conjunctival peritomies at 11 and 1 o'clock in preparation for bimanual vitrectomy.
  - If the surgeon prefers to use a coaxial vitrectomy, a single incision may be adequate.
- Use a 20G or 23G MVR blade (depending on surgeon's preference) to make a limbal incision at 11 and 1 o' clock.
  - If using a bimanual technique, make the incision on the non-dominant hand side first and insert the irrigation to keep the eye firm while making the incision for the vitrector.
  - A marking pen can be used to mark the side of the blade to make finding the small wounds easier. Pay close attention to the exact location and angle of entry with the MVR blade to facilitate insertion of the irrigating cannula and vitrector.
  - The vitrector can be difficult to insert, especially in a 23G opening. A very slight side cut can be made as the MVR blade is withdrawn to slightly enlarge the wound. Care must be taken to not make the opening too large, or the wound will leak, and the chamber will be unstable.
  - Consider pre-placing 9-0 Vicryl sutures across the incisions at the beginning of the case to facilitate efficient closure at the end.

A potential advantage to using the 23G system is less surgical trauma and a more watertight system (more stable anterior chamber) due to smaller wound openings. However, the traditional 20 gauge has been used effectively for many years and in some cases, may have a decreased vitrectomy time. The 20G system can be particularly effective with fibrotic capsules.

Cataract Extraction

- Insert an irrigating cannula and the vitrector into the anterior chamber.
- On IA/cut mode, make an anterior capsulotomy using the vitrector facedown on the capsule (vitrectorhexis).
  - Aim for an anterior capsular opening that is round, measuring ~5-6 mm in diameter.
  - It is important to pay attention to the edges of the capsulotomy. They need to be smooth and round to avoid extension of the capsule during the removal of the lens.
  - To smooth out capsular irregularity, the cut rate should be increased.
  - If there is difficulty cutting the capsule, the cut rate should be decreased and the aspiration increased.
  - In the case of a mature white cataract, trypan blue can be used to improve visualization of the anterior capsule during the capsulotomy (see Chapter 3).
- Consider performing gentle hydrodissection.
  - This may help remove equatorial lens epithelial cells, thereby reducing the incidence of posterior capsule opacification.
  - Hydrodissection is not recommended in cases where there is suspected posterior capsule rupture, in traumatic cataracts with zonular dehiscences, or in mature white cataracts where the nucleus is liquified. Extreme caution needs to be taken when dealing with posterior lenticonus because the thin posterior capsule may break with hydrodisection.

- Use aspiration to remove the lens nucleus and cortex making sure to aspirate all cortex to avoid postoperative intraocular inflammation and reproliferation of lens material. This is particularly important in infants and patients with uveitis. It may be necessary to reverse the positions of the irrigation and the vitrector to reach the subincisional cortex. Lewicky irrigation/suction cannulas are curved and can also be useful for removing subincisional cortex.
- For any child who cannot cooperate for a YAG laser capsulotomy, perform a posterior capsulotomy using the vitrector.
  - Recommended size is ~5 mm to avoid phimosis.
- Switch to cut/IA mode and perform limited anterior vitrectomy, using a high cut rate.
- Remove the irrigating cannula from the anterior chamber, and inject Acetylcholine Chloride 1% (Miochol) (see Chapter 3)
  - A peaked pupil may indicate vitreous prolapse into the anterior chamber; perform further anterior vitrectomy until vitreous is cleared.
- Consider making a peripheral iridotomy to prevent pupillary block (see Chapter 21).
  - Use one of the limbal incisions to make a peripheral iridectomy using the vitrector face down on IA/cut mode, or forceps and vannas scissors.
- Inject a filtered air bubble into the anterior chamber to help reform the chamber see Chapter 3).
  - A displaced or distorted bubble may indicate vitreous prolapse or retained viscoelastic.
  - The presence of the air bubble on postoperative day 1 is a reassuring sign that the chamber is formed if the examination is difficult.

Incision Closure

- Close the limbal incisions with 9-0 Vicryl sutures. Rotate the knots away from the cornea, and make sure the wounds are watertight.
- Close conjunctiva with buried 9-0 Vicryl sutures.
- Inject subconjunctival antibiotic and steroid (see Chapter 3).
- Consider an antibiotic/steroid combination drop or ointment in the inferior conjunctival sac.

> **A Tegaderm over the eye ensures that the lids stay closed.**

- Place a patch and a shield over the operative eye.
- Prescribe an antibiotic/steroid combination drop along with a cycloplegic postoperatively.
- Close postoperative follow-up is recommended to monitor for infection, prescribe aphakic correction, and initiate amblyopia therapy, if indicated.

Suggested Readings

Brambrink AM, et al. Isoflurane- induced apoptosis of oligodendrocytes in the neonatal primate brain. *Ann Neurol.* 2012;72:525-535.

Dave H, et al. Simultaneous versus sequential bilateral cataract surgery for infants with congenital cataracts: visual outcomes and economic costs. *Arch Ophthalmol.* 2010;128(8):1050-1054.

Guo S, et al. Management of the anterior and posterior lens capsules and vitreous in pediatric cataract surgery. *J Pediatr Ophthalmol Strabismus.* 2004;41(6):330-337; quiz 356-357.

Infant Aphakia Study Group. Comparison of contact lens and intraocular lens correction of monocular aphakia during infancy: a randomized clinical trial of HOTV optotype acuity at age 4.5 years and clinical findings at age 5 years. *JAMA Ophthalmol.* 2014;132(6):676-682.

Jeong-Rim Lee JR, Andreas W, Loepke AW. Does pediatric anesthesia cause brain damage? Addressing parental and provider concerns in light of compelling animal studies and seemingly ambivalent human data. *Korean J Anesthesiol.* 2018;71(4):255-273.

Lambert SR, et al. The infant aphakia treatment study: design and clinical measures at enrollment. *Arch Ophthalmol.* 2010;128:21-27.

Lambert SR, Plager DA, Buckley E, et al. The Infant Aphakia Treatment Study: Further on intra and postoperative complications in the intraocular lens group. *J AAPOS.* 2015;19(2):101-103.

Vasavada AR, et al. Randomized, clinical trial of multiquadrant hydrodissection in pediatric cataract surgery. *Am J Ophthalmol.* 2003;135:84-88.

Wilson ME Jr. Anterior lens capsule management in pediatric cataract surgery. *Trans Am Ophthalmol Soc.* 2004;102:391-422.

Wilson ME, Trivedi RH, Pandey SK. *Pediatric Cataract Surgery.* 2014;39-92.

CHAPTER 6

Cataract Surgery With IOL and Management of Posterior Capsule

Elliot C. McKee, MD

PREOPERATIVE CONSIDERATIONS

Cataract extraction with IOL implantation in children is distinguished from that in adults by several logistical, anatomic, and developmental considerations (see Chapter 2):

- General anesthesia is required in nearly all cases.
- The soft lens nucleus allows lens aspiration with a vitrector or irrigation-aspiration handpiece rather than phacoemulsification.
- A high incidence of posterior capsule opacification necessitates the use of a primary posterior capsulotomy unless the patient is able to cooperate with laser capsulotomy.[1–4] There are several methods of posterior capsule management in children, each with benefits and drawbacks (Table 6.1).
    - Children 7 years of age or older may be able to cooperate with laser posterior capsulotomy if needed.
    - Higher laser power is needed for pediatric posterior capsulotomy, and children have a higher incidence of reopacification after capsulotomy by any method.
- Active or uncooperative children require watertight and secure wound construction, usually augmented by sutures.
- An inability to obtain postoperative IOP measurement may lead the surgeon to prophylactically treat postoperative IOP elevations (see Chapter 3).
- Infants <7 months of age are typically left aphakic due to the higher incidence of complications associated with IOL placement in this age group (see Chapter 5).
- IOL power selection is much more challenging in pediatric patients due to the need to balance current visual function needs with anticipated growth of the eye and change in refractive error (see Chapter 4).

TABLE 6.1. Advantages and Disadvantages of Capsulotomy Techniques

Technique	Advantages	Disadvantages
Secondary Laser Posterior Capsulotomy	• Vitrectomy not required • Allows IOL implantation in the lens capsule	• Requires cooperation • Increased need for retreatment compared to adults
Primary Posterior Capsulotomy—Anterior Approach	• Uses device and technique familiar to anterior segment surgeon	• Risk of posterior IOL displacement • Risk of vitreous incarceration in anterior wound
Primary Posterior Capsulotomy—Pars Plana Approach	• Allows IOL implantation in the lens capsule	• Additional surgical time and complexity

SURGICAL PROCEDURE (VIDEOS 6.1, 6.2)

Machine Settings

- There are many different machines that can be used to remove pediatric cataracts, but a vitrector has advantages in young children because it can be used for anterior and posterior capsulotomies, as well as anterior vitrectomy.
- Each machine has different properties, and the specific settings will depend on the machine used, the gauge of the lumen, the unique properties of the cataract, and surgeon preference.
- Vitrector
  - Lumen
    - 20G to 25G lumen is typically adequate for pediatric cataract removal.
    - Larger lumens (with larger openings): remove material more efficiently, but can result in more chamber instability.
    - Smaller lumens: more controlled, but may have more difficulty removing very dense lens material.
    - 23G system can work in most instances.
  - Cut rate
    - Higher vitrectomy cut rates:
      - Smaller and more controlled "bites," which can reduce clogging of the lumen.
      - Less traction of tissues.
      - Smoother capsular openings.
    - Lower cut rates:
      - Tough or fibrotic capsule
      - Larger, denser lenticular fragments.
  - Higher flow rates and higher vacuum can both increase the material that comes to the port.

Incisions

Scleral tunnel incisions are frequently used in young children because they may be made as wide as necessary for IOL insertion and are easily made secure with nonabsorbable suture. Consider clear corneal incisions in older children who are less likely to rub the eye postoperatively and therefore have a lower risk of wound dehiscence.

Scleral Tunnel

- Place a 6-0 Silk traction suture underneath the superior rectus muscle to infraduct the eye.
- Create a superior conjunctival peritomy (at least 6-8 mm). The peritomy will need to be larger if planning pars plana posterior capsulotomy to allow room for the pars plana incision, slightly offset from the limbal incisions and scleral tunnel.

- Use wet-field cautery to provide hemostasis in a zone extending the width of the peritomy and 3-4 mm posterior to the corneal limbus. Ensure hemostasis in the location of the scleral incision, the pars plana incision (if used), and any sclera through which sutures will be passed.
- Use a crescent blade (64 blade) to initiate a superior scleral tunnel. The tunnel must be wide enough to permit entry of the IOL cartridge or folded IOL. A width of 4 mm, depth of 50% of scleral thickness, and location 1-2 mm posterior to the limbus is optimal.
- Tunnel forward in the wound using a 66 blade or bent crescent blade. It is important to maintain a consistent width and depth of the tunnel as it extends anteriorly. Avoid manipulating the anterior lip of the tunnel as this can distort its structure. Avoid entering the anterior chamber while initiating the tunnel, as this will impair anterior chamber stability while removing the cataract.
- Prior to entering the anterior chamber, test both the infusion and the vitrector to ensure proper functioning and allow the exit of air bubbles from the infusion tube.
- Using an MVR blade that matches gauge of vitrector chosen create two small incisions at the corneal limbus to enter the anterior chamber. Consider staining the edges of the blade with a marking pen to allow visualization of the wound location. Usually the first incision is made on the side of the surgeon's nondominant hand, and the infusion cannula is placed into this wound prior to making the second incision on the side of the surgeon's dominant hand. The incisions should be located beyond the nasal and temporal ends of the scleral tunnel. Wound location and angle should be chosen to allow the surgeon a comfortable hand position while operating. The incisions should be small enough to remain watertight when the appropriate instrument is inserted.

Clear Cornea

- A 23G MVR blade or side-port knife is used to create an incision at the limbus on the side of the surgeon's nondominant hand. The incision should be sized to permit the watertight fit of an infusion cannula if such use is planned. The anterior chamber is filled with viscoelastic.
- A clear corneal incision is made with a keratome blade at the temporal limbus.

Capsulorrhexis

The anterior capsule in children is generally thicker and more elastic than adults. This leads to a higher likelihood of peripheral extension of a traditional continuous curvilinear capsulorrhexis (CCC). For this reason vitrectorhexis, a technique in which the vitrector is used facedown on the anterior capsule to create an anterior capsulotomy, is recommended in young children. The optimal anterior capsule opening size is slightly smaller than the diameter of the planned IOL optic. Note that because of the elasticity of the pediatric anterior capsule, the opening will appear larger upon completion of the capsulorrhexis.

Vitrectorhexis

- Insert an irrigation handpiece through the corneal limbal incision on the side of the surgeon's nondominant hand. A self-retaining threaded irrigation cannula or a bimanual irrigation cannula may be used.
- Insert a vitrectomy handpiece through the incision on the side of the surgeon's dominant hand.
- Orient the vitrector handpiece opening posteriorly and place it in contact with the center of the anterior capsule. Engage the capsule with the vitrector on "IA/Cut" setting and move in an outward spiral to create an opening of the desired size. Make the edge of the opening as smooth as possible, and be sure that there are no bridging strands remaining by passing the vitrector over the center capsule and removing it once the capsulotomy is complete. The diameter of the opening should be about 5 mm.

If initial engagement of the capsule is difficult, reducing the cut rate and/or increasing the aspiration can be helpful. An MVR blade may also be used to initiate the capsular opening, followed by enlargement of the opening with the vitrector. If the capsule is very fibrotic, retinal scissors can be used to cut the capsule into pie-shaped wedges that can be more easily engaged with the vitrector.

Manual CCC

- Manual CCC should be performed after injection of viscoelastic into the anterior chamber.
- A CCC is created by initiating a capsular flap with a cystotome or MVR blade, then grasping the flap with small intraocular forceps. The flap is then pulled in a circular manner, using shear and tear forces to guide the curvilinear opening to the correct size. It is often necessary to pull the flap toward the center of the lens capsule at an angle almost perpendicular to the intended path of the tear, as the elasticity of the capsule predisposes the tear to enlarge centrifugally.
- Another technique is the "push-pull" anterior capsulorrhexis described by Nischal (Fig. 6.1). The MVR blade is used to make two stab incisions, one at the inferior edge of the desired capsular opening and another at the superior edge of the desired capsular opening, 4-5 mm apart. Capsulorrhexis forceps are used to grasp the distal edge of the superior opening, and the flap is pulled toward the center, tearing the superior 180 degrees of the capsulorrhexis. The forceps are then used to pull the proximal flap of the inferior opening to tear the inferior portion of the capsular opening.

Cataract Extraction

The vitrector or the irrigation-aspiration handpiece of the phacoemulsification device is used to aspirate the lens cortex and nucleus. As the pediatric lens is soft, phacoemulsification power is rarely, if ever, required. Occasionally, the vitrector cutter is necessary to assist in the fragmentation of calcified lens nucleus or "gummy" lens cortex. The vitrector itself can be used to manually dislodge pieces of cortex adherent to the lens capsule. The infusion cannula can be used to crush and push dense lens material into the vitrector port. The vitrector cutter should always be off when using this maneuver so that the cutter does not strike metal, damaging the vitrector and creating metallic intraocular foreign bodies.

Subincisional cortical material can be separated from the lens capsule by tilting the irrigation device into the lens capsule or by switching the incisions through which the vitrector and irrigation device are inserted.

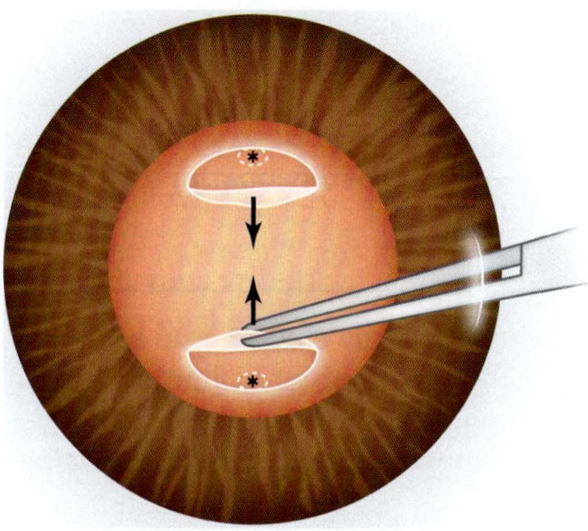

FIGURE 6.1. The 2-incision push-pull technique for capsulorrhexis. The stab incisions (*asterisk*) are made 4-5 mm apart at the proximal and distal ends of the desired capsulorrhexis. The flaps are pulled toward the center to create 180 degrees of the capsulorrhexis at a time.

The subincisional lens material is usually the most difficult to access and remove, and visualization is often challenging. Lewicky cortex extractor cannulas are curved and very maneuverable, making them ideal to remove subincisional lens material. The vitrector can also be used port down, keeping the port just at the edge of the anterior capsule and slightly tipped down during aspiration.

Intraocular Lens Implantation and Posterior Capsulotomy

If a scleral tunnel was initiated earlier in the procedure, it will be opened using a keratome blade of appropriate width for IOL insertion.

IOL Implantation Without Posterior Capsulotomy

- The capsular bag is filled with viscoelastic and a one-piece or three-piece IOL is inserted into the bag. Lenses can be injected or folded (see below).
- The viscoelastic is removed from the capsular bag and anterior chamber using the irrigation-aspiration handpiece or vitrector.
- Intracameral antibiotics, topical antibiotics, and/or topical povidone iodine may be used to reduce the risk of endophthalmitis (see Chapter 3).

IOL Implantation With Primary Posterior Capsulotomy, Anterior Approach

- Enable the vitrector cutter in IA/cut mode.
- With the vitrector facedown, engage the capsule to create a posterior capsulotomy at least 3 mm in diameter.
- Transition to cut/IA mode and perform a limited anterior vitrectomy to prevent vitreous prolapse anterior to the capsular plane. A high cut rate is recommended.
- Preservative-free steroid suspension can be injected into the anterior chamber to visualize any vitreous that may be present in the anterior or posterior chamber (see Chapter 3). Perform additional vitrectomy if needed.
- Inject cohesive viscoelastic such as Provisc or Healon GV into the ciliary sulcus (or lens capsule, if desired) to prepare the space for IOL implantation.
- Sulcus IOL: Insert a three-piece IOL into the ciliary sulcus using a holder-folder or a lens injection cartridge. When using an injection cartridge, care must be taken to ensure proper orientation of the leading haptic. Often, the cartridge must be rotated 90 or even 180 degrees to the surgeon's right to avoid an inverse haptic orientation. The cartridge is then slowly returned to its initial orientation as the lens optic is inserted. The trailing haptic may be left outside the incision initially. McPherson forceps may be used to grasp the trailing haptic and rotate it beneath the proximal iris into the ciliary sulcus.
- Bag IOL: A one- or three-piece IOL can be inserted into the capsular bag. With this technique, there is a higher risk of posterior dislocation of the IOL during insertion, but a lower risk of late IOL subluxation.
- Irrigate the viscoelastic from the ciliary sulcus and anterior chamber using the vitrector, irrigation-aspiration handpiece, and/or anterior chamber irrigation cannula.
- Inject acetylcholine (see Chapter 3) into the anterior chamber to induce pupil constriction, detect residual vitreous in the anterior chamber, and assure stability of the sulcus IOL.

IOL Implantation With Primary Posterior Capsulotomy, Pars Plana Approach

- After completion of lens aspiration, insert the desired IOL into the capsular bag.
- Close the scleral tunnel wound (see below).
- Remove viscoelastic material from the anterior chamber using the vitrector, irrigation-aspiration handpiece, or anterior chamber infusion cannula.
- Maintain the infusion cannula in the limbal wound but consider reducing the infusion rate.

- Using an MVR blade, create a pars plana incision 2-3 mm posterior to the limbus. Point the blade toward the optic nerve until the tip of the blade comes into view and then withdraw the blade. Consider enlarging the external portion of the wound very slightly to make insertion of the vitrector easier.

The recommended incision location is 2 mm posterior to the limbus in patients <1 year of age, 2.5 mm posterior to the limbus in patients 1-4 years of age, and 3 mm posterior to the limbus in patients older than 4 years of age.[4]

- Insert the vitrector handpiece through the incision into the vitreous cavity, pointing posteriorly toward the optic nerve to avoid contact with the IOL. Once the vitrector comes into view, flatten it out to apply the port to the posterior capsule.
- Use the vitrector with a high cut rate to cut a circular opening in the posterior capsule of a diameter 1 mm smaller than that of the IOL optic.

It can be difficult to visualize the posterior capsule at this point in the surgery, as the cornea is often a little hazy. If the opening is difficult to initiate, push up gently on the posterior capsule and lens.

It is uncommon, but possible to *inadvertently* enter the bag between the IOL and posterior capsule. In this case, the port is rotated down to open the capsule and perform a limited vitrectomy.

- Use the vitrector to perform a limited anterior vitrectomy. The port can be slightly rotated to each side, but it is not recommended that the port is advanced far posteriorly.
- Remove the vitrector from the incision. Consider engaging the vitrector cutter at the site of the incision to ensure no vitreous traction to the wound.
- Close the pars plana incision with 8-0 or 9-0 Vicryl suture. A single suture or an "X-" type suture closure can be used.

Wound Closure

Consider injecting sterile air into the anterior chamber to maintain its form during wound closure. In addition, the presence of an air bubble in the anterior chamber at the first postoperative visit is a reassuring sign of a formed chamber in children who are difficult to examine. It may also be helpful to keep the anterior chamber irrigation cannula in place during wound closure to increase globe rigidity.

Scleral Tunnel

- Close the scleral tunnel with interrupted 10-0 nylon and/or 9-0 Vicryl suture and rotate the knots into the sclera. Test the wound for leaks, keeping in mind that the risk of wound dehiscence is higher in children.
- Close the limbal incisions and the conjunctival peritomy with 9-0 or 10-0 Vicryl suture.

Clear Corneal Incision

- Close the incision with a single 10-0 Vicryl suture.
- Consider 10-0 nylon only in those children who can cooperate with suture removal at the slit lamp postoperatively.

POSTOPERATIVE CONSIDERATIONS

- Consider administering intracameral antibiotic, subconjunctival steroid injection, topical IOP-lowering medication, topical steroid, or topical antibiotic (see Chapter 3).
- To avoid a postoperative IOP elevation, consider administering IV acetazolamide (5-10 mg/kg) intraoperatively and prescribing a second dose to administer orally in the evening of the day of surgery (see Chapter 3).
- Cover the eye with a patch and a shield. A transparent adhesive dressing such as Tegaderm may be applied to the skin under the patch to close the eyelids and reduce the drainage from the eye postoperatively.
- Examine the patient within 24 hours to assess for wound dehiscence, IOP elevation, infection, and IOL dislocation.

References

1. Plager DA, Yang S, Neely DE, et al. Complications in the first year following cataract surgery with and without IOL in infants and older children. *J AAPOS*. 2002;6:9-14.
2. Plager DA, Lipsky SN, Snyder SK, et al. Capsular management and refractive error in pediatric intraocular lenses. *Ophthalmology*. 1997;104:600-607.
3. Buckley EG, Klombers LA, Seaber JH, et al. Management of the posterior capsule during pediatric intraocular lens implantation. *Am J Ophthalmol*. 1993;115:722-728.
4. Alexandrakis G, Peterseim MM, Wilson ME. Clinical outcomes of pars plana capsulotomy with anterior vitrectomy in pediatric cataract surgery. *J AAPOS*. 2002;6:163-167.

Suggested Reading

Nischal KK. Two-incision push-pull capsulorhexis for pediatric cataract surgery. *J Cataract Refract Surg*. 2002;28(4):593-595.

CHAPTER 7

Pediatric Cataract With Special Considerations

S. Grace Prakalapakorn, MD, MPH

UVEITIC CATARACT

The pre- and postoperative management of the patient with the uveitic cataract is critical to a good outcome

Preoperative Considerations

- Co-management with a uveitis and/or rheumatology specialist is invaluable. Consider increasing immunomodulating agents prior to surgery.
- On clinical examination:
    - Note other coexisting ocular pathology: band keratopathy, posterior synechiae, glaucoma, macular edema.
    - Note type of cataract (eg, anterior subcapsular, posterior subcapsular).
    - Check for macular edema prior to surgery (perform OCT imaging if possible).
    - Ensure the uveitis is under control before cataract surgery (at least 3 months).
        - Consider starting or increasing steroids (topical and/or oral) in the immediate preoperative period (especially if there is macular edema prior to surgery)[1].

Surgical Considerations

- Small pupils (see Small Pupil section below): try to minimize iris manipulation.
- Consider performing a posterior capsulotomy and anterior vitrectomy at the time of cataract surgery if it is felt that the posterior capsule will soon opacify following surgery (see Chapter 6).
- There are no standard guidelines for IOL implantation in pediatric uveitis.
    - Do not place an IOL in the setting of active inflammation.
    - If able to implant an IOL, try to place it in the capsular bag.
    - Consider an acrylic or heparin surface modified IOL to possibly induce less intraocular inflammation.
- Consider administering IV steroids (communicate with anesthesia team) and also injecting 0.2 mL of 40 mg/mL triamcinolone (ie, Triesence) into the posterior

segment at the end of the case (either through the posterior capsular opening, if there is one, or via a pars plana injection) (see Chapter 3).

Postoperative Considerations

- Taper topical steroids slowly (over many weeks) and maintain patient on a cycloplegic agent until inflammation resolves to prevent the formation of synechiae, posterior capsular opacification, and macular edema.
- Monitor for macular edema (perform OCT imaging if possible).
- Possible complications: recurrent uveitis, hypotony, glaucoma, synechiae, secondary membranes, cystoid macular edema, retinal detachment.

TRAUMATIC CATARACT (see Chapter 26)

Preoperative Considerations

- On clinical examination:
  - Note other coexisting ocular pathology: corneal wound/scar, iris tear, iridodialysis, peaked pupil, posterior synechiae, angle recession, presence of vitreous in the anterior chamber, and vitreous hemorrhage.
  - Note type of cataract, appearance of anterior capsule (may appear fibrotic secondary to trauma), and anterior chamber depth.
  - Check for phacodonesis. If zonules are missing, estimate the missing clock hours and determine if there will be enough structural support to implant a lens.
  - Perform ultrasound prior to surgery to evaluate for possible retinal detachment. If retinal pathology present, consult a retinal specialist prior to proceeding with cataract surgery.

Surgical Considerations

- May be performed through either a limbal or pars plana approach.
- The pupil may not dilate well (see Small Pupil section below).
- If there is a white cataract, consider trypan blue to stain the anterior capsule (see Chapter 3).
- If there is vitreous in the anterior chamber, perform limited anterior vitrectomy before proceeding with the cataract extraction. Use of a cohesive viscoelastic can help tamponade the vitreous.
- If the lens capsule is fibrotic:
  - Attempt to make an incision in the anterior capsule with a cystotome or MVR blade by starting at the edge of the thickened anterior capsule (in normal anterior capsule if possible and not too far peripherally). Make the incision big enough to allow the edge of the anterior capsule to be grasped if planning on performing a manual capsulorrhexis or to allow the vitrector to engage the capsule to start the vitrectorhexis.
  - Intraocular scissors can also be used to cut through the plaque. It is often helpful to cut the capsule into pie-shaped wedges that are easier to engage with the vitrector.

It is not necessary to remove the entire fibrotic capsule, just the portion in the visual axis.

- If there is zonular dehiscence:
  - For mild cases (<4 clock hours) consider the following:
    - Placement of a 3-piece lens in the bag with the haptics oriented in the area of zonular weakness.
    - Placement of a capsular tension ring.

    - Placement of a 3-piece lens in the sulcus with the haptics oriented over the areas of good zonular support.
  - For moderate cases (4-6 clock hours): Consider using a capsular tension ring.
  - For severe cases (>6 clock hours): Consider leaving the child aphakic and using a contact lens (see Chapter 4). If planning lens implantation, may need to consider, iris-fixated or scleral-fixated IOL.

> **If suturing in an IOL, beware of potential suture breakage (avoid using 10-0 polypropylene suture which can degrade and result in spontaneous subluxation of the IOL over time).[2]**

PERSISTENT FETAL VASCULATURE (PFV)

- Previously known as persistent hyperplastic primary vitreous (PHPV)
- Thought to be a result of an arrest of development of the eye wherein vascular structures present during embryological development fail to regress.
- Usually unilateral, but can rarely be bilateral.
- Wide spectrum of disease:
  - Mild cases may present as a Mittendorf dot on the posterior lens capsule and/or a Bergmeister papilla on the optic nerve.
  - Extensive cases may involve a thick vascular stalk connecting the optic nerve to a dense posterior lens plaque/ciliary body and, in severe cases, retinal detachment.

Preoperative Considerations

- On clinical examination:
  - Careful slit lamp examination (may require portable slit lamp): Measure corneal diameter (usually smaller in the eye with the PFV), location and morphology of cataract, elongation of ciliary processes.
  - Perform ultrasound (posterior ± anterior, if indicated) prior to surgery to evaluate the extent of the PFV:
    - Important to note the presence of a stalk and whether/where it attaches (to the optic nerve, the retina, the ciliary body, etc.), whether it is vascularized, and if there is a retinal detachment. In cases in which there is a stalk placing traction on the retina or the ciliary body, consult a retinal specialist before proceeding with the cataract extraction.

> **In PFV the affected eye is often smaller than the unaffected eye, and it may be helpful to document the corneal diameter and an axial length preoperatively. Keratometry measurements may be helpful for postoperative contact lens fitting.**

Surgical Considerations

- The retrolental plaque is usually densest centrally. When performing the posterior capsulotomy, start at the edge of the plaque (in normal posterior capsule if possible and not too peripherally) and proceed circumferentially. Attempt to make an incision in the posterior capsule with a cystotome or MVR blade and have a pair of intraocular scissors available if unable to cut through the plaque. Make the incision big enough to allow you to grasp the edge of the posterior capsule if planning on performing a manual capsulorrhexis or to allow the vitrector to engage the capsule to start the vitrectorhexis.

> **It is not necessary to remove the entire fibrotic capsule, just the portion in the visual axis.**

- Sometimes the vascular stalk can bleed. If the stalk is obviously vascularized, cauterize before cutting. If there is bleeding, increase the infusion rate to tamponade the bleeding.

Postoperative Considerations

- Possible complications: intraocular hemorrhage, ciliary body detachment, glaucoma, retinal detachment, and retinal ischemia.

ECTOPIA LENTIS

- Most common causes of pediatric lens subluxation: Marfan syndrome, homocystinuria, trauma, and simple ectopia lentis
- Spectrum of severity: mild to total lens dislocation
  - In cases of mild lens dislocation, optical correction may be sufficient.
    - Some cases benefit from pupil dilation and use of the aphakic visual axis with aphakic correction.
  - Indications for surgical removal:
    - Unable to attain satisfactory visual function with optical correction.
    - Visual function affected by movement of the dislocated lens.

Preoperative Considerations

- Consider cardiology evaluation (Marfan syndrome), plasma homocysteine levels (homocystinuria), and / or genetics evaluation
- Clinical examination:
  - Check best corrected visual acuity in dilated and undilated states and at both distance and near.
  - Look at the position of the lens in the undilated and dilated state.
  - Check for presence or absence of zonules.
  - Check for phacodonesis.
  - Check refractive error.
    - A partially dislocated lens will induce significant myopic astigmatism.
    - If a lens dislocates out of the visual axis, an aphakic refraction may result in satisfactory visual acuity. Trial of aphakic contact lens can be helpful to predict success of postoperative contact lens use, since IOL implantation can be challenging with lens dislocation (see Chapter 4).

Surgical Procedure (Video 7.1)

- May be performed through either a limbal or pars plana approach.
- In most cases, complete lensectomy is indicated due to poor zonular integrity.
- Very important to keep the anterior chamber stable during the surgery.

> **If the lens is highly mobile, consider placing viscoelastic under the lens or using a second instrument to bring the lens up into the anterior chamber. With the lens in the anterior chamber, also consider constricting the pupil with a miotic in order to perform the lens removal in the anterior chamber.**

> **Since the lens will tend to move away from the vitrectomy handpiece, consider engaging the lens by opening the anterior capsule with an MVR blade or vitrector.**

- If planning a complete lensectomy, work efficiently to remove the lens (consider using a higher gauge vitrector, eg, 20 vs 23 gauge for faster lens removal) before removing the capsular bag.
- Lens implantation is controversial:
  - If planning lens implantation, may need to consider either scleral-fixated or iris-fixated IOL.

Postoperative Considerations

- Bilateral ectopia lentis and lensectomy: optical correction with aphakic glasses (bifocals/progressives) or contact lenses with readers.
- Unilateral ectopia lentis and lensectomy: optical correction with contact lens and glasses with unilateral bifocal.
- If suturing in an IOL, beware of potential suture breakage (avoid using 10-0 polypropylene suture which can degrade and result in spontaneous subluxation of the IOL over time).[2]
- Be aware of the increased risk of retinal detachment in patients with Marfan syndrome.

SMALL PUPIL

Newborns or infants may dilate poorly because the dilator muscle is poorly developed.

Preoperative Considerations

- On clinical examination:
  - Look for the presence of posterior synechiae or a pupillary membrane.
  - Record the size of the dilated pupil

Surgical Considerations

- If unable to instill dilating drops in preoperative area, instill dilation drops after induction (communicate with anesthesia team).
  - For faster action, try placing cotton-tipped applicators soaked in dilation drops in the inferior fornix, but be aware that this can increase the blood pressure and decrease the heart rate in infants (see Chapter 3).
- If dilation still poor, consider:
  - 5% or 10% phenylephrine drops (communicate with anesthesia team).
  - Intracameral preservative-free epinephrine 1:10 000.
  - Intracameral epi-Shugarcaine solution (epinephrine 0.025% and lidocaine 0.75% in fortified balanced salt solution [BSS Plus]).
- If dilation poor secondary to posterior synechiae:
  - Break the synechiae with instrument of choice (iris spatula, cyclodialysis spatula, Sinskey hook, push pull) and try to stretch the pupil with these instruments.
  - Then try to viscodissect and viscodilate the pupil with a cohesive viscoelastic.
  - If unable to dilate using a viscoelastic:
    - Iris hooks (Fig. 7.1):
      - Plan location for placement.
      - Space hooks evenly around the limbus, to allow for good visualization subincisionally and in locations that that do not interfere with infusion, vitrector, or main wound.

Making each stab incision more vertically oriented makes it easier to direct your hook to engage the iris.

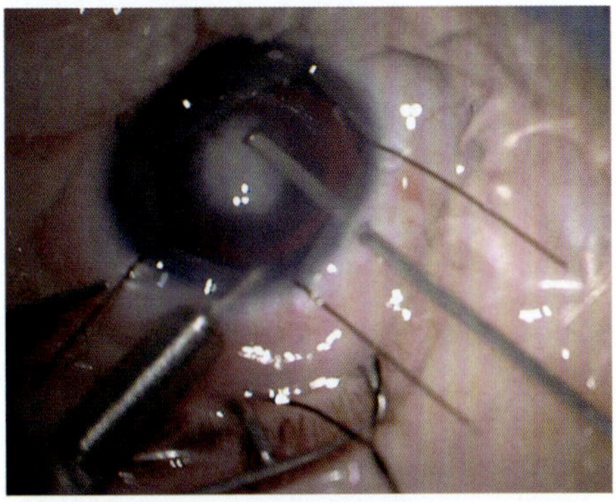

FIGURE 7.1. Iris hooks in a 7-week old infant with small pupil due to pupillary membrane.

- Malyugin ring:
  - Requires at least a 2-mm incision.
  - Requires a second instrument (eg, Sinskey hook or push pull) to help position, insert, and remove the ring.
  - Inserting the ring:
    - Place viscoelastic in the anterior chamber and under the iris without over filling the eye.
    - Position the tip of the injector close to the pupillary margin so the distal scroll can engage the iris directly across from the wound.
    - Continue injecting as the injector is slowly withdrawn. When the lateral scrolls emerge, catch the respective pupillary margins with each.
    - When the last (proximal) scroll is expelled from the injector onto the iris, remove the injector from the eye.
    - Use the second instrument to engage the pupillary margin with the last scroll.
  - Removing the ring:
    - Disengage the distal and proximal scroll from the pupillary margin using a Sinskey hook or other second instrument.
    - Lift up the proximal scroll with the second instrument and engage it with the injector.
    - Retract the ring carefully, using the second instrument to ensure iris tissue does not get caught in the ring.
    - When both lateral scrolls come close to the wound, press down on them with the second instrument (to sandwich the ring between the second instrument and the injector) to guide the ring back into the injector.
- Sphincterectomy (see Chapter 21):
  - Lift up the edge of the pupil with either a second instrument or with a cohesive viscoelastic.
  - Use intraocular scissors to make multiple radial incisions at equal intervals around the pupil margin through the iris sphincter (~0.5 mm).
  - Viscodilate the pupil with a cohesive viscoelastic.
  - After sphincterectomy, pupillary function will be permanently impaired, and there may be increased postoperative intraocular inflammation.

References

1. Bélair ML, Kim SJ, Thorne JE, et al. Incidence of cystoid macular edema after cataract surgery in patients with and without uveitis using optical coherence tomography. *Am J Ophthalmol.* 2009;148(1):128-135.e2.
2. Buckley EG. Hanging by a thread: the long-term efficacy and safety of transscleral sutured intraocular lenses in children (an American Ophthalmological Society thesis). *Trans Am Ophthalmol Soc.* 2007;105:294-311.

Suggested Readings

Leung TG, Lindsley K, Kuo IC. Types of intraocular lenses for cataract surgery in eyes with uveitis. *Cochrane Database Syst Rev.* 2014;(3):CD007284. doi: 10.1002/14651858.CD007284.pub2.

Mehta S, Linton MM, Kempen JH. Outcomes of cataract surgery in patients with uveitis: a systematic review and meta-analysis. *Am J Ophthalmol.* 2014;158(4):676-692.e7.

Phatak S, Lowder C, Pavesio C. Controversies in intraocular lens implantation in pediatric uveitis. *J Ophthalmic Inflamm Infect.* 2016;6:12.

CHAPTER 8

Cataract Surgery Complications

Maria E. Lim, MD

Complications from pediatric cataract surgery are varied and may occur at any point in the intraoperative and postoperative period. Continued long-term followup for aphakic and pseudophakic children is therefore recommended to monitor for these visually significant sequelae.

CAPSULE TEARS

- Anterior capsular tears.
  - Determine the extent of the tear.
    - If the tear extends to the zonules, use microinsional scissors or the vitrector hand piece to truncate the residual capsular flap.
    - Proceed with care aspirating lens material once the residual flap is removed.
  - If attempting a continuous curvilinear capsulorrhexis (CCC), stop, place viscoelastic in the anterior chamber, and use the Little maneuver to pull the capsule centrally to save the CCC (Fig. 8.1). If unsuccessful, try to create a second flap and tear in the opposite direction. Use microincisional scissors to truncate the aborted residual flap.
  - If while creating a vitrectorhexis a "tear-shaped" anterior capsular tear (a tear with a "V" shape pointing peripherally) occurs, proceed with caution to avoid pressure on this area as it may extend peripherally.
- Posterior capsular tears.
  - When there is significant lens material in the capsular bag, attempt to prolapse the lens into the anterior chamber and aspirate from there.
  - Aspirate only when the vitrectomy tip is occluded to avoid aspirating vitreous. Turn the cutter on whenever there is suspicion of vitreous, but be careful not to cut the capsule.
  - Once lens material is cleared, inspect the capsular bag and determine the extent of the posterior capsular tear.
    - If implanting an IOL, an attempt to place the lens in the capsular bag with a small, round posterior capsular tear may be made. Use the vitrector with a high cut rate to even out the edges if they are not smooth.
    - If the tear is large, place a 3-piece sulcus lens or leave the patient aphakic with plans to place a secondary IOL in the future if there is enough support.

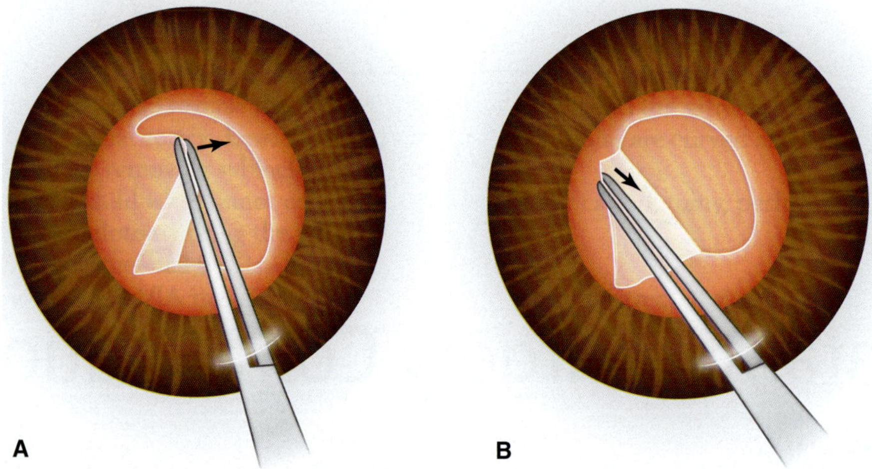

FIGURE 8.1. Schematic showing the Little maneuver, which is used to redirect a continuous curvilinear capsulorrhexis. **A.** First, pull the flap opposite the direction of the rhexis. **B.** Then, pull the flap centrally to redirect the rhexis.

DROPPED LENS

- Very large lens fragments that fall posteriorly should be removed by a vitreoretinal surgeon.
- If lens material falls to the anterior vitreous face, attempt to carefully cut with the vitrector.
- If small fragments fall posteriorly, they can be left and the patient monitored closely as the lens material resorbs.
  - It may take weeks to months for the retained lens material to resorb, depending on the size of the fragment.
  - The patient should be monitored for lens-induced uveitis and secondary glaucoma.
    - The patient can be placed on steroids, both topical and oral (prednisolone 1 mg/kg/day), to treat postoperative inflammation (see Chapter 3).
    - Topical antihypertensives can be added as needed for IOP (see Chapter 3).
  - Refer to a retina specialist to remove lens fragments resulting in severe inflammation, uncontrolled IOP, corneal edema, or cystoid macular edema.[1]

ELEVATED INTRAOCULAR PRESSURE

- Determine the etiology of elevated intraocular pressure. Possible etiologies include inflammation, steroid response, trabeculodysgenesis (especially in congenital cataracts), secondary angle closure from posterior synechiae, and/or vitreous prolapse into anterior chamber.
- Start with topical antihypertensives.
  - Avoid brimonidine in children <2 years old.
  - Use 0.25% timolol in children <6 months age.
- Can also use acetazolamide (5 mg/kg q6h) if refractory to topical medications.
- Consider changing topical steroid (ie, from prednisolone or difluprednate/Durezol) to one that does not result in as much of an elevation in intraocular pressure (ie, fluorometholone). Taper off steroids as soon as possible.
- If patient has secondary angle closure, may need to return to OR for synechiolysis, anterior vitrectomy and/or peripheral iridotomy (PI). PI options include:
  - Awake *laser peripheral iridotomy (LPI)* if patient can cooperate:
    - Pretreat the patient with pilocarpine and apraclonidine.

  - In dark irides, consider pretreating with Argon laser (spot size: 400 µm, duration: 0.2 second, power: 200-300 mW).
  - Apply the iridotomy lens with a coupling agent.
  - Set Yag laser defocus to zero and aim for an iris crypt and iris stroma. Avoid visible iris vessels.
  - Power: 1-6 mJ, pulses per burst: 1-3 (spot size is constant for each laser model).
- *Surgical iridectomy* (see Chapter 21) if unable to cooperated for awake laser PI:
  - Consider preoperative pilocarpine to constrict the pupil.
  - Using a micro-Uttrata through a 20G paracentesis wound, grasp a peripheral piece of iris tissue through the wound and use Vannas scissors to cut this iris tissue. Use a 10-0 Vicryl figure of 8 suture to close the wound.
  - If you prefer to use the vitrector, place the irrigation port through one paracentesis, then use the vitrector through another to aspirate/cut the iris tissue.
- If refractory to conservative management, may require incisional glaucoma surgery (see Section III).

INFECTION

- Carefully examine the anterior chamber, the wound, and the fundus.
  - An examination under anesthesia may be necessary.
  - B-scan ultrasonography can help to determine if vitritis is present.
- If no vitritis, treat with topical fortified vancomycin and tobramycin and monitor daily.
- If there is vitritis, hypopyon, or other signs concerning for endophthalmitis, plan to refer to vitreoretinal specialist for vitreous tap, intravitreal antibiotics, and possible vitrectomy.

VISUAL AXIS OPACITIES

- Visual axis opacities (VAO) are common adverse events of cataract surgery and can be the result of severe capsular phimosis, secondary membrane formation, or cortical proliferation.[2] Uncontrolled postoperative inflammation can predispose a patient to developing VAO. Lensectomy with posterior capsulotomy and anterior vitrectomy (see Chapter 6) should be routinely performed in all children <5 years of age to reduce the incidence of VAO.[3]
- *YAG laser capsulotomy*: cooperative patient and thin membrane.
  - After appropriate pharmacological mydriasis, pretreat the patient with apraclonidine.
  - A capsulotomy lens may or may not be used, depending on patient tolerance.
  - Set defocus with a posterior offset of 250 µm.
  - Power: 1-2 mJ, pulses per burst: 1-2 (spot size is constant for each laser model).
- *Vitrectomy*: if the membrane appears thick or the patient is unable to tolerate YAG capsulotomy.
  - *Anterior vitrectomy*: aphakic or pseudophakic with membranes anterior to the lens.
    - Using a 23G MVR blade, create two paracentesis wounds. Place irrigation through one wound to maintain the anterior chamber. Use the vitrectomy hand piece to aspirate and cut the obscuring membranes.
    - If membranes are too tough for vitrectomy, microincisional scissors or an MVR blade can be used to create flaps in the VAO to widen the opening.

- *Pars plana vitrectomy*: pseudophakic and the VAO is posterior (ie, posterior capsular opacity).
  - For a pars plana approach, use the 23G MVR to create a paracentesis wound and place irrigation.
  - Create a limbal peritomy extending 4 mm posteriorly and cauterize as needed.
  - Using the 23G MVR, enter pars plana at the appropriate distance posterior to the limbus based on patient age, taking care to aim posterior to the IOL (see Chapters 6 and 31). Place the vitrectomy handpiece through the wound, attempt to remove the obstructing membrane.
  - A Sinskey hook or MVR blade can be used to score an opening in the membrane prior to vitrectomy.
- For significant cortical proliferation, use the 23G MVR blade to create a small incision in the Soemmering ring to allow access to the cortical material. Use the vitrectomy handpiece to remove cortical material. Be aware that this material may reproliferate postoperatively.

WOUND LEAKS

- Prevent leaks by suturing all wounds with either 10-0 nylon (corneal sutures will need subsequent removal, while scleral sutures can remain indefinitely) or 9-0 Vicryl and ensure that wounds are watertight.
- Postoperative patients should wear glasses or a shield at all times for a month. This may help to prevent trauma that causes wound leaks.
- If the leak is small, place a bandage contact lens on the eye while treating with topical antibiotics +/− an aqueous suppressant. Follow daily and monitor for infection.
- If the leak is brisk, and/or the anterior chamber is shallow/flat, then return to the operating room to place a suture and reform the anterior chamber.

IOL PROBLEMS

- *Lens removal* due to insufficient capsular support, lens dislocation, or lens intolerance:
  - Prolapse the lens into the anterior chamber and use a dispersive viscoelastic (see Chapter 3) to protect the corneal endothelium.
  - Widen the main wound and use IOL scissors to bisect the lens and create a "Pac-Man" shape (Fig. 8.2A). A Kelman-McPherson forceps may be used to stabilize the lens while cutting.

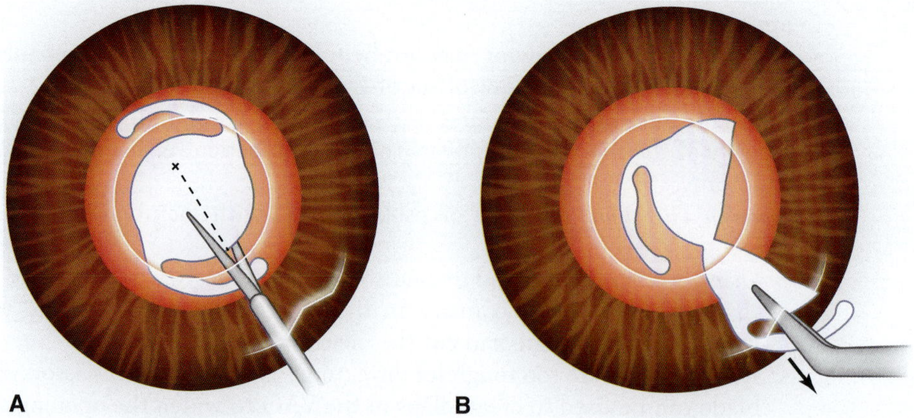

A B

FIGURE 8.2. Schematic showing IOL removal. **A.** Use IOL scissors to cut across the lens to create a Pac-Man shape. **B.** Widen the wound, grasp the optic of the lens with an angled forceps and remove the lens.

  - Using a Kelman-McPherson forceps or similar instrument, grasp the optic near the wound and remove the lens from the anterior chamber (Fig. 8.2B). Suture the enlarged wound with a 10-0 Vicryl figure of 8.
- Decentered or partially subluxed lens in the capsular bag.
  - Viscodissect the capsular bag open and reposition the lens.
- Anteriorly dislocated sulcus lens.
  - If the dislocation is partial and noted incidentally on examination (chronic), it may not cause problems for the patient and can be observed.
  - Conservatively, dilate the pupil and have the patient lie supine to see if the optic will fall back into place.
  - If the haptic is anterior to the iris plane or not amenable to conservative management, return to the OR to reposition the lens.
    - Consider optic capture to prevent further IOL dislocation.
- Posteriorly dislocated lens.
  - Refer to vitreoretinal specialist to remove the lens. In older patients, consider a scleral sutured IOL.
- Chronic inflammation or uveitis-glaucoma-hyphema (UGH) syndrome with a sulcus lens.
  - Immobilize the iris with topical atropine.
  - If refractory to conservative measures, return to the OR to capture the optic on the remaining capsule.

References

1. Borne MJ, Tasman W, Regillo C, et al. Outcomes of vitrectomy for retained lens fragments. *Ophthalmology*. 1996;103:971-976.
2. Infant Aphakia Treatment Study Group; Lambert SR, Lynn MJ, et al. Comparison of contact lens and intraocular lens correction of monocular aphakia during infancy: a randomized clinical trial of HOTV optotype acuity at age 4.5 years and clinical findings at age 5 years. *JAMA Ophthalmol*. 2014;132(6):676-682.
3. Whitman MC, Vanderveen DK. Complications of pediatric cataract surgery. *Semin Ophthalmol*. 2014;29(5-6):414-420.

Section III

Pediatric Glaucoma Surgery

CHAPTER 9

Preoperative Considerations

Amanda L. Ely, MD ● Sharon F. Freedman, MD

PREOPERATIVE CONSIDERATIONS

In an eye with suspected pediatric glaucoma, a full ocular examination is essential to confirm the specific pediatric glaucoma diagnosis, to obtain baseline ocular measurements that will be helpful for future disease management, and to determine which medical and/or surgical therapies are most appropriate to maximize long-term IOP control.

Which Type of Pediatric Glaucoma Does Your Patient Have?

- Determining the specific pediatric glaucoma diagnosis is essential in order to:
  - Counsel the family appropriately on long-term outcomes.
  - Determine which medical and/or surgical therapies are indicated (Fig. 9.1).

When Is Glaucoma Surgery Necessary? Consider Surgery in Patients With:

- Primary congenital glaucoma (PCG).
- Closed angle glaucomas (eg, cicatricial retinopathy of prematurity).
- Progressive IOP–related ocular damage despite maximal tolerated medical therapy.

SURGICAL PLANNING

- Manage patient/parent expectations about the following:
  - Chronic disease management and follow-up.
    - Loss of IOP control can occur even decades after successful glaucoma surgery.
  - Guarded visual prognosis.
  - Likely need for further surgical intervention, including further glaucoma surgery, possible strabismus surgery, and/or possible cataract surgery.
  - Likely need for further medical intervention, including chronic eye drops, glasses, and amblyopia therapy.

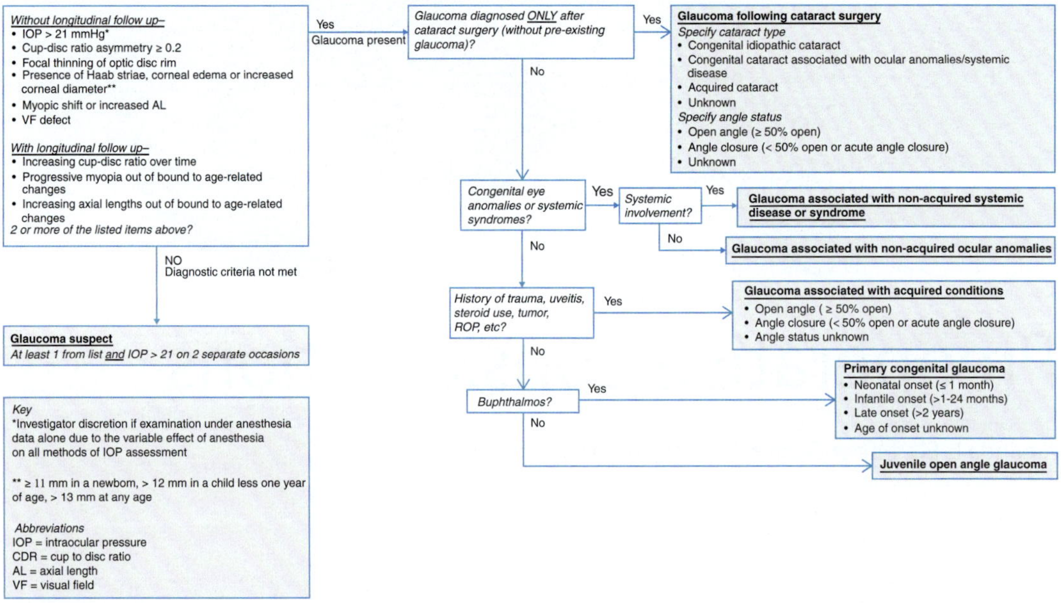

FIGURE 9.1. Classification of childhood glaucomas. Childhood Glaucoma Research Network (CGRN)-World Glaucoma Association algorithm for the classification of childhood glaucoma. IOP = intraocular pressure; ONH = optic nerve head; VF = visual field. (Adapted from Childhood Glaucoma Research Network, courtesy of Ta Chen Peter Chang.)[1]

- Ensure that you have the following equipment/medication:
  - Days to weeks in advance:
    - Specific glaucoma drainage device (GDD) implants (eg, Ahmed FP7 or FP8, Baerveldt 250 or 350) (see Chapter 11).
    - Specific patch graft tissue (eg, sclera, cornea).
    - Special order disposable equipment (eg, illuminated catheter for trabeculotomy, goniotomy lens).
  - Same day:
    - Special pre-op or intraoperative medications (eg, pilocarpine 1% or 2%, apraclonidine 0.5%, sodium chloride 5%, timolol 0.25%, mitomycin C, subconjunctival antibiotic or steroid).
    - Special equipment (eg, Retcam, B-scan ultrasound, anterior chamber maintainer, specific surgical gonioscopy lens).
    - Specific orientation of the microscope (eg, tilt for goniotomy).
- Preoperative medications (to help lower IOP and to clear the cornea preoperatively to facilitate goniotomy), ideally used days before the planned surgery. Consider punctal occlusion in infants to reduce systemic absorption.
  - Beta blocker (eg, timolol 0.25% once daily):
    - Typically first-line and safe for use in infants and toddlers <35 lb.
    - Use with caution, if at all, in those with history of respiratory disorders (eg, asthma, apnea of prematurity).
  - Carbonic anhydrase inhibitor (eg, dorzolamide 2% three times daily):
    - Second line if beta blocker use contraindicated.
    - Caution in neonates <35 weeks postmenstrual age because of the risk for metabolic acidosis.
  - Sodium chloride 5%:
    - Use in conjunction with IOP lowering medications to help lessen corneal edema.

EXAMINATION UNDER ANESTHESIA (EUA)

The EUA is necessary to obtain information that cannot be obtained in the clinic setting. EUA can be performed separately or in conjunction with planned glaucoma surgery.

IOP Measurement

- Preintubation (earlier IOP measurement more accurate):
  - Anesthetic effects on IOP:
    - Mild reduction in IOP: sevoflurane, midazolam, nitrous oxide.
    - Mild elevation in IOP: ketamine.
    - Marked elevation in IOP: laryngospasm, Bells reflex, endotracheal intubation.
- Predilation—Measure IOP before dilation unless dilation is needed for remainder of the EUA or for the procedure to follow.
- Equipment options:
  - Tono-Pen (Reichert, Depew, New York, USA)—accurate and easy to use.
  - Perkins (Clement Clarke Inc., Columbus, OH, USA)—similar accuracy to Tonopen, more cumbersome to use, need fluorescein on ocular surface.
  - Pneumatonometer (Reichert, Depew, New York, USA)—best as confirmatory remeasure, or in settings of opaque or scarred corneas.
  - Rebound tonometer (Icare IC200 [Icare Finland, Helsinki, Finland]) soon to be approved in the United States with ability to be used in a supine patient.

Anterior Segment Examination

- Koeppe Gonioscopy Lens—angle anatomy:
  - Infants with PCG often show a smooth homogenous membrane from iris to Schwalbe's line (Fig. 9.2).
  - The angle normally shows increasing pigmentation with age.
- Portable slit lamp:
  - Corneal examination:
    - Corneal diameter will continue to increase with uncontrolled IOP until approximately age 3 years old.
      - Suspect glaucoma if the corneal diameter is[2,3]:
        - Birth to 6 months: >12 mm (normal 9.5-11.5 mm).
        - 1-2 years: >12.5 mm (normal 10-12 mm).
        - >2 years: >13 mm (normal <12 mm).

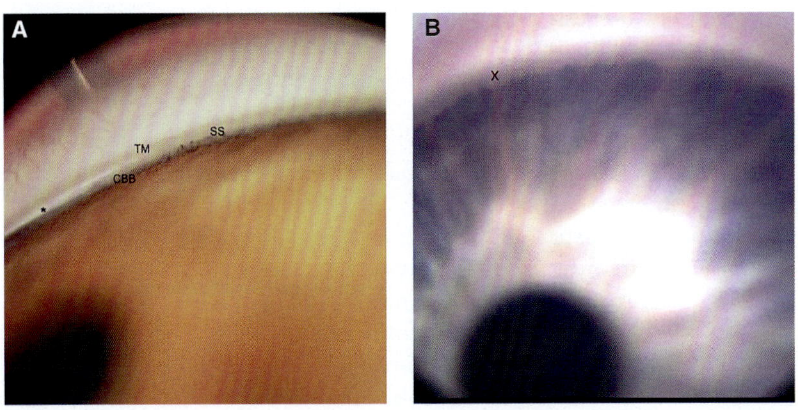

FIGURE 9.2. Angle photos. **A.** Image shows angle anatomy in juvenile open angle glaucoma patient after angle surgery. Note the locations of the tip of the ciliary body band (CBB), the very faint appearing scleral spur (SS), and the trabecular meshwork (TM). Also note the location of a cleft (*asterisk*) created by previous angle surgery. **B.** Image shows the angle anatomy in primary congenital glaucoma. Note the more bland appearing angle features with overlying Barkan's membrane (X).

- Haab striae (breaks in Descemet's membrane)—sign of significant rise in IOP in children <3 years old (can be acute or any time within the first 3 years of life).
- Corneal edema—sign of significantly elevated IOP or severe loss of endothelial cells.
- Posterior embryotoxon (eg, Axenfeld-Rieger syndrome).
- Central corneal opacity with iris or lenticular adhesions (eg, Peters anomaly).
- Anterior chamber examination:
  - Depth: Assess whether the chamber is deep enough for a GDD.
  - Look for iris abnormalities including stromal hypoplasia, complete vs partial aniridia, ectropion uveae, corectopia, etc.
  - Lenticular examination: clear, opaque, zonular support, etc.

Cycloplegic Retinoscopy

- Haab striae can cause irregular astigmatism, and chronically elevated IOP can cause progressive myopia (both may be amblyogenic)

Ophthalmoscopy

- Optic nerve:
  - Document cupping, pallor, size.
  - 28-D or 30-D lens will minimize appearance of cupping. The nerve is best viewed with a direct ophthalmoscope through Koeppe gonioscopy lens.
- Retina—indirect ophthalmoscopy to ensure retinal integrity.

Do NOT dilate the operative eye if planning to do angle surgery under the same sedation.

Ultrasonography

- Pachymetry—measure central corneal thickness:
  - Avoid "adjusting" measured IOP based on this number.
  - Normative data[4]:
    - 6-23 months: 538 ± 40 μm.
    - 2-4 years old: 546 ± 41 μm.
    - Adult norms by 5-9 years of age.
  - Thinner corneal thickness in PCG (stretched cornea).
  - Thicker in aniridia and glaucoma following cataract surgery (GFCS) (likely acquired due to corneal pathology).
  - Thicker with corneal edema, even if subclinical.
- Axial length—will continue to lengthen with uncontrolled IOP until approximately 10 years of age.
  - Immersion—best.
  - Contact A-scan—may give falsely low axial length due to operator indentation of cornea.
  - Normative data[5]:
    - 0-12 months: 21.1-22.5 mm.
    - 13-24 months: 22.5-22.9 mm.
    - 25-48 months: 22.9-25.1 mm.
  - Need an axial length ≥21 mm for GDD. For eyes < 21mm, either trim back of plate or place it closer to limbus than standard 7-8 mm (see Chapter 11).
    - people.duke.edu/~freed003/GDDCalculator[6]
- Confirm patency of GDD if bleb not well seen. B-scan ultrasound evaluation may be helpful when the GDD tube cannot be seen because of opaque corneas, or the bleb was not visualized.[7]
- Confirm status of retina if there is a poor view to posterior segment.

Photography

- Retcam photos (Clarity Medical Systems, Inc., Pleasanton, CA, USA)—for future comparison of optic nerve cupping and morphology.
  - The Retcam can also be used for imaging of the anterior segment and angle. For anterior segment photos, the lens is cleaned using alcohol to ensure a clear image and held above the surface of the eye focusing up until a clear anterior segment can be seen. For angle photos, a generous amount of a viscous material (best is clear gel, any viscoelastic may also be used) is applied to the concave portion of the lens, which is then placed directly on the ocular surface angled toward the corneal limbus of the desired angle location. The focus can then be adjusted for clarity of the angle image.
- OCT (optical coherence tomography) imaging—if available, this is the most accurate for long-term comparison.
  - Published normative pediatric data for Spectralis SD-OCT device (Heidelberg Engineering, Heidelberg, Germany).[8]
    - Global mean peripapillary retinal nerve fiber layer thickness—107.6 μm.

References

1. Weinreb RN, Grajewski AL, Papadopoulos M, Grigg J, Freedman SF. *Childhood Glaucoma: The 9th Consensus Report of the World Glaucoma Association*. Amsterdam, The Netherlands: Kugler Publications; 2013.
2. Kiskis AA, Markowitz SN, Morin JD. Corneal diameter and axial length in congenital glaucoma. *Can J Ophthalmol.* 1985;20(3):93-97.
3. Becker B, Shaffer RN. *Diagnosis and Therapy of the Glaucomas*. St. Louis, MO: CV Mosby; 1965.
4. Hussein MA, Paysse EA, Bell NP, et al. Corneal thickness in children. *Am J Ophthalmol.* 2004;138(5):744-748.
5. Cronemberger S, Calixto N, Milhomens TGA, et al. Effect of intraocular pressure control on central corneal thickness, horizontal corneal diameter, and axial length in primary congenital glaucoma. *J AAPOS*. 2014;18:433-436.
6. Margeta MA, Kuo AN, Proia AD, Freedman SF. Staying away from the optic nerve: a formula for modifying glaucoma drainage device surgery in pediatric and other small eyes. *J AAPOS*. 2017;21(1):39-43.
7. Baig NB, Lin AA, Freedman SF. Ultrasound evaluation of glaucoma drainage devices in children. *J AAPOS*. 2015;19(3):281-284. https://doi.org/10.1016/j.jaapos.2015.02.001
8. El-Dairi MA, Asrani SG, Enyedi LB, Freedman SF. Optical coherence tomography in the eyes of normal children. *Arch Ophthalmol.* 2009;127(1):50-58.

CHAPTER 10

Angle Surgery

Brenda L. Bohnsack, MD, PhD

PREOPERATIVE CONSIDERATIONS

Angle surgery is highly effective in many forms of glaucoma that affect children, often providing long-term and in many cases lifetime IOP control. However, the success of angle surgery is dependent on the type of childhood glaucoma and the angle configuration (see Chapter 9).

- Primary congenital glaucoma (PCG): Angle surgery is the mainstay of PCG (70%-90% success rate) and should be the first surgical approach in these cases.[1-7]
- Juvenile open angle glaucoma (JOAG): Angle surgery has been shown to effectively control IOP in 50%-70% of cases of JOAG.[8-12] Similar to PCG, angle surgery should be considered as a first surgical approach in JOAG.
- Glaucoma following cataract surgery (GFCS): In GFCS, if the angle is open, then angle surgery should be the first surgical approach and can be effective in obtaining IOP control.[8,11,13] However, if the angle is closed, then angle surgery is less likely to be successful and there is the risk of disinsertion of the iris root at the time of surgery.
- Uveitic glaucoma: Uveitic glaucoma is often mixed-mechanism, and the angle configuration preoperatively is important to assess. In eyes with an open-angle and good preoperative inflammation control, angle surgery is successful in 60%-80% of cases.[14-17]
- Sturge-Weber glaucoma: Glaucoma in Sturge-Weber syndrome can be due to goniodysgenesis and/or increased episcleral venous pressure. In eyes with goniodysgenesis as evidenced by an open angle with immature trabecular meshwork and dysplastic iris insertion, angle surgery may be effective in controlling IOP.[18-20] However, the presence of a choroidal hemangioma in these eyes should be evaluated preoperatively given the increased risk of suprachoroidal hemorrhage due to hypotony.[21,22] An *ab externo* approach has increased the risk of hypotony; thus, an *ab interno* approach may be the safer option in eyes with choroidal hemangiomas.

SURGICAL APPROACHES

Angle surgeries are categorized by the surgical approach (*ab externo*, *ab interno*) and the amount of angle treated. The 180-degree trabeculotomy and 180-degree goniotomy have been the traditional angle surgeries employed for over 70 years.[23-27] However, in the last 25 years, many studies have shown that 360-degree trabeculotomy (*ab externo* or *ab interno*) may yield higher success rates and longer IOP control.[8,9,11,28-31] Nonetheless, in eyes with congenital anomalies or previous surgeries, the suture or catheter may not be able to be passed 360 degrees and a 180-degree approach may be required.

Ab Externo Approach

Advantages: Does not require gonioscopic view; may be combined with trabeculectomy.

Disadvantages: Requires conjunctival incision; longer operating time compared to *ab interno* approach.

Ab Interno Approach

Advantages: Preservation of conjunctiva; shorter operating time compared to *ab externo* approach.

Disadvantages: Requires clear cornea for gonioscopic view.

SURGICAL PROCEDURES

Ab Externo Approach

- Place partial-thickness 7-0 Vicryl traction sutures at the superior and inferior limbus. Rotate the eye superonasally to expose the inferotemporal quadrant (Figs. 10.1A).
- Create a 3-clock hour conjunctival peritomy inferotemporally with Westcott scissors. Bluntly and sharply dissect off Tenon capsule. Use Wet-Field cautery for hemostasis (Figs. 10.1A and B, 10.2A and B).
- Using a combination of a 7515 blade and mini-crescent blade, create a 3-mm triangular scleral flap with 75% depth that extends beyond the limbus just into the clear cornea (Figs. 10.1C and 10.2C).
- Reflect the scleral flap over the cornea and identify the approximate location of Schlemm canal, which is "where blue and white meet" just posterior to the limbus. NOTE: Especially in buphthalmic or microphthalmic eyes, Schlemm canal may be shifted more posteriorly or anteriorly than the anticipated location due to stretching of the sclera or abnormalities in development of the cornea, scleral, and angle structures.
- Carefully dissect in the anticipated location of Schlemm canal with a 7515 blade. The main landmark is the circumferential scleral fibers, which are the bed of Schlemm canal. Look for an egress of aqueous humor to identify the canal (Figs. 10.1D and 10.2D).
- Use a 7515 blade to create a paracentesis. Inject viscoelastic into the anterior chamber and specifically into the angle (Figs. 10.1E and 10.2E).
- Canalization of Schlemm canal and trabeculotomy.
  - VIDEO **180-degree trabeculotomy *ab externo* with Harms trabeculotomes** (Video 10.1):
    - Insert the lower arm of the Harms trabeculotome "to the right" in a counterclockwise fashion in Schlemm canal (Fig. 10.1F). Once the lower arm of the trabeculotome has been completely advanced, then carefully rotate the arms of the trabeculotome toward the anterior chamber until the lower arm has incised the trabecular meshwork and is in the anterior chamber (Fig. 10.1G). Withdraw the trabeculotome.
    - Repeat this process with the trabeculotome "to the left" in the clockwise direction (Fig. 10.1H and I).

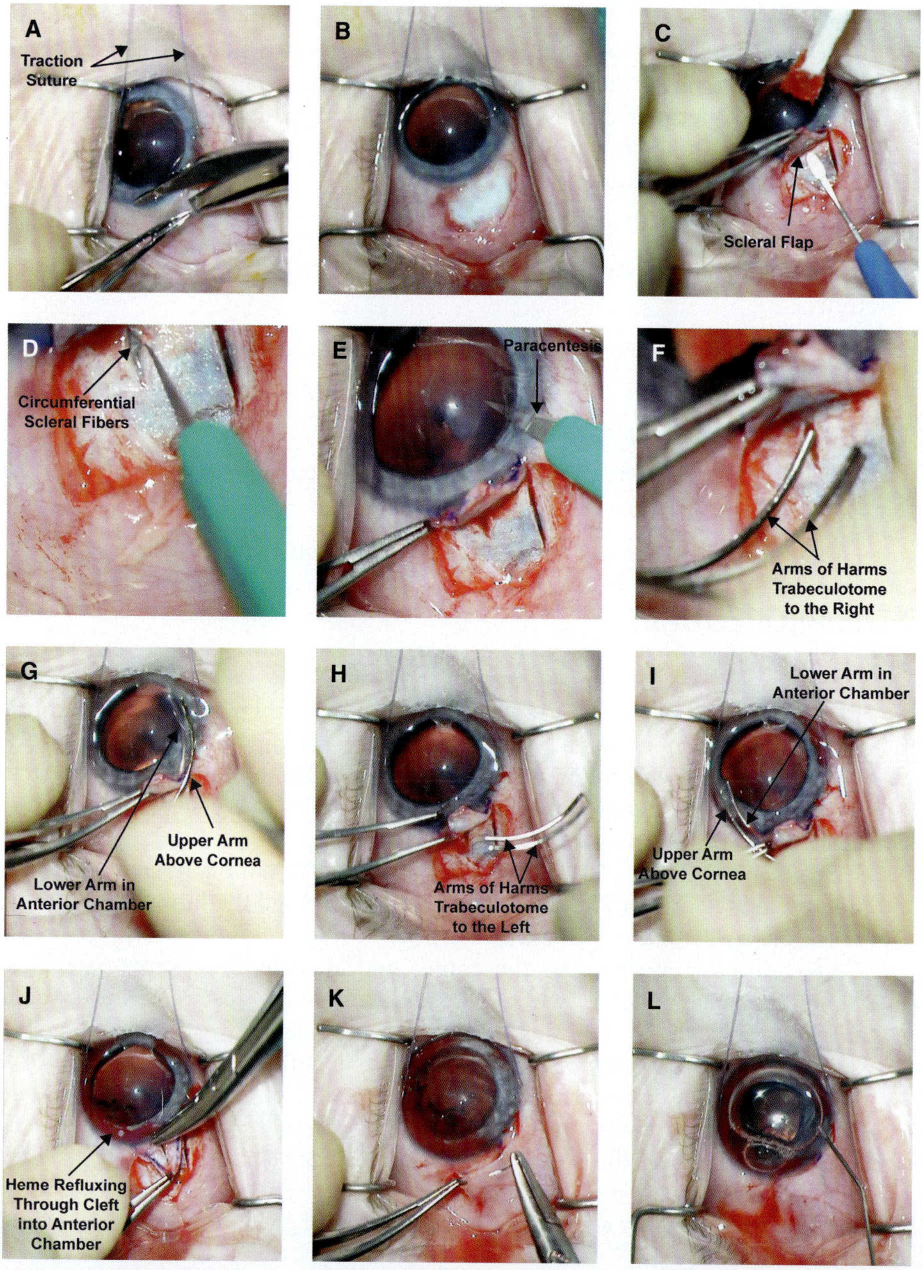

FIGURE 10.1. 180-degree trabeculotomy *ab externo* with Harms trabeculotomes. **A.** Following placement of partial-thickness 7-0 Vicryl sutures at the superior and inferior limbus, the eye is rotated superonasally to expose the inferotemporal quadrant. A 3-clock hour peritomy is created with Westcott scissors. **B.** Dissection of Tenon insertion followed by Wet-Field cautery is used to prepare the inferotemporal quadrant. **C.** A 75% depth scleral flap is created with a combination of a 7515 blade and a micro-crescent blade. The flap is reflected over the cornea to expose the anticipated area of Schlemm canal, "where blue and white meet." **D.** A 7515 blade is used to carefully dissect down to the circumferential scleral fibers, which are the bed of Schlemm canal. An egress of aqueous humor demarcates Schlemm canal. **E.** A 7515 blade is used to create a paracentesis, and viscoelastic is injected into the anterior chamber. **F.** The lower arm of the Harms trabeculotome to the right is inserted into Schlemm canal. The upper arm of the trabeculotome indicates the location of the lower arm. **G.** After completely advancing the trabeculotome into Schlemm canal, the lower arm is rotated into the anterior chamber. **H.** The lower arm of the Harms trabeculotome to the left is inserted into Schlemm canal. **I.** The trabeculotome is then rotated into the anterior chamber. **J.** Heme refluxes into the anterior chamber through the cleft. The scleral flap is closed with 10-0 Vicryl suture. **K.** The conjunctiva is closed with 10-0 Vicryl suture. **L.** Balanced salt solution is irrigated through the paracentesis to remove the viscoelastic. Filtered air is injected into the anterior chamber.

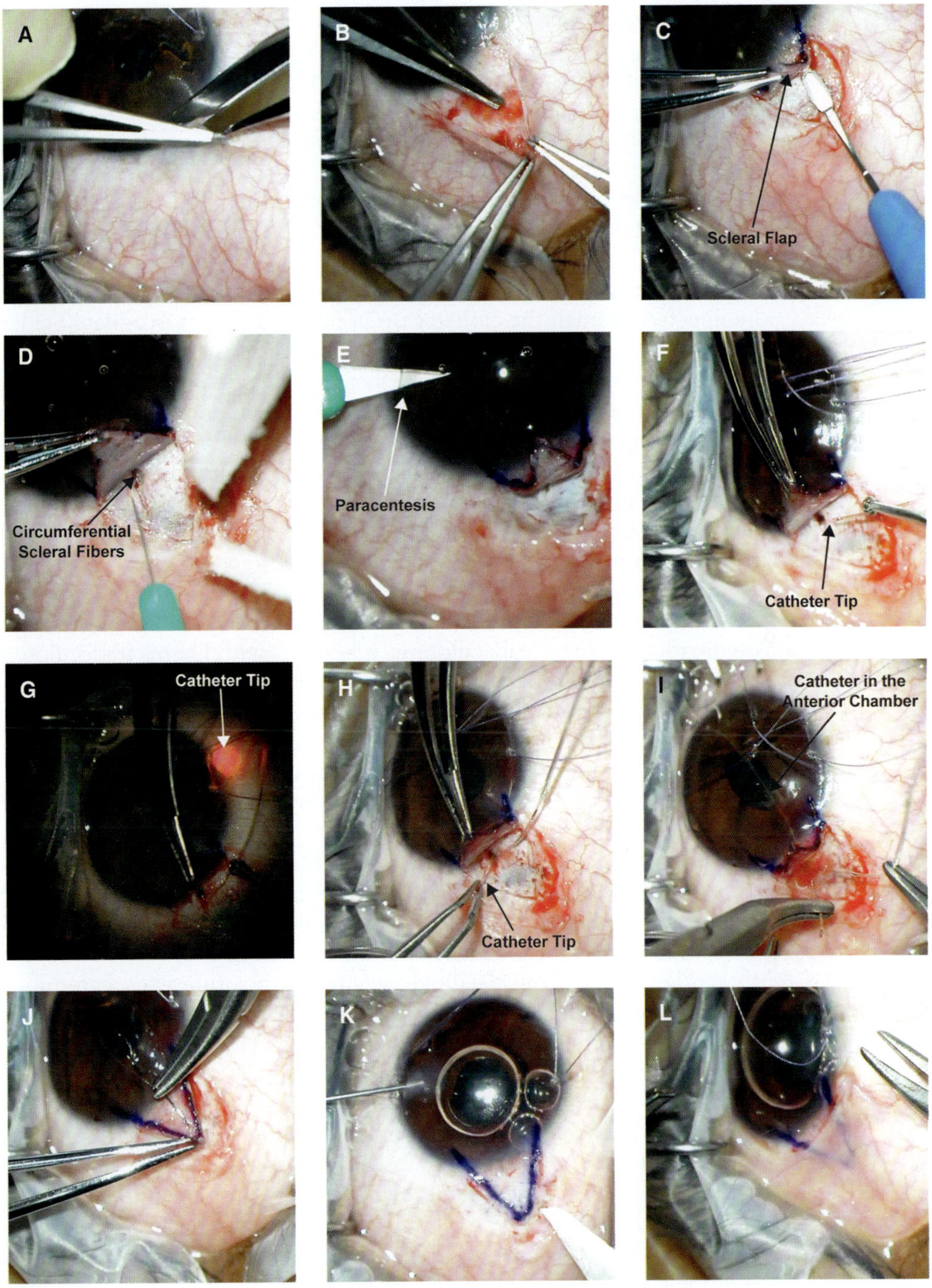

FIGURE 10.2. 360-degree trabeculotomy *ab externo* with an illuminated microcatheter. **A.** A 3-clock hour peritomy is created with Westcott scissors in the inferotemporal quadrant. **B.** Dissection of Tenon insertion followed by Wet-Field cautery is used to prepare the inferotemporal quadrant. **C.** A 75% depth scleral flap is created with a combination of a 7515 blade and a micro-crescent blade. The flap is reflected over the cornea to expose the anticipated area of Schlemm canal, "where blue and white meet." **D.** A 7515 blade is used to carefully dissect down to the circumferential scleral fibers, which are the bed of Schlemm canal. An egress of aqueous humor demarcates Schlemm canal. **E.** A 7515 blade is used to create a paracentesis, and viscoelastic is injected into the anterior chamber. **F.** The tip of the illuminated microcatheter is carefully inserted into Schlemm canal. **G.** The catheter is advanced while observing the lighted catheter tip. **H.** After traveling 360 degrees, the catheter tip is retrieved under the scleral flap. **I.** Both ends of the catheter are grasped with needle drivers, and the catheter is pulled through the trabecular meshwork into the anterior chamber. **J.** The scleral flap is closed with 10-0 Vicryl suture. **K.** Balanced salt solution is irrigated through the paracentesis to remove the viscoelastic. Filtered air is injected into the anterior chamber. **L.** The conjunctiva is closed with 10-0 Vicryl suture.

- **360-degree trabeculotomy *ab externo* with an illuminated microcatheter (Video 10.2):**
    - Assemble the illuminated microcatheter with attachment of viscoelastic as per manufacturer's instructions.
    - Insert the illuminated microcatheter into Schlemm canal (Fig. 10.2F). Use care to avoid bending the catheter. Carefully advance the catheter, visualizing the light at the tip of the catheter at all times (Fig. 10.2G). After traveling 360 degrees, retrieve the catheter from under the scleral flap (Fig. 10.2H).
    NOTE:
        - If the catheter is unable to be advanced, a small amount of viscoelastic can be injected through the catheter tip in order to try to viscodilate Schlemm canal. This may allow for further advancement of the catheter.
        - If the catheter will not advance further or is directed posteriorly into a collecting channel, withdraw the catheter from Schlemm canal and attempt canalization in the opposite direction.
        - If the catheter can be advanced >180 degrees, but not 360 degrees, the end of the catheter can be retrieved by cutting down through the sclera over the lighted tip. Once the catheter end is retrieved, then proceed with pulling the catheter through the trabecular meshwork and then removing the catheter from the anterior chamber.
        - If the catheter cannot be advanced >180 degrees from either side, then proceed with traditional trabeculotomy *ab externo* with Harms trabeculotomes.
    - With gentle traction from needle drivers on both ends of the catheter, carefully pull the catheter through the trabecular meshwork into the anterior chamber and then remove the catheter from the anterior chamber (Fig. 10.2I).
- **360-degree trabeculotomy *ab externo* with a suture:**
    - Blunt the tip of a 5-0 Prolene suture by heating with a disposable low-temperature cautery.
    - Insert the blunted end of the suture into Schlemm canal. Place a gonioprism on the cornea to visualize the blue suture in Schlemm canal. Carefully advance the suture while directly visualizing the angle. After traveling 360 degrees, retrieve the suture from the incision under the scleral flap.
    - With gentle traction from needle drivers on both suture ends, carefully pull the suture through the trabecular meshwork into the anterior chamber. Once the suture has incised the trabecular meshwork, remove the suture from the anterior chamber.
    NOTE:
        - If the suture is unable to be advanced, there may be stenosis of Schlemm canal. Withdraw the suture and attempt canalization going in the opposite direction.
        - If the suture does not continue to travel through Schlemm canal despite advancing the suture at the incision, the suture has been directed posteriorly into a collecting channel. Retract the suture from Schlemm canal, and attempt canalization in the opposite direction.
        - If the suture is unable to be advanced 360 degrees in either direction, then proceed with 180-degree trabeculotomy *ab externo* with Harms trabeculotomes.

- Close the scleral flap 9-0 or 10-0 Vicryl or nylon suture (Figs. 10.1J and 10.2J). Then close the overlying conjunctiva with 9-0 or 10-0 Vicryl suture (Figs. 10.1K and 10.2L).
- Remove viscoelastic from the anterior chamber with balanced salt solution through the paracentesis. Inject filtered air into the anterior chamber (Figs. 10.1L and 10.2K).
- If needed, close the paracentesis with 10-0 Vicryl or nylon suture. Remove the traction suture.

Ab Interno Approach

180-Degree Nasal Goniotomy

- Instill one drop 2% pilocarpine and one drop 0.5% iopidine into the operative eye.
- With the surgeon sitting temporally, rotate the patient's head away from the surgeon. Tilt the microscope 45 degrees toward the surgeon.
- If using a Barkan or Swan Jacob gonioprism, place locking curved forceps at Tenon insertion superiorly and inferiorly. These forceps will be used by the assistant to rotate the eye to enlarge the cleft superiorly and inferiorly. If using a gonioprism with which the surgeon is able to stabilize and rotate the globe (ie, Volk Vold VVG lens), there is no need for the forceps or an assistant.
- Place viscoelastic on the cornea followed by the gonioprism. Adduct the eye to visualize the angle structures (Fig. 10.3A).

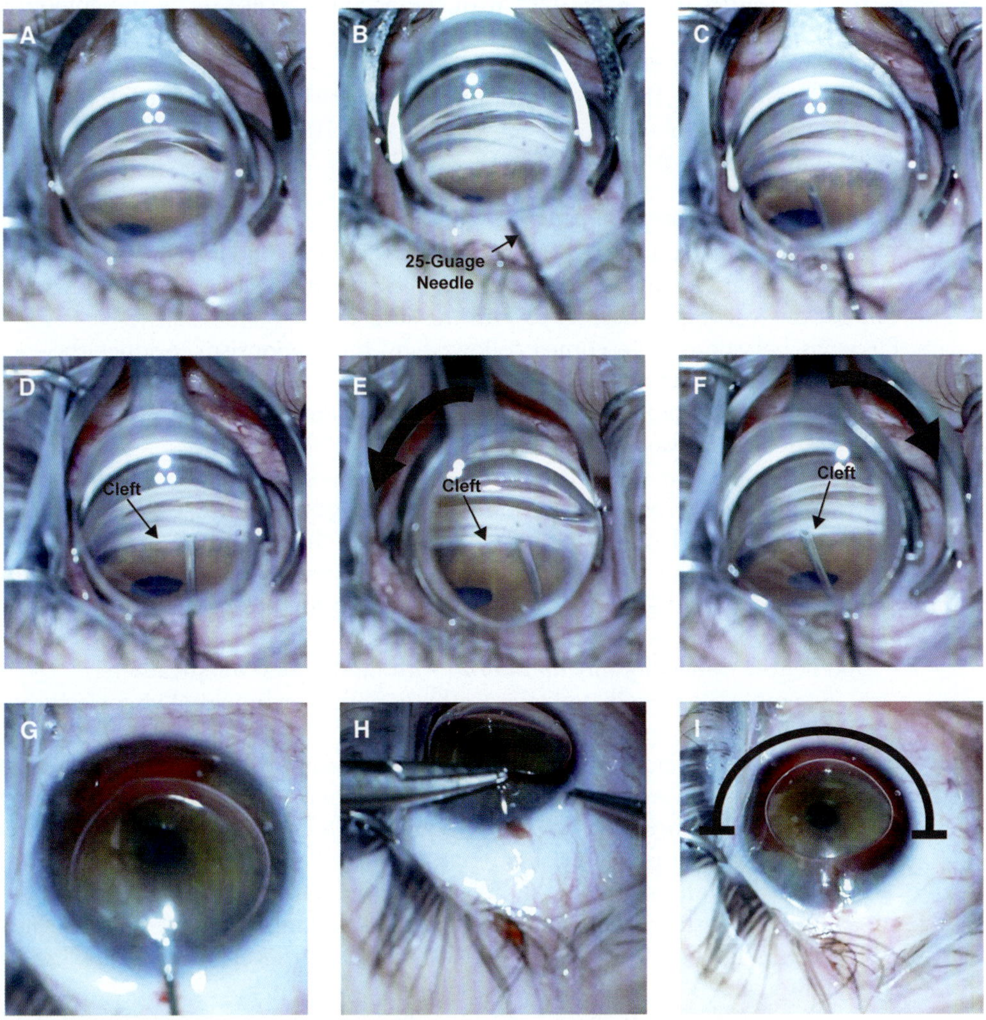

FIGURE 10.3. 180-degree nasal goniotomy. **A.** The Volk Vold VVG gonioprism, which allows the surgeon to adduct and rotate the eye, is placed on the cornea. **B.** A 25G needle is inserted into the anterior chamber just anterior to the temporal limbus. **C.** The needle is carefully passed through the anterior chamber. **D.** The needle is used to engage the nasal anterior trabecular meshwork to create a cleft. **E.** The eye is rotated counterclockwise to extend the cleft inferiorly. **F.** The eye is then rotated clockwise to extend the cleft superiorly for a total of 120-180 degrees. **G.** After the needle is withdrawn from the eye, heme is seen emanating from the cleft. Filtered air is injected into the anterior chamber. **H.** The incision is closed with a 10-0 Vicryl suture. **I.** The suture is buried to complete the surgery. The final cleft is ~180 degrees.

VIDEO
- Goniotomy with a 25G needle (Video 10.3) or goniotomy knife:
  - Incision:
    - **Goniotomy with a 25G needle**: Attach a 1.5-in 25G needle on a vial of viscoelastic if the pupil is undilated or on a syringe with Miochol if the pupil is dilated. Insert the needle just anterior to the temporal limbus into anterior chamber (Fig. 10.3B). If the pupil is dilated, inject Miochol into the anterior chamber to constrict the pupil. Carefully advance the needle across the anterior chamber (Fig. 10.3C).
    - **Goniotomy with a goniotomy knife**: Use a 7515 blade to create a paracentesis just anterior to the temporal limbus. Inject viscoelastic into the anterior chamber. Insert the knife through the incision into the anterior chamber. Carefully advance across the anterior chamber.
  - Engage and incise the anterior trabecular meshwork with the needle or knife to create a cleft (Fig. 10.3D). The iris plane will lower as the cleft is created. Rotate the eye (either by the assistant with the Moody forceps or by the gonioprism) counterclockwise (Fig. 10.3E) and then clockwise (Fig. 10.3F) to extend the cleft inferiorly and superiorly.
  - Carefully remove the needle from the anterior chamber. Inject filtered air into the anterior chamber through the incision (Fig. 10.3G). Close the incision with a 10-0 nylon or 10-0 Vicryl suture (Fig. 10.3H).

360-Degree Trabeculotomy Ab Interno

- Instill one drop 2% pilocarpine and one drop 0.5% iopidine into the operative eye.
- With the surgeon sitting temporally, rotate the patient's head away from the surgeon. Tilt the microscope 45 degrees toward the surgeon.
- Place viscoelastic on the cornea followed by the gonioprism. Adduct the eye to visualize the angle structures.
- With a 7515 blade, create a paracentesis just anterior to the temporal limbus. Inject viscoelastic into the anterior chamber.
- Insert either a 1.5-in 25G needle or a goniotomy knife through the incision and carefully advance across the anterior chamber. Engage and incise the anterior nasal trabecular meshwork creating ~1- to 2-clock hour cleft (Fig. 10.4A).
- Carefully remove the needle or knife from the anterior chamber. Inject additional viscoelastic in order to maintain chamber and decrease bleeding from the cleft.
- Canalization of Schlemm canal and trabeculotomy.
  - **360-degree trabeculotomy *ab interno* with illuminated microcatheter:**
    - Assemble the illuminated microcatheter with attachment of viscoelastic as per manufacturer's instructions.
    - With a 7515 blade, create a second paracentesis either superiorly or inferiorly (Fig. 10.4B). Insert suture through the superior or inferior paracentesis into the anterior chamber. Insert a 23G Grieshaber forceps or DORC retinal forceps through the temporal incision.
    - Place the gonioprism on the cornea to visualize the angle. Using the forceps, direct the catheter into the cleft created in the nasal trabecular meshwork (Fig. 10.4C). Carefully advance the catheter while visualizing the lighted tip.
    - After traveling 360 degrees, retrieve the catheter from the cleft with the forceps. With gentle traction on both catheter ends (one in the anterior chamber with the forceps and the other outside the eye), carefully pull the catheter through the trabecular meshwork into the anterior chamber. Remove the catheter from the anterior chamber.

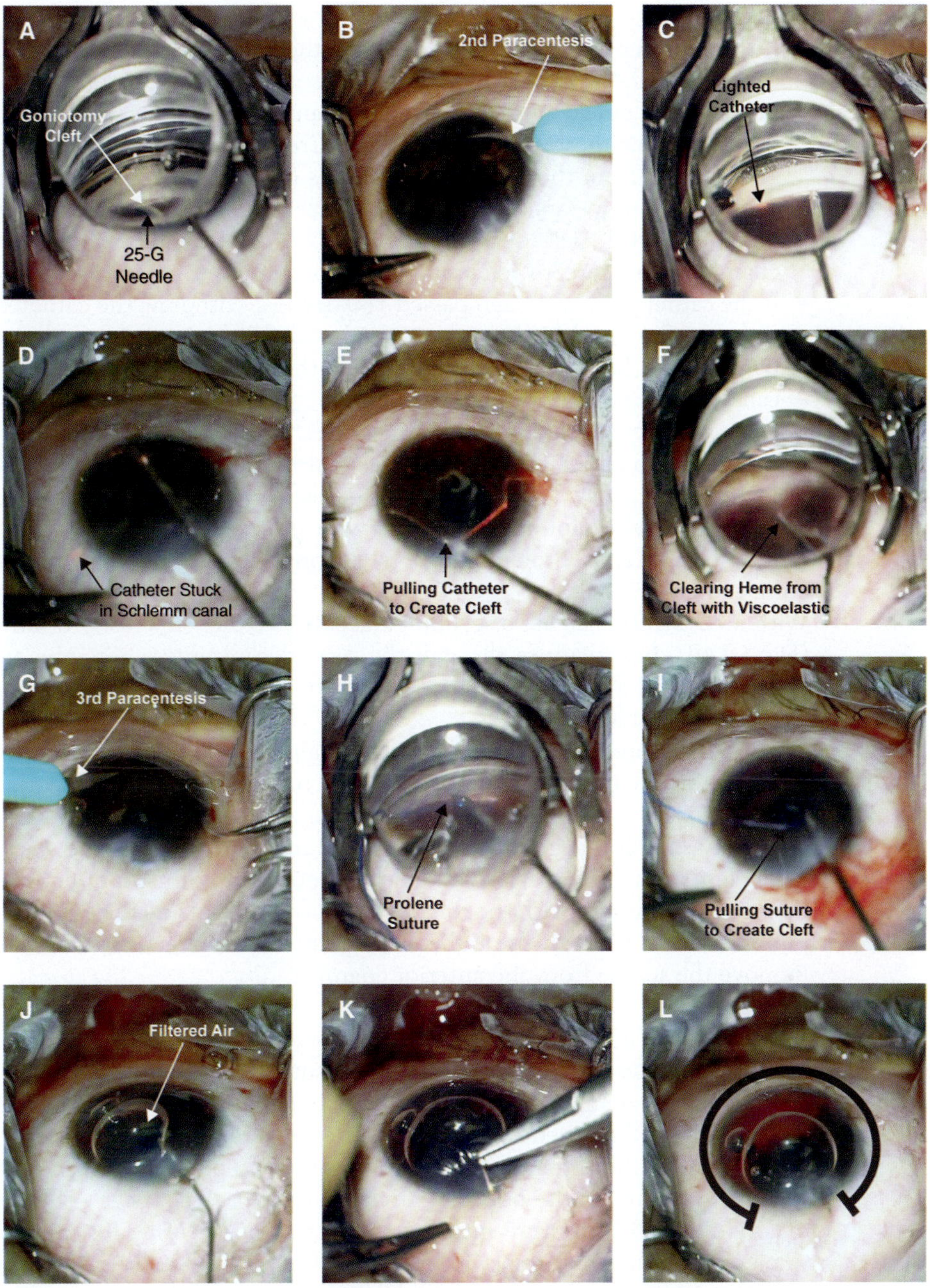

FIGURE 10.4. Trabeculotomy *ab interno* with illuminated catheter and Prolene suture. **A.** Following creation of a paracentesis temporally and deepening of the anterior chamber with viscoelastic, the Volk Vold VVG gonioprism is placed on the cornea. A 25G needle is inserted through the paracentesis and used to create a 1-clock hour nasal cleft in the anterior trabecular meshwork. **B.** A second paracentesis is created superiorly. **C.** The illuminated catheter is placed through the superior paracentesis. DORC retinal forceps or Grieshaber forceps are placed through the temporal paracentesis and used to cannulate Schlemm canal with the catheter. **D.** The catheter would not advance after ~5 clock hours. **E.** The forceps are used to create the cleft by carefully pulling the catheter through the trabecular meshwork into the anterior chamber. The catheter is removed from the eye. **F.** Viscoelastic is injected into the angle to clear the heme to revisualize the nasal cleft. **G.** A third paracentesis is created inferiorly. **H.** The blunt-ended Prolene suture is placed through the inferior paracentesis. The forceps are used to cannulate and advance the Prolene suture through Schlemm canal. **I.** After ~180 degrees, the forceps are used to carefully pull the suture through the trabecular meshwork into the anterior chamber. **J.** Filtered air is injected into the anterior chamber to tamponade the refluxing blood. **K.** The paracenteses are closed with a 10-0 Vicryl sutures. **L.** The final cleft is ~300 degrees.

NOTE:

- If the catheter is unable to be advanced, there may be stenosis of Schlemm canal (Fig. 10.4D). If the catheter has passed ~180 degrees, the catheter can be carefully pulled into the anterior chamber using the forceps, opening the trabecular meshwork (Fig. 10.4E). Create a third paracentesis that is 180 degrees from the second paracentesis (Fig. 10.4G). Insert the catheter through the new paracentesis, and canalize Schlemm canal in the opposite direction. After ~180 degrees, carefully pull the catheter into the anterior chamber using forceps to complete a trabeculotomy.
- If the catheter has not been passed 180 degrees, withdraw the catheter from the eye. Create a third paracentesis that is 180 degrees from the second paracentesis. Insert the catheter through the new paracentesis and attempt canalization in the opposite direction.
- If the catheter is unable to be advanced 180 degrees in either direction, then proceed with either 180-degree nasal goniotomy or traditional trabeculotomy *ab externo* with Harms trabeculotomes.

- **For 360-degree trabeculotomy *ab interno* with suture:**
  - Blunt the tip of a 5-0 Prolene suture by heating with a disposable low-temperature cautery.
  - With a 7515 blade, create a second paracentesis either superiorly or inferiorly (Fig. 10.4B). Insert suture through the second paracentesis into the anterior chamber. Insert a 23G Grieshaber forceps or DORC retinal forceps through the temporal incision.
  - Place the gonioprism on the cornea to visualize the angle. Using the forceps, direct the suture into the cleft created in the nasal trabecular meshwork. Carefully advance the suture while directly visualizing the angle.
  - After traveling 360 degrees, retrieve the suture from the opposite side of the nasal cleft with the forceps. With gentle traction on both suture ends (one in the anterior chamber with the forceps and the other outside the eye), carefully pull the suture through the trabecular meshwork into the anterior chamber. Remove the suture from the anterior chamber.

    NOTE:
    - If the suture is unable to be advanced, there is stenosis of Schlemm canal. If the suture has passed ~180 degrees, the suture can be carefully pulled into the anterior chamber using the forceps, opening the trabecular meshwork. Create a third paracentesis that is 180 degrees from the second paracentesis (Fig. 10.4G). Insert the suture through the new paracentesis, and canalize Schlemm canal in the opposite direction (Fig. 10.4H). After ~180 degrees, carefully pull the suture into the anterior chamber using forceps to complete the trabeculotomy (Fig. 10.4I).
    - If the suture has not been passed 180 degrees, withdraw the suture from the eye. Create a third paracentesis that is 180 degrees from the second paracentesis. Insert the suture through the new paracentesis, and attempt canalization going in the opposite direction.
    - If the suture is unable to be advanced in either direction, then proceed with either 180-degree nasal goniotomy or 180-degree trabeculotomy *ab externo* with Harms trabeculotomes.
- Remove the viscoelastic by irrigating the anterior chamber with balanced salt solution. Inject filtered air into the anterior chamber through the paracentesis (Fig. 10.4J).
- Close the paracenteses with a 10-0 nylon or 10-0 Vicryl suture (Fig. 10.4K).

POSTOPERATIVE CONSIDERATIONS

Complications (see Chapter 15)

- Hyphema:
  - Most eyes will have transient hyphemas that spontaneously resolve within 1 week.
  - Especially in aphakic or pseudophakic eyes undergoing 360-degree angle surgery, nonclearing heme within the vitreous cavity may necessitate vitrectomy 1-2 months postoperatively.[8,32]
- Cyclodialysis cleft:
  - Prolonged postoperative hypotony may be due to inadvertent cyclodialysis cleft formation. Gonioscopy may be difficult due to patient's age and hypotony. If patient is able to tolerate, obtain ultrasound biomicroscopy or anterior segment OCT to confirm the diagnosis.
  - Many cyclodialysis clefts will spontaneously close within the first postoperative month and may be able to be observed during this time.
  - If the cleft does not spontaneously close, then surgical closure of the cleft is indicated.[33]

References

1. Anderson DR. Trabeculotomy compared to goniotomy for glaucoma in children. *Ophthalmology*. 1983;90(7):805-806.
2. Barkan O. Surgery of congenital glaucoma: review of 196 eyes operated by goniotomy. *Am J Ophthalmol*. 1953;36(11S):1523-1534.
3. Bowman RJ, Dickerson M, Mwende J, Khaw PT. Outcomes of goniotomy for PCG in East Africa. *Ophthalmology*. 2011;118(12S):236-240.
4. Broughton WL, Parks MM. An analysis of treatment of congenital glaucoma by goniotomy. *Am J Ophthalmol*. 1981;91(5):566-572.
5. Huang JL, Huang JJ, Zhong YM, et al. Surgical outcomes of trabeculotomy in newborns with PCG. *Chin Med J (Engl)*. 2016;129(18):2178-2183.
6. Khalil DH, Abdelhakim MA. Primary trabeculotomy compared to combined trabeculectomy-trabeculotomy in congenital glaucoma: 3-year study. *Acta Ophthalmol*. 2016;94(7):e550-e553.
7. Mendicino ME, Lynch MG, Drack A, et al. Long-term surgical and visual outcomes in PCG: 360 degrees trabeculotomy versus goniotomy. *J AAPOS*. 2000;4(4):205-210.
8. Dao JB, Sarkisian SRJ, Freedman SF. Illuminated microcatheter-facilitated 360-degree trabeculotomy for refractory aphakic and juvenile open-angle glaucoma. *J Glaucoma*. 2014;23(7):449-454.
9. Grover DS, Smith O, Fellman RL, et al. Gonioscopy assisted transluminal trabeculotomy: an ab interno circumferential trabeculotomy for the treatment of PCG and juvenile open angle glaucoma. *Br J Ophthalmol*. 2015;99(8):1092-1096.
10. Kjer B, Kessing SV. Trabeculotomy in juvenile open-angle glaucoma. *Ophthalmic Surg*. 1993;24(10):663-668.
11. Lim ME, Dao JB, Freedman SF. 360-degree trabeculotomy for medically refractory glaucoma following cataract surgery and juvenile open-angle glaucoma. *Am J Ophthalmol*. 2017;175:1-7.
12. Yeung HH, Walton DS. Goniotomy for juvenile open-angle glaucoma. *J Glaucoma*. 2010;19(1):1-4.
13. Bothun ED, Guo Y, Christiansen SP, et al. Outcome of angle surgery in children with aphakic glaucoma. *J AAPOS*. 2010;14(3):235-239.
14. Bohnsack BL, Freedman SF. Surgical outcomes in childhood uveitic glaucoma. *Am J Ophthalmol*. 2013;155(1):134-142.
15. Freedman SF, Rodriguez-Rosa RE, Rojas MC, Enyedi LB. Goniotomy for glaucoma secondary to chronic childhood uveitis. *Am J Ophthalmol*. 2002;133(5):617-621.
16. Ho CL, Wong EY, Walton DS. Goniosurgery for glaucoma complicating chronic childhood uveitis. *Arch Ophthalmol*. 2004;122(6):838-844.

17. Wang Q, Wang J, Fortin E, Hamel P. Trabeculotomy in the treatment of pediatric uveitic glaucoma. *J Glaucoma*. 2016;25(9):744-749.
18. Iwach AG, Hoskins HDJ, Hetherington JJ, Shaffer RN. Analysis of surgical and medical management of glaucoma in Sturge Weber syndrome. *Ophthalmology*. 1990;97(7):904-909.
19. Wu Y, Yu R, Chen D, et al. Early trabeculotomy ab externo in treatment of Sturge-Weber Syndrome. *Am J Ophthalmol*. 2017;182:141-146.
20. Olsen KE, Huang AS, Wright MM. The efficacy of goniotomy/trabeculotomy in early-onset glaucoma associated with the Sturge-Weber syndrome. *J AAPOS*. 1998;2(6):365-368.
21. Celebi S, Alagöz G, Aykan U. Ocular findings in Sturge-Weber syndrome. *Eur J Ophthalmol*. 2000;10(3):239-243.
22. Shihab ZM, Kristan RW. Recurrent intraoperative choroidal effusion in Sturge-Weber syndrome. *J Pediatr Ophthalmol Strabismus*. 1983;20(6):250-252.
23. Barkan O. Goniotomy for congenital glaucoma; urgent need for early diagnosis and operation. *J Am Med Assoc*. 1947;133(8):526-533.
24. Barkan O. Goniotomy for the relief of congenital glaucoma. *Br J Ophthalmol*. 1948;32(9):701-728.
25. Scheie HG. Goniotomy and the treatment of congenital glaucoma. *Am J Ophthalmol*. 1950;33(6):977-979.
26. McPherson SDJ, McFarland D. External trabeculotomy for developmental glaucoma. *Ophthalmology*. 1980;87(4):302-305.
27. Luntz MH. Congenital, infantile, and juvenile glaucoma. *Ophthalmology*. 1979;86(5):793-802.
28. Shakrawal J, Bali S, Sidhu T, Verma S, Sihota R, Dada T. Randomized trial on illuminated-microcatheter circumferential trabeculotomy versus conventional trabeculotomy in congenital glaucoma. *Am J Ophthalmol*. 2017;180:158-164.
29. Neustein RF, Beck AD. Circumferential trabeculotomy versus conventional angle surgery: comparing long-term surgical success and clinical outcomes in children with PCG. *Am J Ophthalmol*. 2017;183:17-24.
30. Girkin CA, Rhodes L, McGwin G, Marchase N, Cogen MS. Goniotomy versus circumferential trabeculotomy with an illuminated microcatheter in congenital glaucoma. *J AAPOS*. 2012;16(5):424-427.
31. Shi Y, Wang H, Yin J, et al. Microcatheter-assisted trabeculotomy versus rigid probe trabeculotomy in childhood glaucoma. *Br J Ophthalmol*. 2016;100(9):1257-1262.
32. Bothun ED, Groth SL, Freedman SF. Vitreous hemorrhage after trabeculotomy in aphakic eyes. *J AAPOS*. 2013;17(3):307-308.
33. Berk TA, An JA, Ahmed IIK. Inadvertent cyclodialysis cleft and hypotony following ab-interno trabeculotomy using the Trabectome device requiring surgical repair. *J Glaucoma*. 2017;26(8):742-746.

CHAPTER 11

Glaucoma Drainage Device Surgery

Ann Shue, MD • Sharon F. Freedman, MD

PREOPERATIVE CONSIDERATIONS

- Assess status of the conjunctiva.
- Decide type of glaucoma drainage device (GDD)—based on level of IOP and glaucoma severity.
  - Valved: Provides immediate IOP lowering, for refractory moderate to severe glaucoma, or if there is concern for low aqueous production as in uveitic glaucoma or after cycloablation. Avoid in Sturge-Weber–associated glaucoma.
  - Nonvalved: 5-6 week delay in IOP lowering, for refractory moderate to severe glaucoma, or in cases where immediate IOP reduction may pose risk (eg, Sturge-Weber–associated cases).
- Determine placement of tube—Assess anterior chamber depth, lens status, and if vitrectomized.
  - May need retina surgeon to perform vitrectomy for pars plana tube or anterior chamber in aphakic eye with high risk for forward vitreous movement.
- Determine location of plate—Superior temporal and inferior nasal are preferred first and second-choice locations, respectively, followed by inferior temporal and superior nasal.[1] In some cases, inferior nasal may be preferred for first GDD, to leave room for a superior trabeculectomy or larger nonvalved GDD in superior quadrants when the patient is older.
- Manage patient expectations about IOP control:
  - With valved devices, there may be a hypertensive phase in 2-4 weeks.
  - With nonvalved devices, IOP likely will remain unchanged for 5-6 weeks.
- Discuss risks of infection in short- and long-term, hypotony, elevated IOP, and need for additional surgery. Discuss that the goal of surgery is not to improve vision, but to preserve remaining vision. There is risk of further damage to vision or to the eye. There is a small possibility of inducing strabismus with or without diplopia, or worsening known strabismus.

SURGICAL PLANNING

- Let the OR team know which materials are needed:
  - Patch graft: Recommend scleral patch graft for superior GDDs and corneal patch graft for inferior GDDs (for cosmesis).
  - GDD: Valved (Ahmed FP7, Ahmed FP8) or nonvalved (Molteno, Baerveldt 250 mm^2 or 350 mm^2).[2]

> **Ahmed FP7 and Baerveldt (250 and 350 mm^2) are the most commonly used GDDs in children. Pediatric Molteno and Ahmed implants are available (Ahmed Model S3 and FP8, Molteno M1); however, adult size implants are preferred when possible. Silicone Ahmed implants have been shown to have better long-term IOP control compared to polypropylene Ahmed models, but the outcome is unlikely to be determined by implant type, thus choice of implant depends on clinical scenario, availability, and surgeon's experience.**

  - Instruments:
    - Sutures:
      - Dyed, polyglactin 6-0 on a spatulated needle (for tube ligature in nonvalved GDDs).
      - Dyed, polyglactin 7-0 on a spatulated needle.
      - Dyed, polyglactin 8-0 on tapered round needle.
      - Nylon 8-0 and 9-0 suture.
    - Needles: hypodermic 30 gauge × 1/2" and hypodermic 23 gauge × 1".
    - Sodium hyaluronate.
    - Locking hemostat.
    - 0.12 forceps.[2]
    - Blunt Westcott scissors.
    - Needle driver, locking (2) for nonvalved implant.
    - Tenotomy hooks (2), large muscle hooks (2).
    - Nugent forceps.
    - Paracentesis blade.
    - AC maintainer (recommended in Sturge Weber glaucoma and other cases at high risk for damage if IOP spikes from retained viscoelastic).
    - Smooth curved forceps (2).
    - Needle driver, locking or nonlocking, to close conjunctiva.
  - Medications:
    - Povidone-iodine 5%.
    - Balanced salt intraocular solution (BSS).
    - Bupivacaine 0.75%, preservative-free.
    - Cefazolin 200 mg/mL subconjunctival injection (vancomycin 25 mg/mL if patient allergic to penicillin).
    - Dexamethasone 10 mg/mL, preservative-free injection.
    - If implanting a nonvalved GDD, recommend glaucoma medications including timolol if no contraindication, dorzolamide, apraclonidine for younger patients, brimonidine for older patients, and acetazolamide IV.
    - Antibiotic-steroid ointment.
- If eye is small, measure axial length and horizontal corneal diameter. Use the Freedman-Margeta calculator available online (http://people.duke.edu/~freed003/GDDCalculator/) to determine if GDD needs to be trimmed posteriorly to avoid optic nerve-plate touch.[3]

VIDEO SURGICAL PROCEDURE: GLAUCOMA DRAINAGE DEVICE IMPLANTATION WITH PATCH GRAFT (VIDEO 11.1)

- Standard prep and drape for intraocular surgery, recommend drape to keep eyelashes out of surgical field.

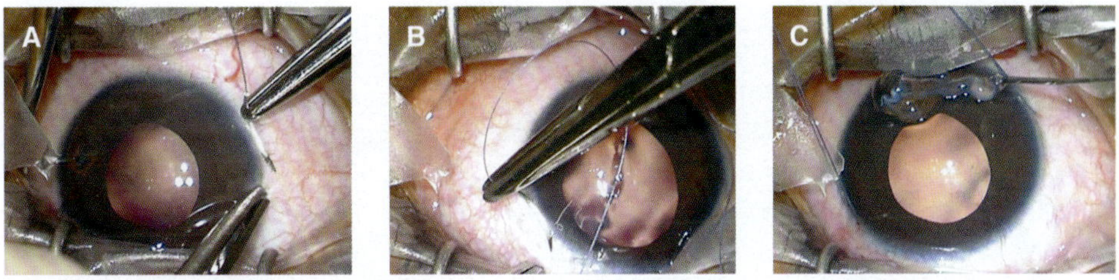

FIGURE 11.1. Limbal traction suture placement for adequate quadrant exposure and avoidance of corneal damage from corneal traction suture. **A.** 7-0 double (or single)-armed polyglactin suture needle partial-thickness pass at limbus ~90 degrees from the quadrant of GDD implantation (superotemporal in this case). **B.** After suture has been pulled to approximately the midway point of the suture, the same or other suture end can be passed partial-thickness at the limbus 180 degrees from the original pass. **C.** The two suture ends have been pulled up along with the central portion of the suture between the two limbal passes until they are approximately even. The ends have been tied, and the suture needles cut off. A locking hemostat has been clamped to the suture ends to maintain the position of the eye in the opposite quadrant of the GDD implantation. Viscoelastic has been instilled generously on cornea to prevent corneal abrasion as eye is manipulated.

- Place traction suture—pass 7-0 double-armed polyglactin suture partial-thickness at limbus about 90 degrees from quadrant of implantation on either side (Fig. 11.1).
- After positioning eye with traction suture and locking hemostat to expose quadrant of implantation, surgeon and assistant each lift the conjunctiva with 0.12 or Bishop-Harmon forceps 7-8 mm posterior to and parallel to the limbus. Conjunctiva will fold perpendicular to the limbus in between the forceps (Fig. 11.2A).

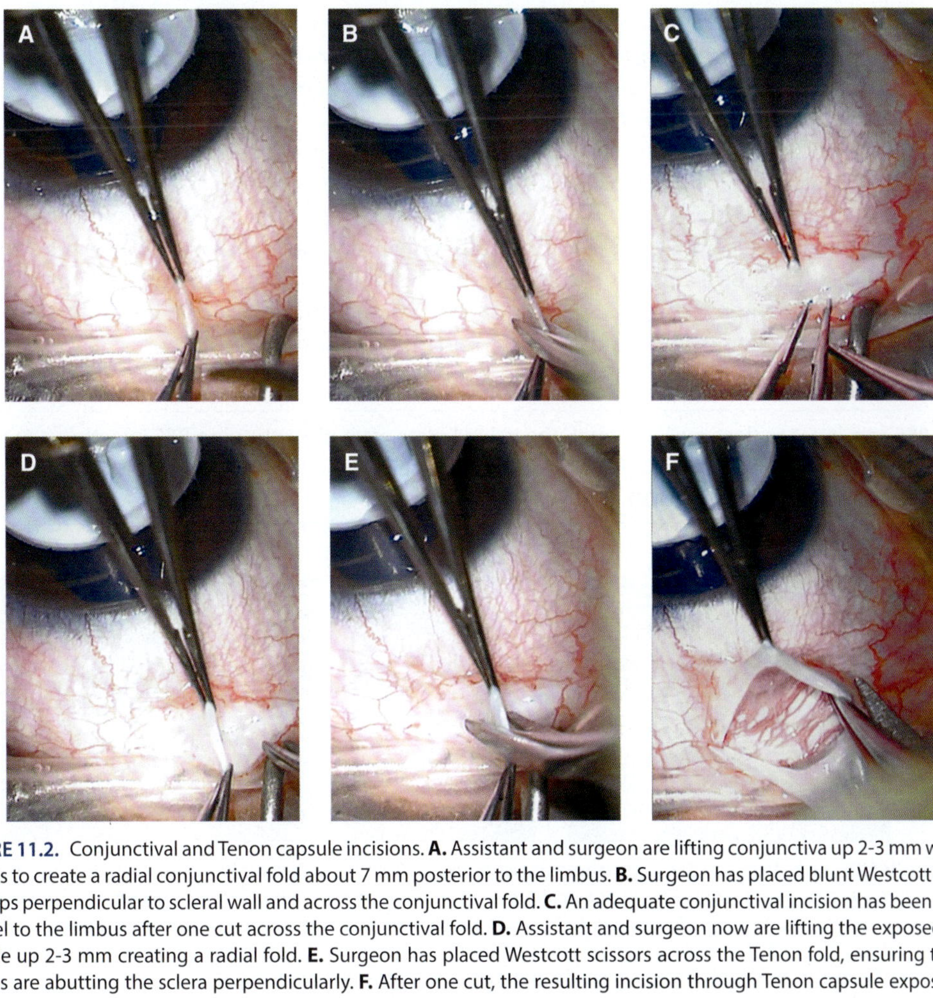

FIGURE 11.2. Conjunctival and Tenon capsule incisions. **A.** Assistant and surgeon are lifting conjunctiva up 2-3 mm with two forceps to create a radial conjunctival fold about 7 mm posterior to the limbus. **B.** Surgeon has placed blunt Westcott scissors with tips perpendicular to scleral wall and across the conjunctival fold. **C.** An adequate conjunctival incision has been created parallel to the limbus after one cut across the conjunctival fold. **D.** Assistant and surgeon now are lifting the exposed Tenon capsule up 2-3 mm creating a radial fold. **E.** Surgeon has placed Westcott scissors across the Tenon fold, ensuring the scissor tips are abutting the sclera perpendicularly. **F.** After one cut, the resulting incision through Tenon capsule exposes bare sclera. Assistant and surgeon continue to lift up the cut edges to facilitate extension of the incision with the Westcott scissors.

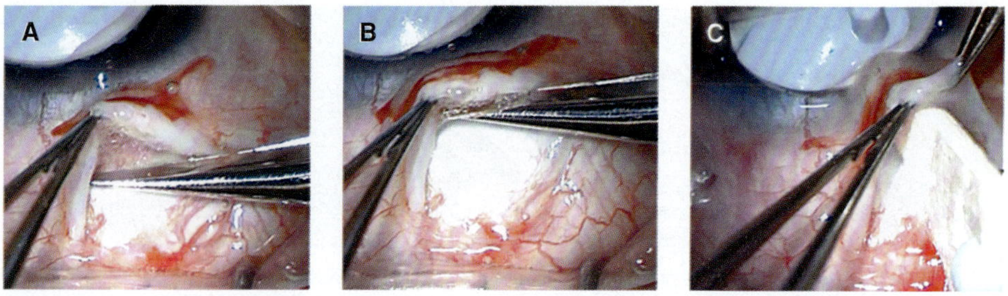

FIGURE 11.3. Gentle anterior dissection of Tenon tissue to limbus in preparation for tube placement. **A, B.** Closed blunt Westcott scissors being used with one edge pushing Tenon insertion anteriorly on sclera. **C.** Dry sponge also being used to push remaining adhesions anteriorly until bare sclera is visualized up to limbus.

- With Westcott scissors perpendicular to the sclera wall, cut across the conjunctival fold between the forceps to create an incision parallel to the limbus (Fig. 11.2B and C).
- Repeat the previous two steps to create a Tenon capsule layer incision identical to the conjunctival incision (Fig. 11.2D-F).

Recommend limbal-based incision (fornix incision) in children to decrease tube exposure risk and potentially preserve limbal stem cells.

- Use a toothed forceps to lift the posterior edge of the Tenon capsule incision and blunt Westcott scissors to dissect posteriorly until there is sufficient space for the GDD plate to lie on the sclera; consider micro Westcott scissors to sharply dissect Tenon capsule from sclera if scarring is encountered, with care to preserve Tenon capsule and the conjunctival flap.
- Next, use forceps and closed Westcott scissors, with or without a Weck-Cel sponge, to push the Tenon capsule adhesions anteriorly until the sclera is bare up to the limbus (Fig. 11.3).
- Prepare GDD: flush device (insert 27G cannula on BSS syringe into tube tip and inject until BSS streams through plate (Fig. 11.4). For valved GDD, ensure that BSS stops flowing through the valve outlet almost immediately when injection stops. Then remove syringe and set plate aside in antibiotic soak.

If BSS continues to flow easily through the valved plate after discontinuing BSS injection, the valve mechanism of the particular GDD is inadequate (especially in cases where hypotony poses extra risk). Obtain and test a new GDD.

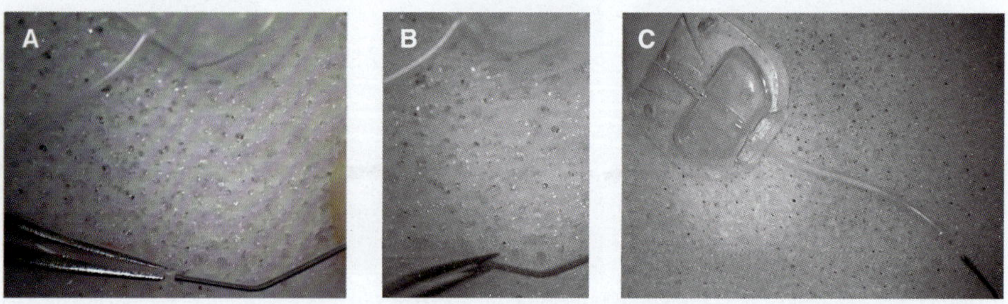

FIGURE 11.4. Priming valved glaucoma drainage device (GDD) and flushing nonvalved GDD before implantation. **A.** Tube held steady close to proximal tube end with fine forceps, while 27G cannula on a syringe filled with BSS is inserted into tube. **B.** Since in **A**, the cannula is barely within the tube, the forceps are placed across the tube and cannula and force-slide tube further distal on the cannula. **C.** A stream of BSS ejects from the distal valve outlet as BSS is injected through the tube indicating the valve is now primed.

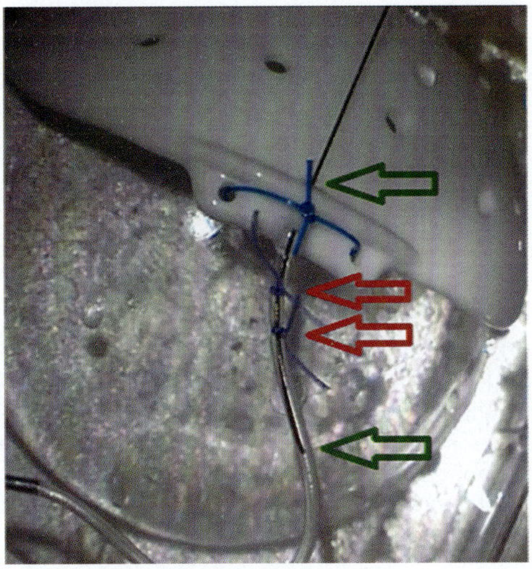

FIGURE 11.5. Preparation of Baerveldt 250 or 350 mm^2 before implantation in Sturge-Weber pediatric glaucoma patient. Tube is ligated with two, instead of the traditional single, 6-0 polyglactin suture tied around proximal tube in 2-1-1-1 fashion (*red arrows*). Before securing the ligating sutures, a 5-0 nylon suture was inserted through the plate aperture to create a ripcord (insertion and suture end shown with *green arrows*). The ripcord may be omitted if spontaneous tube opening is acceptable.

- For nonvalved GDD, keep the syringe on the tube after confirming flow. Ligate the tube with a 6-0 polyglactin suture in 2-1-1-1 fashion using two locking needle holders. (In Sturge-Weber patients, recommend double ligation with two separate sutures, and consider a ripcord to open the tube earlier than the anticipated spontaneous opening) (Fig. 11.5). Knot should be tied ~2 mm anterior to plate. Attempt to push BSS through syringe to confirm complete ligation. Cut tails to 1-2 mm long. Set plate aside in antibiotic soak.
- Soak the patch graft in antibiotic bath as well.
- If the eye is short, trim the posterior plate the calculated amount according to the Freedman-Margeta online calculator[3] (see "Surgical Planning" section above) using calipers and Stevens scissors (Fig. 11.6).
- Hook rectus muscles in the intended quadrant of GDD placement, first with a tenotomy hook, then with a large hook. Have the assistant hold large hooks to expose the quadrant in which the GDD will be implanted (Fig. 11.7).
- Place the GDD with forceps (ie, Nugent forceps, nonserrated or serrated smooth forceps) (Fig. 11.8).

Do not crush valve on Ahmed. For Baerveldt, ensure wings are underneath muscles by pulling forward on plate until stopped by muscle insertions.

- Secure plate eyelets to scleral wall adjacent to muscle insertions with 8-0 nylon ~7-8 mm posterior to limbus.[4] Bury tails in eyelets (Fig. 11.9).

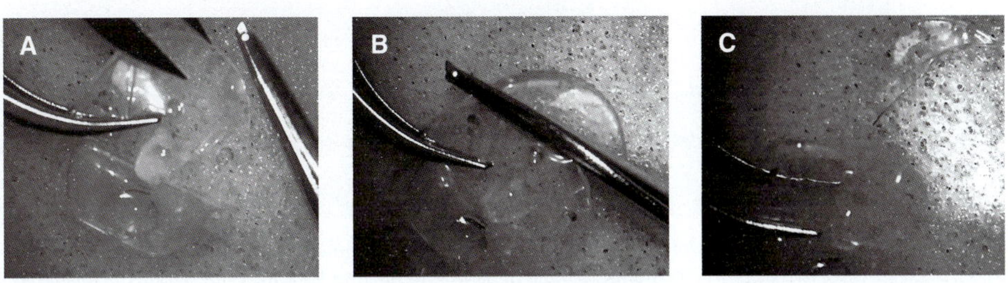

FIGURE 11.6. Trimming posterior portion of a glaucoma drainage device for implantation into an eye with short axial length (18.77 mm) in 2-month-old patient with congenital glaucoma associated with Axenfeld-Rieger syndrome with an aniridic phenotype. **A.** Calipers set to calculated amount to trim according to the Freedman-Margeta online calculator and placed from posterior edge of plate. **B.** Stevens scissors are used to cut the silicone Ahmed glaucoma valve to trim the posterior portion that was measured. **C.** The trimmed plate and separated posterior portion that will be discarded.

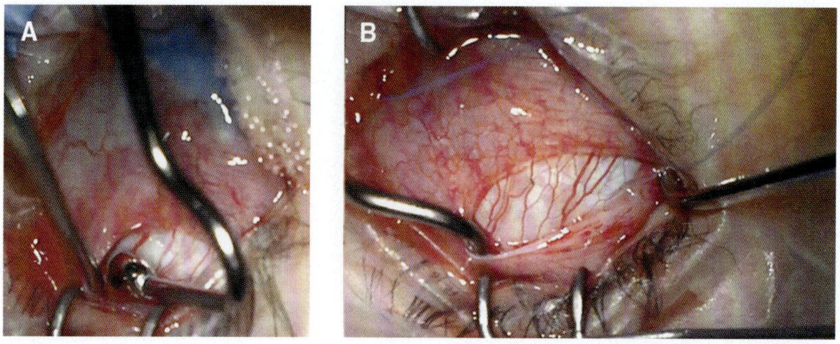

FIGURE 11.7. Exposure of quadrant with muscle hooks to facilitate GDD plate placement in pediatric patients who tend to have more Tenon capsule tissue than adult patients. **A.** The superior rectus muscle has been hooked by a small muscle hook first, and now a larger Jameson muscle hook is being inserted to fully isolate the muscle and the small hook will be removed. **B.** The same has been done with the lateral rectus muscle which is now isolated on a square muscle hook. The bare sclera of the superotemporal quadrant is now well-exposed while an assistant holds both hooks.

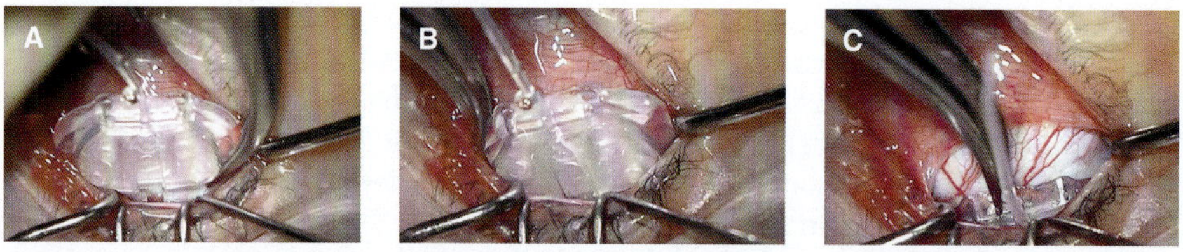

FIGURE 11.8. One method for placement of the Ahmed glaucoma valve plate. **A.** The plate is held on one side of the valve, avoiding damage to the valve itself, and pushed posteriorly into the sub-Tenon space. **B.** The other side of the plate is pushed posteriorly. **C.** The anterior edge of the plate is pushed posteriorly to ensure the plate slides back and the anterior edge of the plate is ~7-8 mm posterior to the limbus.

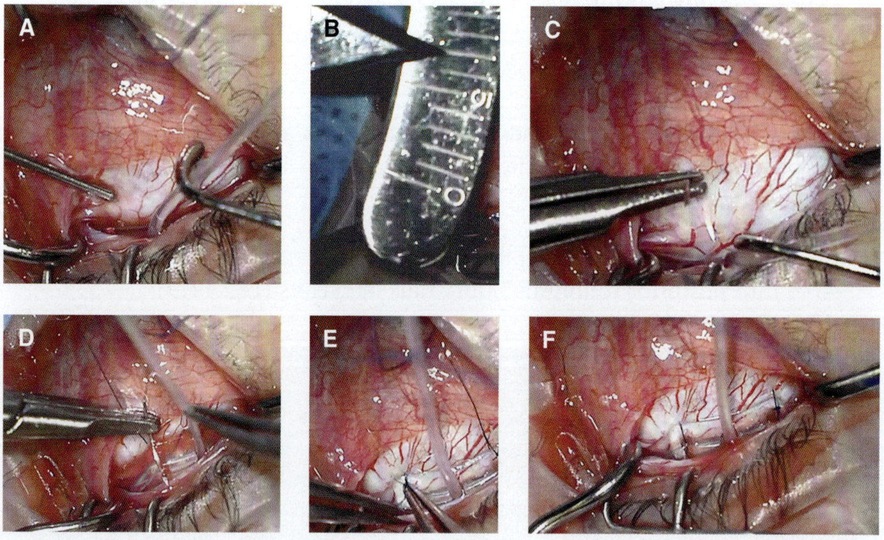

FIGURE 11.9. Securing plate to scleral wall. **A.** Wet-field cautery to maintain hemostasis in anticipation of suture needle passes. **B.** Calipers set to mark 7 mm posterior to the limbus where the anterior plate edge should be located (7-8 mm posterior to the limbus is appropriate, but 8 mm is preferred if possible). **C.** 8-0 nylon suture is used to secure the plate to the scleral wall. A partial-thickness scleral pass is made 7 mm posterior to the limbus, just adjacent to the superior rectus muscle temporal insertion (seen anterior to muscle hook). **D.** After completing the scleral pass, the needle is passed through the superior eyelet of the plate with care not to pierce through the plate. **E.** After securing both eyelets, the knots are rotated into the eyelet. **F.** Both knots and tails have been rotated and are hidden in the eyelets to prevent conjunctival erosion over the plate.

When passing the suture needle through the eyelet, take care to pass through the eyelet and not through plate itself so the suture knot can be rotated into the eyelet. This can be double checked by wiggling the needle as it is passed through the eyelet or pass the needle backward to avoid piercing the plate.

- Trim the tube to appropriate length so tube extends ~2 mm from the limbus if in the anterior chamber and beyond the pupillary margin if in the sulcus or pars plana. Use 0.12 forceps to hold the tube tip and position tube in an elongated but neutral configuration and cut bevel with Westcott scissors—bevel up for anterior chamber and sulcus (to avoid occlusion by a Soemmering ring), bevel down for pars plana (Fig. 11.10).
- Create a paracentesis at temporal side to allow for chamber reformation during tube insertion. (The paracentesis will be more difficult to create later when the eye is soft). In a Sturge-Weber patient, use the paracentesis to insert an anterior chamber maintainer to avoid a postoperative IOP spike due to retained viscoelastic[5] (Fig. 11.11).

Use a marking pen to mark tips of blade or needles entering the eye to help identify incisions efficiently.

- Prepare 30G and 23G hypodermic needles for sclerostomy; 30 gauge on an empty syringe, and 23 gauge on a viscoelastic syringe. For a more ergonomic hand position when creating the sclerostomy, bend the needles with a hemostat (or non-cutting side of scissors behind hinge) placed near the needle hub and rotate the hemostat so

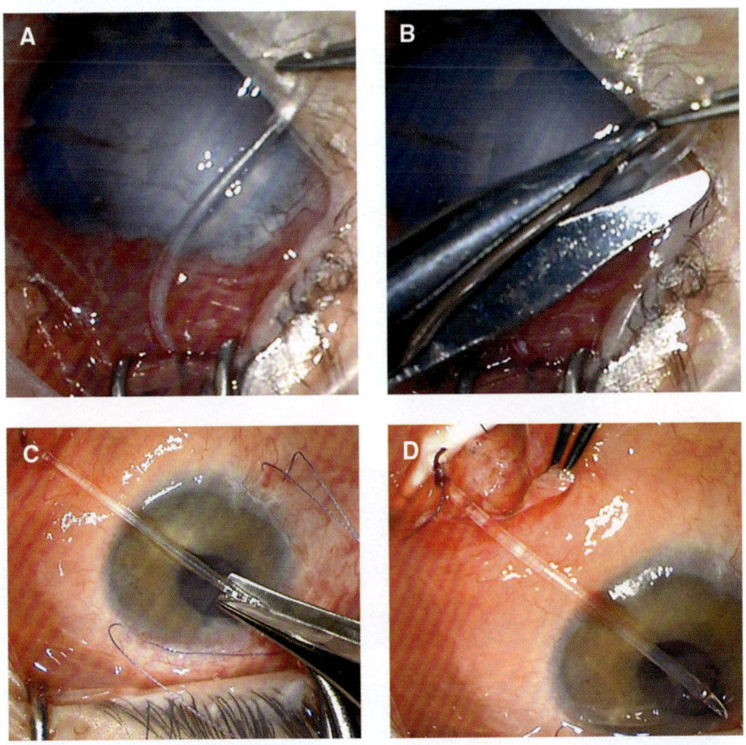

FIGURE 11.10. Trimming the tube to appropriate length and with a bevel. **A.** Due to aniridic phenotype and possible limbal stem cell deficiency in this patient, the plan is to insert the tube in an oblique direction over the zonular fibers to avoid central corneal decompensation. Thus, the tube is held by forceps simulating the path the tube will enter the eye, prior to tube trimming. **B.** While maintaining the position, the tube will enter the eye with forceps, Westcott scissors are used to trim from the distal-to-proximal direction, from above the tube, to create a bevel pointing up at the tube tip and a tip that will extend 2-3 mm into the eye after insertion. **C.** Due to aphakia, the tube will be inserted through the pars plana in this eye. The tube tip is cut from the proximal-to-distal direction, from above the tube, to create a bevel down tip. **D.** A downward bevel prevents iris blockage of the tube. The tube is also sufficiently long for the tube tip to be visualized in the pupil after insertion.

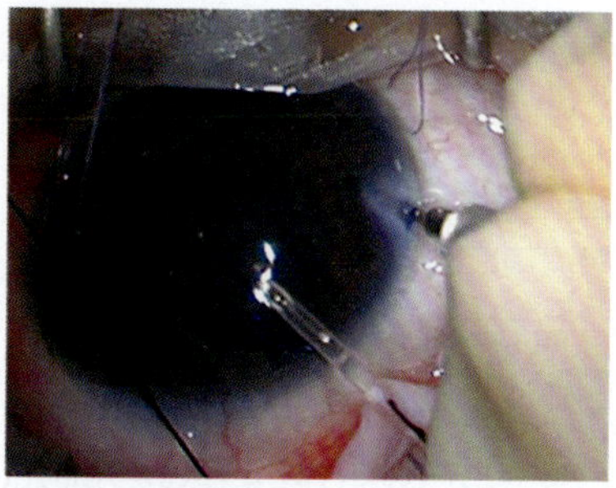

FIGURE 11.11. Insertion of 27G anterior chamber (AC) maintainer in a Sturge-Weber pediatric glaucoma patient to avoid use of viscoelastic. Insert the AC maintainer by rotating it back and forth between fingers to maintain a tight fit and prevent wound leakage during surgery.

the needle tip, with bevel up, moves ~30 degrees up from its original position and the needle develops an angle of ~150 degrees. For an inferonasal GDD, one must bend needles 90 degrees with the angle ~5-6 mm posterior to the needle tip to allow needle placement in the smaller inferonasal working space. Mark needle tips for efficient identification of incisions.

- Use 30 gauge first to enter eye. Use 0.12 forceps to lift Tenon tissue and conjunctiva to expose limbus and stabilize eye while advancing needle through previously cleared limbus (Fig. 11.12A and B).

Use a 30G hypodermic "finder needle" first when creating the sclerostomy to find the best location for tube entrance. The needle can be used to enter the eye several times without consequence until the desired entrance is found. Generally, aim toward the center of the anterior chamber. For aniridic patients, due to increased likelihood of corneal decompensation, aim parallel to the lens edge in peripheral anterior chamber and overlying zonular fibers to prevent potential tube-related corneal opacification near the visual axis.[2]

- Once the desired location is found with 30G needle, use a 23G needle on viscoelastic syringe (unless have infusion in eye to maintain IOP and chamber depth) and enter through same location to create the sclerostomy, ensuring the tip is not touching cornea or iris. Inject a small amount of viscoelastic when removing the needle from the eye (Fig. 11.12C and D).
- Insert the tube tip into the sclerostomy using a tube inserter and forceps or two 0.12 forceps (Fig. 11.13).

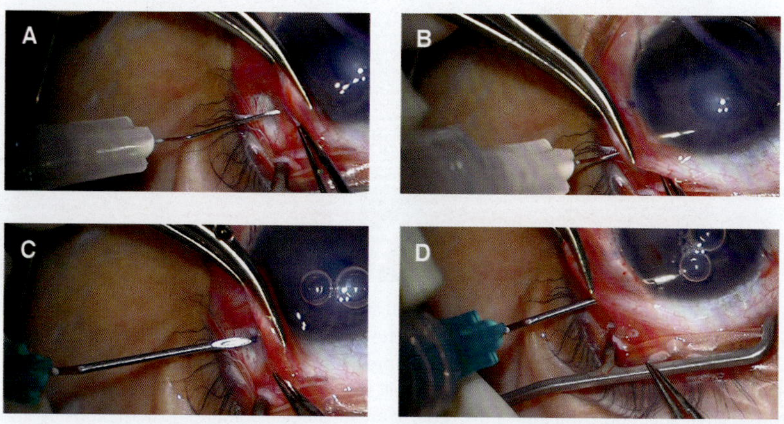

FIGURE 11.12. Creating the sclerostomy in pediatric glaucoma. **A, B.** A 30G finder needle marked with surgical marking pen is first used to enter the anterior chamber to establish the ideal sclerostomy location. **C, D.** The sclerostomy is then enlarged with a 23G needle, also marked with surgical marking pen, to facilitate tube insertion.

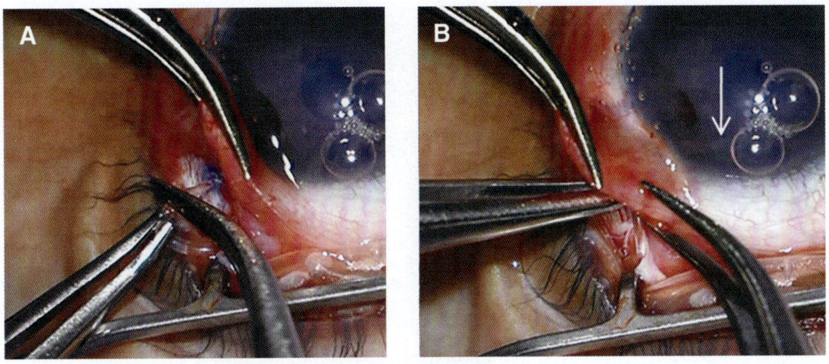

FIGURE 11.13. Insertion of tube into anterior chamber. **A.** A tube inserter forceps with grooves within the blunt tips is used to push the tube tip into the sclerostomy. Another forceps is used to bend the tube tip and guide it down into the sclerostomy. **B.** The tube tip (white arrow) is seen extending ~2.5 mm into the anterior chamber, without corneal or iris touch. In children, caution and time should be taken to ensure as much distance from the iris and cornea as possible.

- Ensure tube tip in good position (not close to cornea and not touching iris if in anterior chamber). Take the time needed to adjust position or shorten tube length.

Tube-cornea and tube-iris touch are less tolerated in children compared to adults. Iritis and corectopia can occur with iris touch.[2] However, often in young children, the tube will seem to migrate anteriorly once the IOP is reduced and the eye wall presumably shrinks, so would prefer "deep" tube in AC in most cases.

If the tube tip is too long it may bend up or down and touch the cornea or retina, if in pars plana, with external pressure on the eye, especially in buphthalmic eyes with thin sclera walls.

- Secure the tube to sclera with a 9-0 nylon figure-of-8 suture across the tube (Fig. 11.14).
- In nonvalved GDD, may create 3-4 venting slits in tube anterior to ligation with needle of 9-0 nylon (Fig. 11.15). Do not create venting slits in Sturge-Weber glaucoma patients.
- Place patch graft over tube with aim to cover tube entry site into eye. Recommend trimming anterior corners of sclera patch graft to create round corners. Do not cover ligating suture (Fig. 11.16).

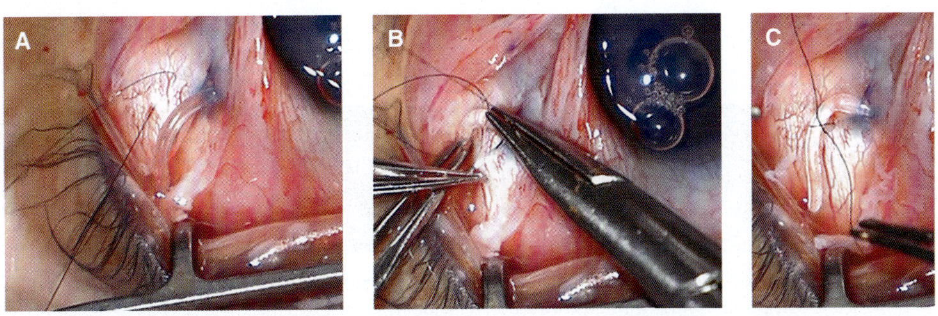

FIGURE 11.14. Securing tube on scleral wall. **A.** Beginning of figure-of-8 suture with one partial-thickness scleral pass parallel to the tube. (Note: scleral thinning is seen as bluish areas in this buphthalmic eye). **B.** Second scleral pass on other side of tube. A C-shape curve is maintained in the tube's path before entering the eye to allow easier tube revision in the case of tube retraction, which can be seen with eye growth in a child. **C.** The figure-of-8 suture is tightened and completed so the tube lays flat.

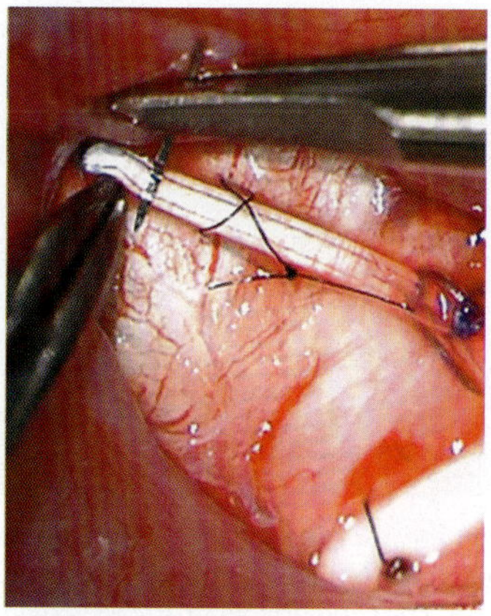

FIGURE 11.15. Venting slits in a ligated nonvalved GDD (avoid in Sturge-Weber glaucoma patients). The 9-0 suture needle that had been used to secure the tube to the scleral wall is now used to pierce through the tube proximal to the ligating suture to allow some egress of fluid before tube opening. This is repeated to create 3-4 slits. Some surgeons may enlarge the slit by sliding the needle to the side of the puncture; however, this may be uncontrolled and could lead to hypotony.

- Suture patch graft with 6-0 or 7-0 polyglactin suture on one or both sides to scleral wall; pass needle partial-thickness through sclera first, then full thickness through the patch graft. Sometimes, if the patch graft seems stable in position, suturing is not needed (Fig. 11.17).
- Close the Tenon capsule incision with a running 8-0 polyglactin suture on a round tapered (BV) needle. Use fine curved nontoothed forceps to handle the tissue and needle (Fig. 11.18). Before complete closure, inject bupivacaine (0.75%) diffusely into the sub-Tenon space with a blunt cannula.

When closing Tenon and conjunctival incisions, take a smaller anterior bite and a larger posterior bite to pull the incision posteriorly toward the fornix.

- Close the conjunctival incision with same running 8-0 polyglactin on a round tapered needle (Fig. 11.19).
- If Ahmed valve GDD implanted, inject a medium-sized air bubble into the anterior chamber to help maintain anterior chamber if hypotony occurs due to overfiltration on postoperative day 1. It is acceptable to intentionally leave a small amount of viscoelastic in the anterior chamber at the close of surgery as well.

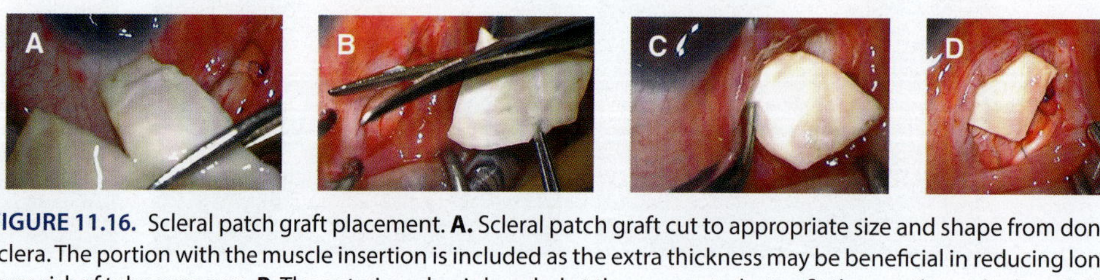

FIGURE 11.16. Scleral patch graft placement. **A.** Scleral patch graft cut to appropriate size and shape from donor sclera. The portion with the muscle insertion is included as the extra thickness may be beneficial in reducing long-term risk of tube exposure. **B.** The anterior edge is beveled at the corners to better fit the curvilinear limbus. **C.** The patch graft is placed over the tube and pushed anteriorly up to the limbus. **D.** Final placement of the graft after further trimming, ensuring the ligating suture is not covered, which could hinder suture absorption.

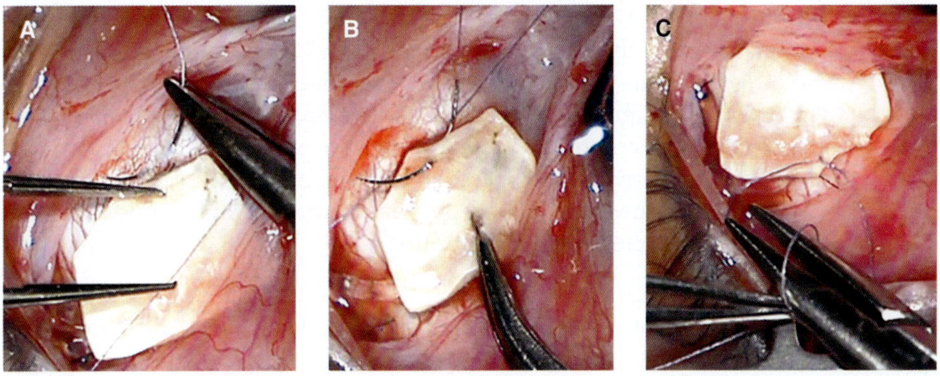

FIGURE 11.17. Securing the patch graft. **A.** Partial thickness scleral pass after visualizing ideal placement of graft and moving graft slightly aside. **B.** Then, full-thickness pass through the patch graft. **C.** Finally, securing the suture with a 2-1-1 knot. This patch graft was secured with two sutures; some grafts do not need any sutures or may be stable with one suture.

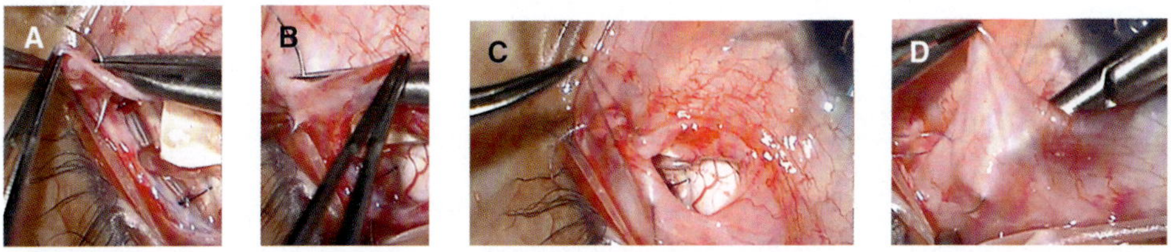

FIGURE 11.18. Tenon capsule and conjunctival (double-layer) closure. **A, B.** The Tenon incision is being closed with an 8-0 polyglactin suture on a round tapered needle in a running fashion starting from one end of the incision with each bite beginning on the anterior wound edge **(A)**, followed by draping of the posterior wound edge over the needle tip with fine forceps to complete the bite **(B)**. **C.** The suture is pulled taut to ensure complete apposition of the wound edges. **D.** Large posterior bites like this may help bring the incision more posteriorly which may reduce the risk of postoperative exposure and infection.

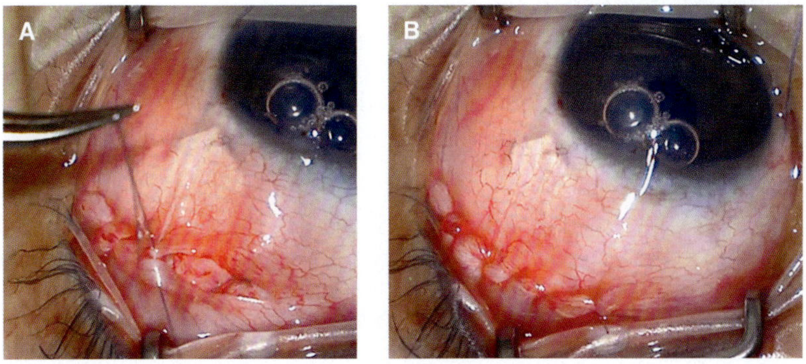

FIGURE 11.19. Conjunctival closure. **A.** Using the same technique as in Figure 11.18 for the Tenon wound closure, the conjunctiva is closed in running fashion with an 8-0 polyglactin suture on a round tapered needle. The suture is pulled taut after each pass to ensure complete apposition of the wound edges. A round tapered needle is preferred to minimize conjunctival injury and possible wound leakage through suture sites. **B.** The wound closure is complete.

- If nonvalved GDD implanted, flush the viscoelastic from the eye with BSS on a cannula through the paracentesis to avoid an IOP spike on postoperative day 1, or use infusion via an anterior chamber maintainer during the case to avoid all use of viscoelastic (see above). If no contraindication, give IV acetazolamide (5 mg/kg × 1 dose) near the end of the case or prescribe one dose to take at home the evening of the surgery to avoid postoperative IOP spike.
- Close the paracentesis with 10-0 polyglactin or, in an older child, 10-0 nylon. Rotate the knot to the scleral side and/or bury it.

To facilitate burying of knots, tie using 2-1-1 and when tightening the second throw, stop just before knot becomes round. On the third throw, tighten the knot.

- Inject subconjunctival antibiotic and steroid. May instill drop of dilute povidone-iodide on the ocular surface.
- Instill IOP-lowering drops if nonvalved GDD implanted. Instill cycloplegic in most cases (atropine if no contraindication).
- Instill ointment on surface, then place an eye patch and shield for overnight.

POSTOPERATIVE CONSIDERATIONS

- General postoperative regimen includes antibiotic and cycloplegic drops for 1 week, and a topical steroid taper for 4-8 weeks.
- If the anterior chamber is shallow: Rule out choroidal effusions or hemorrhage with dilated fundus examination or B-scan ultrasonography. Increase strength and/or frequency of cycloplegic eye drop if no contraindications, and observe closely. Refill anterior chamber with viscoelastic if lens-cornea touch is present. Involve a retinal specialist if a choroidal hemorrhage occurs.
- In Ahmed GDD, the hypertensive phase may be mitigated or avoided by using glaucoma drops in the first week after surgery to keep IOP below 10-15 mm Hg.[6]
- Consider adding topical nonsteroidal anti-inflammatory drop 1-4 times a day in postoperative period and long-term.[7]
- Patency of tube may be checked by performing B-scan ultrasonography of the quadrant where the plate is located (by placing the probe across from the quadrant) and looking for fluid surrounding the GDD plate.[8]

References

1. Rachmiel R, Trope GE, Buys YM, Flanagan JG, Chipman ML. Intermediate-term outcome and success of superior versus inferior Ahmed Glaucoma Valve implantation. *J Glaucoma*. 2008;17(7):584-590.
2. Weinreb RN, Grajewski AL, Papadopoulos M, Grigg J, Freedman SF. *Childhood Glaucoma: The 9th Consensus Report of the World Glaucoma Association*. Netherlands: Kugler Publications; 2013:270.
3. Margeta MA, Kuo AN, Proia AD, Freedman SF. Staying away from the optic nerve: a formula for modifying glaucoma drainage device surgery in pediatric and other small eyes. *J AAPOS*. 2017;21(1):39-43.e1.
4. O'Malley Schotthoefer E, Yanovitch TL, Freedman SF. Aqueous drainage device surgery in refractory pediatric glaucomas: I. Long-term outcomes. *J AAPOS*. 2008;12(1):33-39.

5. Chang L, Mruthyunjaya P, Rodriguez-Rosa RE, Freedman SF. Postoperative cilioretinal artery occlusion in Sturge Weber-associated glaucoma. *J AAPOS*. 2010;14(4):358-360.
6. Pakravan M, Rad SS, Yazdani S, Ghahari E, Yaseri M. Effect of early treatment with aqueous suppressants on Ahmed glaucoma valve implantation outcomes. *Ophthalmology*. 2014;121(9): 1693-1698.
7. Scott GR, Weizer JS, Moroi SE, et al. Can topical ketorolac 0.5% improve the function of Ahmed(R) glaucoma drainage devices? *Ophthalmic Surg Lasers Imaging*. 2011;42(3):190-195.
8. Baig NB, Lin AA, Freedman SF. Ultrasound evaluation of glaucoma drainage devices in children. *J AAPOS*. 2015;19(3):281-284.

CHAPTER 12

Trabeculectomy

Brenda L. Bohnsack, MD, PhD

PREOPERATIVE CONSIDERATIONS

Trabeculectomy surgery has been a mainstay for refractory glaucoma in children and adults since the 1960s.[1,2] While trabeculectomy surgery can provide excellent IOP control, careful preoperative screening is required to identify good surgical candidates.[2] In children, cooperation with slit lamp examinations for monitoring of the bleb is required. In addition, a preoperative conversation with the patient and family about the lifelong risk of infection due to trauma and even swimming is important. This, combined with the introduction of glaucoma drainage devices (see Chapter 11), has made trabeculectomy a less common surgery in the pediatric population.[3]

The morphology of the trabeculectomy bleb is important to understand.[4] A diffuse, slightly elevated bleb with microcysts and low conjunctival vascularization is desirable for IOP control and less risk of leaks. In contrast, a focal, highly elevated vascular bleb is likely to be encapsulated and not provide adequate IOP control. An elevated, thin cystic bleb at or near the limbus is caused by scarring posterior to the scleral flap and is at higher risk for leak and infection, which can be visually devastating.[5] Much attention has been directed at intraoperative factors that influence bleb morphology in order to improve the functionality and longevity of the trabeculectomy.

- Intraoperative antifibrotic medications: The use of antifibrotics, namely mitomycin C (MMC) and 5-fluorouracil (5FU), has become standard with trabeculectomy surgery. While many studies show better long-term IOP control with MMC, these blebs tend to have more early postoperative complications.[6-9] The traditional method of application consists of sponges soaked in MMC (0.2-0.4 mg/mL) or 5FU (50 mg/mL), which are applied for 1-5 minutes to the prepared scleral bed prior to creation of the flap.[10-12] Increased time of MMC exposure in adults may lead to complications such as cataract formation; however, the data in children are limited.[13] MMC (0.2 mg/mL) can also be injected (0.1 mL) sub-Tenon's prior to conjunctival incision in the desired area of the bleb. This approach may encourage a diffuse, posterior low-lying bleb.[14,15] More recently the collagen matrix, Ologen (Aeon Astron), has been used to augment trabeculectomy surgery either as a substitute for or with low-dose MMC. The collagen matrix is placed under and posterior to the scleral flap and is hypothesized to prevent fibroblast organization and subsequent scar formation. Limited studies show that Ologen has similar efficacy to MMC in obtaining IOP control.

- Conjunctival incision: Fornix-based and limbus-based incisions are the typical approaches for glaucoma surgery.[16] Limbus-based incisions (conjunctival incisions made in the fornix) produce more avascular, thin cystic blebs that are localized at the limbus and prone for infection.[17] However, fornix-based incisions (conjunctival incisions made at the limbus) are at higher risk for early bleb leaks.[18] A hybrid approach may be used by creating the conjunctival incision ~2-3 mm posterior to the limbus, which promotes posterior filtration by decreasing flow anterior to the suture line and has less early wound leaks.
- Tenonectomy: Removal of Tenon capsule anterior and posterior to the scleral flap aims to prevent encapsulation and formation of the "ring of steel" (dense scarring above the flap/sclerostomy, which limits aqueous diffusion).[19,20]

VIDEO SURGICAL PROCEDURE (VIDEO 12.1)

Trabeculectomy With MMC (Fig. 12.1)

- For subconjunctival injection of MMC: Mix 1 mL of MMC (0.5 mg/mL) with 1 mL of lidocaine (2%) for a final concentration of 0.2 mg/mL of MMC and 1% lidocaine. Inject 0.1 mL of MMC and lidocaine mixture sub-Tenon's in the area of the anticipated bleb, ~6 mm posterior to the superior limbus. Use a cotton-tipped applicator to spread the MMC and lidocaine mixture (Fig. 12.1).
- Place a partial-thickness 7-0 Vicryl traction suture at or just posterior to the superior limbus to expose the superior conjunctiva.
- Conjunctival incision:
    - Limbus-based: With Westcott scissors, incise the conjunctiva, followed by Tenon capsule ~8 mm posterior to the superior limbus. Dissect anteriorly to 0.5-1 mm posterior to the limbus.
    - Fornix-based: With Westcott scissors, create a peritomy superiorly for ~3 clock hours. Dissect posteriorly to expose the anterior 3-4 mm of sclera.
    - Hybrid incision: With Westcott scissors, incise the conjunctiva 2-3 mm posterior to the limbus. Sharply dissect Tenon tissue anteriorly to 0.1-1 mm posterior to the limbus.
- Use Wet-Field cautery to obtain hemostasis and prepare the scleral bed.
- For sponge-applied MMC: Soak four to six sponges (~2 × 2 mm) in MMC (0.2-0.4 mg/mL). Apply sponges to the clean scleral bed in the area of the desired bleb for 1-5 minutes (surgeon preference). Irrigate the entire ocular surface (cornea, conjunctiva, exposed sclera) with balanced salt solution at least 2-3 times.
- Scleral flap creation:
    - With a 7515 blade, create a scleral flap (~3 × 1.5 mm) that is 75% depth and extends anteriorly to 0.5 mm posterior to the limbus.
    - Alternatively, use a crescent blade to create a 3-mm wide scleral tunnel starting ~3 mm posterior to the limbus and advancing to 0.5 mm posterior to the limbus. Open the sides of the tunnel with Vanass scissors.
- With a 7515 blade, enter into the anterior chamber under the flap, ~0.5-1 mm posterior to the limbus. Enlarge the sclerostomy with a Kelly punch.
- Insert tying or Colibri forceps through the sclerostomy and pull out a small amount of peripheral iris. Excise with Vanass scissors to create the peripheral iridectomy.
- Loosely suture the scleral flap along each edge with an interrupted 10-0 nylon.
- Create a temporal paracentesis with a 7515 blade.
- Injected balanced salt solution into the anterior chamber through the paracentesis in order to gauge flow from under the scleral flap. Adjust flow with removal of or placement of additional 10-0 nylon sutures as needed.
- Secure the conjunctival incision with a continuous closure using 8-0 Vicryl suture on a BV needle.

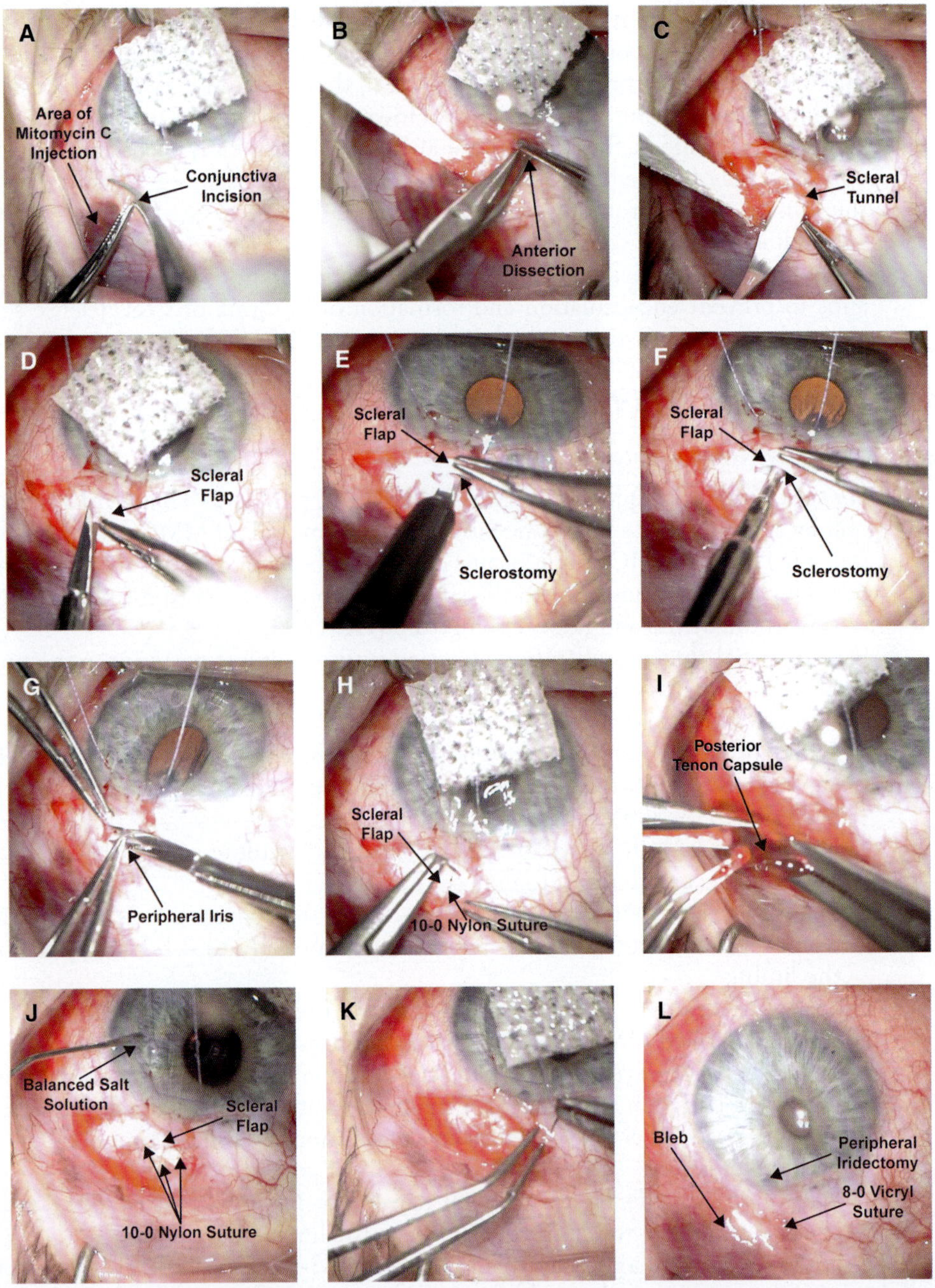

FIGURE 12.1. Trabeculectomy with subconjunctival injection of MMC and tenonectomy. **A.** A 7-0 Vicryl suture is placed superiorly and used to infraduct the eye to expose the superior conjunctiva. The area of the preoperative MMC sub-Tenon injection is evident by subconjunctival hemorrhage superiorly. Westcott scissors are used to incise the conjunctiva ~2-3 mm posterior to the limbus. **B.** Dissection is carried anteriorly to 0.5 mm posterior to the limbus. **C.** A crescent blade is used to create a 75% depth, 3-mm wide scleral tunnel that starts 2-3 mm posterior to the limbus and extends to 0.5 mm posterior to the limbus. **D.** The sides of the scleral tunnel are opened with Vanass scissors. **E.** A sclerostomy under the scleral flap is created with a 7515 blade. **F.** The sclerostomy is enlarged with a Kelly punch. **G.** A peripheral iridectomy is created using forceps and Vanass scissors. **H.** The scleral flap is loosely closed with interrupted 10-0 nylon sutures along each edge. **I.** Posterior Tenon capsule is dissected and brought anteriorly. The tissue is clamped with a hemostat and excised with Westcott scissors. **J.** Balanced salt solution is injected through a paracentesis and flow from under the scleral flap is observed. Sutures are added or removed to adjust flow. **K.** The conjunctiva is closed with a running 8-0 Vicryl suture on a BV needle. **L.** Following conjunctiva closure, a bleb forms superiorly.

POSTOPERATIVE CONSIDERATIONS (SEE CHAPTER 15)

Bleb Management

Bleb management plays a crucial role in the postoperative success of patients who have undergone trabeculectomy surgery.

- Suture removal: At the time of surgery, the flow from the trabeculectomy is adjusted by placement of sutures to tighten or loosen the scleral flap. Aqueous humor outflow can continue to be adjusted postoperatively by removal of the sutures; however, the timing depends on the use of intraoperative antifibrotic medications and surgeon preference.[21-23]
  - In eyes treated with MMC, studies have shown that suture lysis can be done as late as 5 months posttrabeculectomy but is most commonly done between 1 day and 2 months. Early suture lysis within the first week may cause hypotony, especially with intraoperative MMC. In 5FU-treated eyes, suture lysis is typically performed within the first 2-3 weeks postoperatively.
  - The diode or argon laser (200-400 mW with 50-100 μm spot size) along with a lens that compresses the blood vessels (ie, Ritch or Hoskins lens) are most commonly used for suture lysis. A second approach is to place releasable sutures at the time of surgery, which are exposed at the limbus for easy access.[24]
- Postoperative antifibrotic injections:
  - With signs of bleb failure (ie, increased vascularization) in adults, 0.1 mL of 5FU (50 mg/mL) can be subconjunctivally injected inferiorly for up to 2 months in the postoperative period to inhibit wound healing. This is less commonly performed in children due to faster scarring and limited in-clinic cooperation.
  - Alternatively, 0.1 mL of MMC (0.2-0.4 mg/mL) can be injected in and around the bleb to help prevent scarring and is usually done in association with needling (see below).[12,25-27]
- Bleb needling: Needling involves the mechanical disruption of scar tissue and Tenon capsule within the bleb and is performed in failing blebs to encourage additional flow into the subconjunctival space.[25-28] Further needling can be done in thin, cystic elevated blebs that are at high risk for infection in order to encourage posterior flow and create a more diffuse, less elevated bleb. Although needling can be done in clinic for adults, it is often performed in the operating room for children.
  - A 23G or 25G needle on balanced salt solution is often used, but some surgeons prefer a blade (ie, MVR).
  - The needle or blade is inserted in a biplanar fashion first through the conjunctiva and then through Tenon capsule ~8 mm posterior to the scleral flap to limit postneedling leaks. The needle or blade is carefully advanced and used to disrupt scar tissue and Tenon capsule, which is limiting flow posterior to the scleral flap.
  - This is often augmented by preneedling injection of MMC.
- Bleb revision: An in-depth surgical revision of the bleb is done to more aggressively remove scar tissue and Tenon encapsulation in a failing bleb or reinforce a thin bleb prone to leaks and infection.
  - Surgical removal of scar tissue: Opening of the bleb and exposure of the sclera often through the original conjunctival incision allows for greater removal of scarring and encapsulation tissue but requires resuturing of the conjunctiva. If minimal aqueous humor is observed flowing from the scleral flap, an MVR blade or needle can be used to carefully reopen the sclerostomy under the flap. This is often paired with preoperative MMC injection.[29]
  - Reinforcement of bleb: Recurrent bleb leaks, especially in thin and cystic limbal blebs, may lead to ill-formed and weak granulation tissue within the bleb conjunctiva. The granulation tissue and thin, avascular conjunctiva should be excised

and healthy superior conjunctiva then advanced to the limbus.[30] However, depending on the redundancy and laxity of the conjunctiva, this approach may result in upper eyelid ptosis. Conjunctival relaxing incisions extending into the fornix may release tension and minimize ptosis. A second technique is to use an autograft from the inferior conjunctiva. In general, a conjunctival graft should be twice the size of the area that needs coverage. In addition, care should be taken to maintain the orientation of the conjunctival graft such that the original side closest to the limbus remains closest to the limbus. The conjunctival graft is secured with horizontal mattress sutures along each edge.[31]

Postoperative Infections

It is estimated that over 20% of patients with trabeculectomies may experience a bleb leak in the first 5 years with 0.5%-7% developing infection.[32-34] Without immediate diagnosis and treatment, blebitis can have visually devastating consequences. Children need to be able to cooperate with slit lamp examinations as recognition of bleb leaks, and management with a bandage contact lens and aqueous suppression is imperative. In addition, frequent follow-up and aggressive treatment with topical antibiotics if blebitis develops, and intravitreal cultures and antibiotics if endophthalmitis occurs, are critical.[32,33]

References

1. Cairns J. Trabeculectomy. Preliminary report of a new method. *Am J Ophthalmol.* 1968;66:673-679.
2. Chang I, et al. Surgical management of pediatric glaucoma. *Dev Ophthalmol.* 2017;59: 165-178.
3. Kwon YH, et al. Surgical outcomes of trabeculectomy and glaucoma drainage implant for uveitic glaucoma and relationship with uveitis activity. *Clin Exp Ophthalmol.* 2017;45: 472-480.
4. Wells AP, et al. A pilot study of a system for grading of drainage blebs after glaucoma surgery. *J Glaucoma.* 2004;13:454-460.
5. Morita K, et al. In vivo confocal microscopy and ultrasound biomicroscopy study of filtering blebs after trabeculectomy: limbus-based versus fornix-based conjunctival flaps. *J Glaucoma.* 2012;21:383-391.
6. Cabourne E, et al. Mitomycin C versus 5-fluorouracail for wound healing in glaucoma surgery. *Cochrane Database Syst Rev.* 2015;(11):CD006259.
7. De Fendi LI, et al. Mitomycin C versus 5-fluorouracil as an adjunctive treatment for trabeculectomy: a meta-analysis of randomized clinical trials. *Clin Exp Ophthalmol.* 2013;41: 798-806.
8. Kim HY, et al. Long-term comparison of primary trabeculectomy with 5-fluorouracil versus mitomycin C in West Africa. *J Glaucoma.* 2008;17:578-583.
9. Palanca-Capistrano AM, et al. Long-term outcomes of intraoperative 5-fluorouracil versus intraoperative mitomycin C in primary trabeculectomy surgery. *Ophthalmology.* 2009;116: 185-190.
10. Flynn WJ, et al. Mitomycin trabeculectomy: the microsurgical sponge difference. *J Glaucoma.* 1995;4:86-90.
11. Mora JS, et al. Trabeculectomy with intraoperative sponge 5-fluorouracil. *Ophthalmology.* 1996;103:963-970.
12. Freedman SF, et al. Mitomycin C-augmented trabeculectomy with postoperative wound modulation in pediatric glaucoma. *J AAPOS.* 1999;3:117-124.
13. Robin AL, et al. A long-term dose response study of mitomycin in glaucoma filtration surgery. *Arch Ophthalmol.* 1997;115:969-974.
14. Pakravan M, et al. Mitomycin C-augmented trabeculectomy: subtenon injection versus soaked sponges: a randomised clinical trial. *Br J Ophthalmol.* 2017;101:1275-1280.
15. Khouri AS, et al. Intraoperative injection vs sponge-applied mitomycin C during trabeculectomy: one-year study. *J Curr Glaucoma Pract.* 2017;11:101-106.

16. Al-Haddad CE, et al. Fornix-based versus limbal-based conjunctival trabeculectomy flaps for glaucoma: findings from a Cochrane Systemic Review. *Am J Ophthalmol.* 2017;174: 33-41.
17. Solus JF, et al. Comparison of limbus-based and fornix-based trabeculectomy: success, bleb-related complications, and bleb morphology. *Ophthalmology*. 2012;119:703-711.
18. Wells AP, et al. Cystic bleb formation and related complications in limbus- versus fornix-based conjunctival flaps in pediatric and young adult trabeculectomy with mitomycin C. *Ophthalmology*. 2003;110:2192-2197.
19. Miller KN, et al. A comparison of total and partial tenonectomy with trabeculectomy. *Am J Ophthalmol.* 1991;111:323-326.
20. Awadein A, El Sayed YM. Excision of Tenon capsule in pediatric trabeculectomy: a controlled study. *J Glaucoma*. 2016;25:39-44.
21. Pappa KS, et al. Late argon laser suture lysis after mitomycin C trabeculectomy. *Ophthalmology*. 1993;100:1268-1271.
22. Aykan U, et al. Laser suture lysis or releasable sutures after trabeculectomy. *J Glaucoma*. 2007;16:240-245.
23. Savage JA, et al. Laser suture lysis after trabeculectomy. *Ophthalmology*. 1988;95: 1631-1638.
24. Duman F, et al. Comparison of 3 different releasable suture techniques in trabeculectomy. *Eur J Ophthalmol.* 2016;26:307-314.
25. Mercieca K, et al. Trabeculectomy bleb needling and antimetabolite administration practices in the UK: a glaucoma specialist national survey. *Br J Ophthalmol.* 2018;102:1244-1247.
26. Lin S, et al. Long-term outcome of mitomycin C-augmented needle revision of trabeculectomy blebs for late trabeculectomy failure. *Eye (Lond)*. 2018;32:1893-1899.
27. Liu W, et al. Comparison of subconjunctival mitomycin C and 5-fluoruracil injection for needle revision of early failed trabeculectomy blebs. *J Ophthalmol.* 2016;2016:3762674.
28. Than JYL, et al. Factors predicting the success of trabeculectomy bleb enhancement with needling. *Br J Ophthalmol.* 2018;102:1667-1671.
29. Nikita E, Murdoch I. Same-site surgical revision of failed trabeculectomy blebs with mitomycin C augmentation: long-term follow-up. *Eye (Lond)*. 2018;32:352-358.
30. Bashford KP, et al. Bleb revision for hypotony maculopathy after trabeculectomy. *J Glaucoma*. 2004;13:256-260.
31. Schnyder CC, et al. Free conjunctival autologous graft for bleb repair and bleb reduction after trabeculectomy and nonpenetrating filtering surgery. *J Glaucoma*. 2002;11:10-16.
32. Waheed S, et al. Bleb-related ocular infection in children after trabeculectomy with mitomycin C. *Ophthalmology*. 1997;104:2117-2120.
33. DeBry PW, et al. Incidence of late-onset bleb-related complications following trabeculectomy. *Arch Ophthalmol.* 2002;120:297-300.
34. Kim EA, et al. Long-term bleb-related infections after trabeculectomy: incidence, risk factors, and influence of bleb revision. *Am J Ophthalmol.* 2015;159:1082-1091.

CHAPTER 13

Cyclodestructive Procedures

Sara Fransen Grace, MD

PREOPERATIVE CONSIDERATIONS

Determine if transscleral diode cyclophotocoagulation (TDC) or endoscopic diode cyclophotocoagulation (ECP) is indicated for the patient. TDC is used for phakic eyes with refractory glaucoma or eyes that are not suited to undergo incisional surgery. ECP should be reserved for eyes that are aphakic or pseudophakic in which external landmarks are not easily identified and an endoscopic view is needed. ECP can be performed concurrently with other intraocular procedures (ie, vitrectomy and posterior capsule membranectomy to clear an opacified visual axis).[1,2]

Preoperative Examination

- Evaluate for scleral thinning as TDC can induce further thinning with possible staphyloma and perforation.
- If the ciliary processes cannot be identified well by external landmarks or transillumination, ECP is preferred to TDC.
- Evaluate for inflammation. Success rates for these procedures are lower in uveitic eyes.
- Due to the risk of sympathetic ophthalmia (however low), cyclodestructive procedures should be avoided in eyes with NLP vision.[3]

Preoperative Counseling

Discuss the following with the patient's family to ensure an understanding of the postoperative course:

- Treatment may need to be titrated over several sessions to obtain adequate IOP control while avoiding hypotony and vision loss.
- Topical glaucoma therapy may still be necessary.
- Eyes with multiple prior surgeries or previous TDC/ECP are at increased risk for complications (hypotony, cataract, choroidal/retinal detachment, inflammation).

SURGICAL PROCEDURE

Transscleral Diode Cyclophotocoagulation

TDC Equipment

- 0.3 Toothed forceps.
- Diode laser (810 nm) with G-probe.

- No sterile preparation is needed. Place an eyelid speculum.
- Stabilize/manipulate the eye with 0.3 forceps.
- Apply the G-probe footplate to the limbus and adjust footplate as needed. When the limbus cannot be clearly identified due to buphthalmos or anatomic abnormalities, use transillumination through the pupil to look for the junction of light and dark areas indicating the scleral spur and anterior attachment of the uvea. The footplate should be applied at the junction.
- Start with 1500 mW spot[1] at 200 ms duration, listening for a faintly audible pop and titrate up to not more than 2000 mW (and not <1500 mW) per application. If a loud pop is heard, titrate down until the pop is barely discernable. Applications should be spaced ½ G-probe width apart.
- In eyes without glaucoma drainage devices, treat up to three quadrants for a first treatment, never 360 degrees. Spare the 3- and 9-o'clock meridians due to the entrance of the long ciliary nerves.
- Limit application to two quadrants if there is a preexisting glaucoma drainage device and do not treat in any areas with preexisting glaucoma devices or scleral thinning. To avoid hypotony, it is best to leave one quadrant untreated. If repeat treatment is needed, do not treat >180 degrees in one session.

Endoscopic Diode Cyclophotocoagulation

ECP Equipment

- Operating microscope.
- Display monitor.
- MVR blade or 20G or 23G trocar needle for pars plana incision (same size as endoscopic probe).
- Viscoelastic (Healon) or AC maintainer.
- Mechanical vitrector (if pars plana approach and no prior vitrectomy).
- Diode laser (810 nm).
- Endoscopic probe, 20G or 23G, straight or curved.
- 8-0 Vicryl suture (pars plana incision) or 10-0 Vicryl suture (limbal incision).
- Intracameral epinephrine (if patient not already dilated from concurrent procedure).

After completion of any concurrent intraocular procedures, dilate pupil (if not already dilated) with intracameral epinephrine.

- Bring endoscopic probe onto field and adjust focus and orientation for display monitor.
- Pars plana approach: If infusion not already in place, use AC maintainer or viscoelastic to keep eye formed. Use appropriate gauge trocar or MVR blade to make pars plana incision (approach from limbus: 0-1 year: 1.5 mm, 1-2 years: 2 mm, 2-4 years: 2.5 mm, >4 years: 3 mm). Perform anterior vitrectomy.
- Limbal approach: Use AC maintainer or viscoelastic to maintain AC. Inflate ciliary sulcus with viscoelastic to aid visualization. Anterior vitrectomy not needed.
- Under direct microscopic visualization, introduce the endoscopic probe into the eye and position the tip posterior to the iris on the side across from the point of entry. Look at monitor and retract or advance probe so that several ciliary processes are visible.
- Start with 150 mW* power on the continuous setting until shrinkage and whitening occurs without rupturing the ciliary processes or causing bubbles (titrate higher or lower as needed to induce effect). Treat 120-180 degrees depending on patient's preoperative IOP and history. A second incision may be necessary

*The above initial power settings are based on those of Sharon Freedman, MD. Initial power settings may vary according to the surgeon and experience.

to access a greater number of ciliary processes (can exchange irrigation and laser ports).

- Irrigate out any viscoelastic/remove AC maintainer and close incisions.

In both TDC and ECP, consider sub-Tenon bupivacaine (0.75%) and triamcinolone. Intravenous ketorolac and dexamethasone can help with postoperative pain and inflammation control. Advise patients to take oral NSAIDs and Tylenol postoperatively.

POSTOPERATIVE CARE

Postoperative Drop Regimen

- Topical atropine 1% once daily for 2 weeks then taper.
- Prednisolone acetate (Pred Forte) 1% or dexamethasone 4-6 times daily for 2 weeks then taper.
- Resume preoperative glaucoma medications as needed.
- Examine the patient on post-op day 1 and post-op week one to measure IOP and assess for intraocular complications. Rexamine the patient after the tapering of steroid drops.
- In uncooperative pediatric patients, use B-scan ultrasonography to rule out posterior complications like excessive inflammation or choroidal effusions secondary to hypotony.
- Delay repeat laser at least 8 weeks to discern outcome of initial procedure and allow inflammation to subside.

References

1. Chang TC, Joos K. Cyclodestruction. In: Grajewski AL, Bitrian E, Papadopoulos M, Freedman SF, eds. *Surgical Management of Childhood Glaucoma: Clinical Considerations and Techniques*. Cham, Switzerland: Springer International Publishing; 2018:129-135.
2. Bock CJ, Freedman SF, Buckley EG, et al. Transscleral diode laser cyclophotocoagulation for refractory pediatric glaucomas. *J Pediatr Ophthalmol Strabismus*. 1997;34(4):235-239.
3. Aujla JS, Lee GA, Vincent SJ, et al. Incidence of hypotony and sympathetic ophthalmia following trans-scleral cyclophotocoagulation for glaucoma and a report of risk factors. *Clin Exp Ophthalmol*. 2013;41(8):761-772.

CHAPTER 14

Glaucoma Surgery: Special Cases

Amanda L. Ely, MD • Sharon F. Freedman, MD

Despite the considerable surgical approaches to childhood glaucoma, there are those "special cases" that require individually tailored, and sometimes out-of-the-box management.

ANIRIDIA WITH EARLY-ONSET GLAUCOMA (OR PHENOTYPICALLY SIMILAR ANTERIOR SEGMENT DESPITE NON-ANIRIDIC GENOTYPE)

- These cases fall under the diagnostic category of secondary glaucoma with nonacquired, mainly ocular anomalies[1] (see Chapter 9).
- Technical challenges include minimal iris tissue, a shallow anterior chamber, and often corneal opacity.
- Recommendations to avoid early disasters:
    - SLOW DOWN and see if you can temporize with medications long enough to allow a little eye growth, management of family expectations, and formulation of a plan.
        - Remember this is a journey, and careful is better than fast.
        - Discuss this approach with the family, who must travel this long road with you.
    - Begin with sodium chloride 5% (if there is corneal edema), and medical therapy tailored to patient age/health (eg, topical beta blocker at low dose, topical carbonic anhydrase inhibitor despite the corneal edema, and prostaglandin; possible use of apraclonidine, oral acetazolamide, or even brimonidine [for older/larger children only]).
- Surgical considerations and adaptations (provided medical therapy and close monitoring have proven inadequate to control the IOP, as evidenced by significant ocular enlargement and/or optic nerve cupping when the latter can be visualized).
    - *Angle surgery* (see Chapter 10)—(unlikely to work despite technical success):
        - Consider only if anterior chamber depth is moderate to deep and the view is adequate.
        - Trabeculotomy is recommended over goniotomy, with great caution to avoid injuring "naked" lens.
    - *Filtration surgery* (see Chapter 12):
        - Not recommended except for older and very cooperative children with extremely close follow-up, given great propensity for flat chamber and resultant corneal and lens damage.

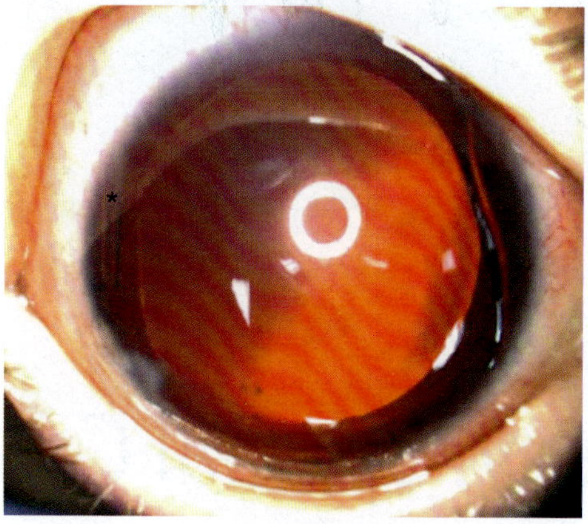

FIGURE 14.1. Baerveldt implant with sulcus tube placement in aniridia. (*Asterisk* notes location of temporally placed tube.)

- *Glaucoma drainage device surgery* (see Chapter 11):
  - Consider only if anterior chamber depth is moderate to deep.
  - Place tube over zonules in the sulcus if possible, to minimize damage to very vulnerable cornea. Expect long-term lens changes which are manageable (Fig. 14.1).
- *Cycloablation (transscleral)* (see Chapter 13):
  - Consider only if other options not feasible, very conservatively, to "buy time."
  - Consider reducing energy and extent of treatment.

ANTERIOR SEGMENT DYSGENESIS WITH CORNEAL OPACITY AND COMPROMISED ANTERIOR CHAMBER (eg, PETERS ANOMALY OR SIMILAR CASES)

- These cases similarly constitute secondary glaucoma with nonacquired, mainly ocular anomalies[1] (see Chapter 9).
- Technical challenges include the lack of visualization of the anterior chamber and suspected lack of normal anterior chamber to provide "working room" for typical surgical procedures.
- Recommendations to avoid early disasters—same as for Aniridia above.
- Surgical considerations and adaptations.
  - *EUA-only*:
    - Strongly consider in order to perform ultrasound biomicroscopy to better delineate anterior chamber depth, presence/location of iridocorneal adhesions, and presence/location of the crystalline lens (Fig. 14.2).
  - *Angle surgery* (see Chapter 10): Often technically impractical/ill-advised.
  - *Cycloablation* (see Chapter 13):
    - Reasonable as initial therapy in some of these cases, cautiously, and to buy time, but beware of the impossible task of gaining IOP control if there truly is no outflow; one may see an IOP reduction right after treatment, followed by return to prelaser high IOPs.
  - *Glaucoma drainage device surgery* (see Chapter 11): often impractical due to lack of a space to place the tube.
  - *Optical iridectomy* (see Chapter 21):
    - Consider if there could be a visual axis through native cornea (may not help with glaucoma surgery but may dramatically aid visual development).
  - *Lensectomy/anterior vitrectomy* (see Chapter 5):
    - Consider to make room for endoscopic laser cycloablation and later pars plana vitrectomy (by a vitreoretinal surgeon) for possible pars plana tube placement if the view is adequate for an anterior segment approach.

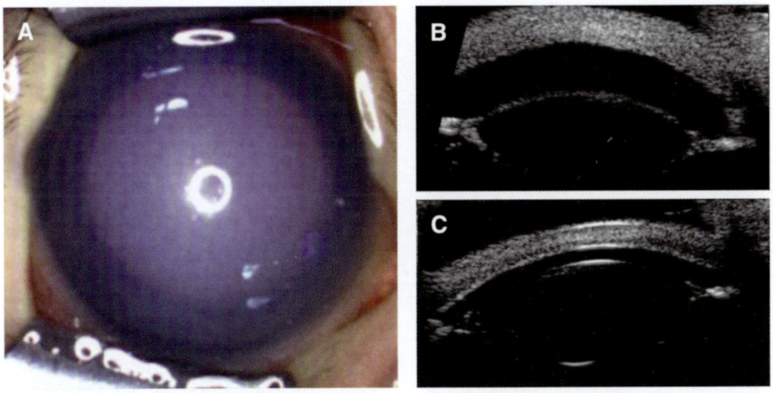

FIGURE 14.2. Ultrasound biomicroscopy (UBM) images of glaucoma in suspected aniridia. **A.** Right eye of an infant born with cloudy corneas, high intraocular pressure, and no visible iris, believed to be aniridia, but found later to be Axenfeld-Rieger variant. Preoperative UBM imaging **(B)** shows absence of iris, deep anterior chamber, and thickened cornea. Postoperatively after Ahmed glaucoma drainage device placement **(C)**, the UBM image demonstrates shallowing of the anterior chamber and improvement in corneal thickness.

- *Corneal transplant* (see Chapter 19):
  - Can be considered in such cases, but would function as a "space-making" procedure rather than an optical treatment, as typically the lens must be removed in these cases.
  - Prognosis for a corneal transplant to remain clear is very guarded and should be presented to the family as such.
- *Pars plana lensectomy/vitrectomy* (see Chapter 31):
  - Consider whether a more aggressive procedure such as this would allow later glaucoma drainage device surgery and/or endoscopic cycloablation by making room.
  - May require an endoscopic approach for the lensectomy/vitrectomy and must have a very experienced retinal surgeon as partner (especially if endoscopic view is necessary).

EYES WITH GLAUCOMA IN SETTING OF ELEVATED EPISCLERAL VENOUS PRESSURE (USUALLY PORT WINE MARK-ASSOCIATED, WITH OR WITHOUT TRUE STURGE WEBER SYNDROME)

- These cases are secondary glaucomas associated with predominantly nonacquired features that may be ocular (in the case of isolated port wine mark and associated ipsilateral glaucoma) or systemic (in case of associated leptomeningeal hemangioma with seizures/developmental delay; these may have either ipsilateral or bilateral glaucoma).[1]
- The special considerations for glaucoma surgery are related to the presence of choroidal hemangioma and associated elevated episcleral venous pressure as cause for the glaucoma.
- The optimal management of these patients depends upon the presentation of the glaucoma and its severity. In birth- or infant-onset glaucoma, there may be an element of abnormal angle development, while in childhood-onset glaucoma, the mechanism is assumed to be strictly elevated episcleral venous pressure.
- Medical therapy is usually recommended first, even in infant-onset cases.
- If the medical therapy is inadequate to reduce the intraocular pressure, and especially to clear the corneal edema and slow ocular enlargement in infant-onset cases, surgery is indicated.
- Surgical considerations and adaptations:
  - The goal of surgery in these cases is to avoid unnecessary intraocular pressure fluctuations, especially hypotony, in the intraoperative and perioperative period, since choroidal expansion and even choroidal hemorrhage are possible in this setting.

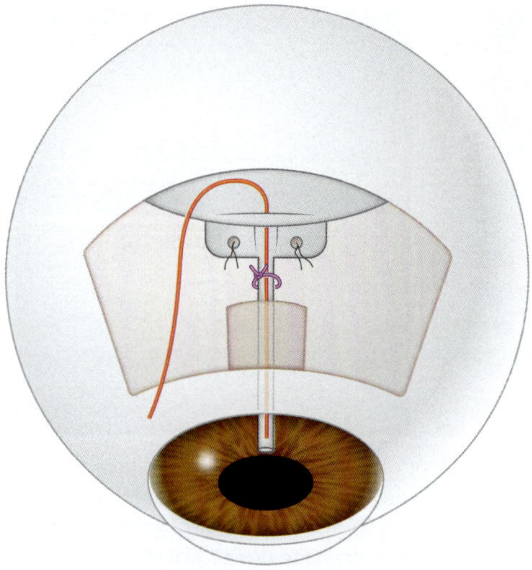

FIGURE 14.3. Ripcord suture for Baerveldt implant in Sturge Weber (*red line* represents 5-0 nylon suture within tube, *purple* represents overlying dissolvable suture ligature). Note this implant was placed via a fornix incision. Note the pathway of the "rip cord" nylon passed within the tube with tail then passed beneath conjunctiva to the temporal limbus allowing easy access for later removal.

- *Angle surgery* (see Chapter 10):
  - Goniotomy or trabeculotomy can be effective. It is important to maintain intraoperative IOP at reasonable levels throughout the surgery and to not leave any wound leak at the end of the case.
  - Goniotomy is more conducive to this pressure stability and is recommended, provided the corneal clarity allows for it.
- *Trabeculectomy* (see Chapter 12): is not recommended in this setting, especially in infant eyes where scleral rigidity is lower.
- *Glaucoma drainage device surgery* (see Chapter 11): can be safely performed, but several modifications are recommended.
  - Non-valved drainage devices (eg, Baerveldt rather than Ahmed) are preferred, with double ligature of the tubing and no venting slits.
  - An anterior chamber maintainer is recommended during the tube insertion, avoiding any viscoelastic which may cause a very high pressure spike the next day, and has been reported, rarely, to cause cilioretinal artery occlusion.[2]
  - In cooperative children, or those with high risk of serous chorioretinal detachment after tube opening, a rip cord (Fig. 14.3) may be placed (5-0 nylon inside the tube with an encircling 6-0 polyglactin suture). The rip cord can then be removed in the operating room along with anterior chamber reformation at just under 6 weeks when spontaneous tube opening is expected.

References

1. Weinreb RN, Grajewski AL, Papadopoulos M, Grigg J, Freedman SF. *Childhood Glaucoma: The 9th Consensus Report of the World Glaucoma Association*. Amsterdam, The Netherlands: Kugler Publications; 2013.
2. Chang L, Mruthyunjaya P, Rodriguez-Rosa RE, Freedman SF. Postoperative cilioretinal artery occlusion in Sturge Weber-associated glaucoma. *J AAPOS*. 2010;14(4):358-360. doi: 10.1016/j.jaapos.2010.04.014.

Suggested Readings

Go MS, Barman NR, House RJ, Freedman SF. Home tonometry assists glaucoma drainage device management in childhood glaucoma. *J Glaucoma*. 2019;28:818-822. doi: 10.1097/IJG.0000000000001322.

Ozgonul C, Besirli CG, Bohnsack BL. Combined vitrectomy and glaucoma drainage device implantation surgical approach for complex pediatric glaucomas. *J AAPOS*. 2017;21(2):121-126. doi: 10.1016/j.jaapos.2017.02.001.

CHAPTER 15

Glaucoma Surgery: Postoperative Management, Complications, and Prognosis

Jing Jin, MD, PhD

Throughout this section, glaucoma surgery success is defined as IOP ≤ 21 mm Hg with or without medication, stable optic disc appearance and refraction, or no need for further glaucoma surgery.[1]

ANGLE SURGERY (GONIOTOMY OR TRABECULOTOMY) (SEE CHAPTER 10)

- Postoperative management:
  - Patient should be kept quiet with head elevated for 24-48 hours with the operative eye shielded at all times.
  - Postoperative medication regimen:
    - 1% Pilocarpine twice a day for 2-4 weeks.
    - Antibiotic/steroid drop or ointment 4 times per day for 1 week.
    - Closely monitor IOP in follow-up period. May need examination under anesthesia to ensure adequate pressure control.
- Complications:
  - Inadequate IOP control. The patient may require further surgery and should be monitored at regular intervals even if IOP is controlled in the immediate perioperative period.
  - Hyphema:
    - Common with angle surgery.
    - Usually resolves spontaneously within 1 week.
    - Nonclearing vitreous hemorrhage may necessitate vitrectomy in the first or second month postoperatively. Pseudophakic or aphakic eyes undergoing 360-degree angle surgery are at highest risk for this complication.
  - Lens damage, cataract:
    - Patients with aniridia who have an exposed lens are at high risk for this complication.

- Iridodialysis.
- Cyclodialysis cleft:
  - May result in prolonged postoperative hypotony.
  - Cleft can be confirmed with ultrasound biomicroscopy or anterior segment OCT as gonioscopy may be challenging.
  - Many clefts will close spontaneously within the first month. If the cleft does not close, surgical closure of the cleft is indicated.
- Peripheral anterior synechiae.
- Retinal detachment.
- Endophthalmitis.

- Prognosis:
  - Success rate in infants who present between 3 months and 1 year of age with primary congenital glaucoma is reported to be 70%-80%.
  - The success rate for 360-degree trabeculotomy is greater than traditional trabeculotomy.[2]
  - For glaucoma associated with childhood uveitis, goniotomy has a reported success rate (final IOP $\leq$ 21 mm Hg) of up to 75%.[3]

GLAUCOMA DRAINAGE DEVICE (SEE CHAPTER 11)

- Postoperative management:
  - Dress the eye with atropine and antibiotic/steroid ointment. Apply a light gauze dressing and protective shield.
  - Atropine twice daily for 2-4 weeks.
  - Antibiotic/steroid drop or ointment for 4-8 weeks on a tapering schedule.
- Complications:
  - Tube related:
    - Misdirection of tube in anterior chamber with corneal touch/decompensation. May require tube repositioning or removal.
    - Tube erosion through sclera and conjunctiva. May need to place a patch graft over the tube.
    - Tube blockage by blood, iris, or vitreous. Blood blockage may dissolve with time. Iris and vitreous blockage may be cleared with laser or surgery.
  - Scar tissue and fibrosis around the plate may form a thick dome-shaped bleb and cause elevated IOP. May require needling of the bleb or surgical excision of the capsule.
  - Endophthalmitis.
  - Suprachoroidal hemorrhage.
  - Hyphema:
  - Strabismus (see Chapter 59).
    - Patients undergoing Baerveldt drainage device placement are at higher risk given the size of the plate and proximity to rectus muscles.
  - A hypertensive phase may develop after implant of a glaucoma drainage device. Management options include:
    - Aqueous suppressant.
    - Inflammation control.
  - Early hypotony and flat chamber:
    - Suture ligation after Baerveldt or Molteno placement.
- Prognosis:
  - Reported success rates are highly variable and range from 31.3% to 97.2%.
  - Many children require IOP lowering medications after surgery.[1]

TRABECULECTOMY (SEE CHAPTER 12)

- Postoperative management:
  - Dress the eye with atropine and antibiotic/steroid ointment. Apply a light gauze dressing and protective shield.
  - Atropine twice daily for 2-4 weeks.
  - Antibiotic/steroid drop or ointment 4-8 weeks on a tapering schedule.
- Complications:
  - Flat anterior chamber:
    - Wound leak: Confirm with Seidel test.
      - Initiate antibiotic topically and place bandage contact lens.
      - Close follow-up to monitor for signs of blebitis.
      - May require repair of leak if no resolution with conservative measures.
    - Excessive filtration:
      - Place a pressure patch.
      - If anterior chamber fails to reform in 2-3 days, then:
        - If no large choroidal detachment is present, consider deepening anterior chamber with viscoelastic.
        - If large choroidal detachment is present, consider draining the fluid with the assistance of a vitreoretinal surgeon, then reform anterior chamber with balanced salt solution.
    - Corneal edema secondary to endothelial failure may result.
  - Deep chamber and high IOP: This may indicate the need for suture lysis or may suggest bleb encapsulation that can lead to bleb failure.
    - Consider digital pressure, laser suture lysis, needling the encapsulated bleb, surgical revision of bleb.
  - Blebitis: the rate of infection in children is greater than in adults and can be as high as 6.7%.[4] If untreated, blebitis can be visually devastating.
    - Topical antibiotics should be initiated immediately.
    - Follow closely to monitor for improvement or development of endophthalmitis.
    - Obtain intravitreal culture and administer intravitreal antibiotics if suspecting endophthalmitis.
  - Hyphema.
- Prognosis:
  - Reported success rates range from 55.3% to 92.3%.[1]
  - Higher failure rates are associated with aphakia/pseudophakia (60% vs 24% in phakic eyes) and younger age (88% in patients under 1 year vs 29% in age 1-17 years).[4,5]

CYCLODESTRUCTIVE PROCEDURE (TRANSSCLERAL CYCLOPHOTOCOAGULATION) (SEE CHAPTER 13)

- Postoperative management:
  - Consider subconjunctival injection of steroid and bupivacaine at the end of procedure.
  - Antibiotic/steroid ointment: 4-8 weeks on a tapering schedule.
  - Topical atropine 1%.
- Complications:
  - Hypotony:
    - Treatment may be reduced to 180 degrees in patients judged to be at risk for hypotony.[6]
  - Uveitis.
  - Phthisis.

  - Blindness.
  - Sympathetic ophthalmia in the fellow eye: extremely rare.
- Prognosis:
  - Transscleral diode laser cyclophotocoagulation for refractory primary congenital glaucoma or secondary glaucoma has reported success rate of 62%-66% with one treatment. The success rate increases to 72%-79% after multiple treatments.[7,8]

References

1. Chen TC, Chen PP, Francis BA, et al. Pediatric glaucoma surgery: a report by the American Academy of Ophthalmology. *Ophthalmology*. 2014;121(11):2107-2115.
2. Giangiacomo A, Beck A. Pediatric glaucoma: review of recent literature. *Curr Opin Ophthalmol*. 2017;28(2):199-203.
3. Freedman SF, Rodriguez-Rosa RE, Rojas MC, Enyedi LB. Goniotomy for glaucoma secondary to chronic childhood uveitis. *Am J Ophthalmol*. 2002;133(5):617-621.
4. Giampani J, Borges-Giampani AS, Carani JC, Oltrogge EW, Susanna R. Efficacy and safety of trabeculectomy with mitomycin C for childhood glaucoma: a study of results with long-term follow-up. *Clinics (Sao Paulo)*. 2008;63(4):421-426.
5. Beck AD, Wilson WR, Lynch MG, Lynn MJ, Noe R. Trabeculectomy with adjunctive mitomycin C in pediatric glaucoma. *Am J Ophthalmol*. 1998;126(5):648-657.
6. Pastor SA, Singh K, Lee DA, et al. Cyclophotocoagulation: a report by the American Academy of Ophthalmology. *Ophthalmology*. 2001;108(11):2130-2138.
7. Autrata R, Rehurek J. Long-term results of transscleral cyclophotocoagulation in refractory pediatric glaucoma patients. *Ophthalmologica*. 2003;217(6):393-400.
8. Kirwan JF, Shah P, Khaw PT. Diode laser cyclophotocoagulation: role in the management of refractory pediatric glaucomas. *Ophthalmology*. 2002;109(2):316-323.

Section IV

Pediatric Cornea Surgery

CHAPTER 16

Corneal Limbal Dermoids

Bradley P. Barnett, MD, PhD • Matthew S. Ward, MD • Natalie A. Afshari, MD

PREOPERATIVE CONSIDERATIONS

- In many instances, limbal dermoids can be managed conservatively with topical lubrication and occasional epilation.
- Surgical excision may be considered in cases of:
  - A lesion causing visual changes either by encroaching on visual axis or inducing high cylinder. Children may be at risk for deprivation and/or refractive amblyopia.
  - A lesion that causes discomfort.
  - A lesion that is cosmetically disfiguring.
- The potential benefits of surgery must be carefully weighed against potential surgical complications and scar formation. The family should be included in medical decision-making via the informed consent process.
- A thorough medical and family history is necessary with referral to a pediatrician who specializes in genetics if the dermoid is thought to be syndromic in nature.

Limbal dermoids are known to be associated with Goldenhar syndrome.

- If a limbal dermoid appears to only involve superficial structures, B-scan ultrasonography can be performed to confirm.
- If the lesion appears to extend into the lateral canthus or into the conjunctival fornix, MRI imaging may be necessary. It is not uncommon for these deep lesions to be interconnected with orbital fat and connective tissue adjacent to extraocular muscles, necessitating an orbital surgeon for the excision.

SURGICAL PROCEDURE (FIG. 16.1 AND VIDEO 16.1)

- Mark the border of the dermoid with a fine marking pen.
- In the subconjunctival space peripheral to the lesion, inject ~0.1 cc of preservative-free lidocaine 0.75% with epinephrine.
- Using Westcott scissors, perform a conjunctival peritomy along the border of the lesion.

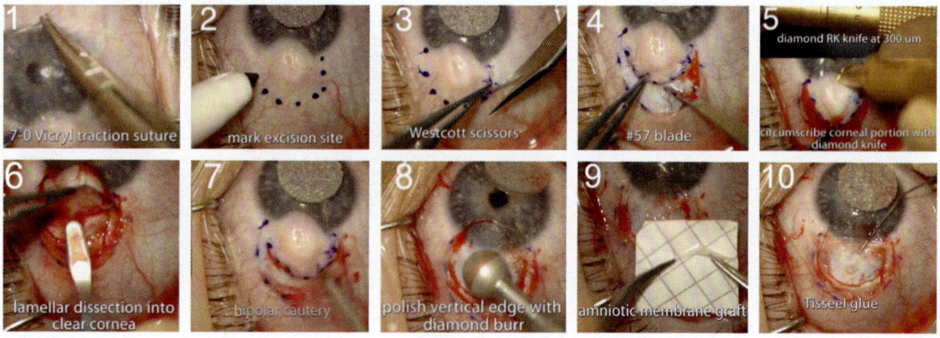

FIGURE 16.1. Step by step limbal dermoid excision. (Modified from https://www.youtube.com/watch?v=TBfPJOFHLEw by Dr. Matt Ward, Riverwoods Eye Center, Provo, UT.)

- Starting peripherally in the area of peritomy, perform a lamellar dissection of the lesion using a crescent blade knife to the edge of the cornea.
- With a diamond RK knife set at 300 μm, circumscribe the corneal portion of the lesion.
- Using a crescent blade, continue the previously dissected scleral portion of the lesion into the clear cornea until the lesion is completely excised.
- Remove any residual dermoid fibers from the corneal stroma using a longitudinal planar dissection with a straight beaver blade knife.
- Achieve hemostasis by judicious use of bipolar cautery.
- In order to achieve a smooth corneal surface bed, use a fine diamond burr to remove ~20% of corneal stromal tissue in the area of the limbal dermoid.
- Using calipers, measure the size of the corneal defect as well as the total defect including bare sclera.
- Trim amniotic membrane to the size of the measured corneal defect (see Chapter 20).
- With the cut amniotic membrane oriented stromal side down, place the amniotic membrane in place thereby filling the corneal defect.
- Affix the amniotic membrane to the corneal defect by applying Fibrin glue (eg, Tisseel, Baxter Inc., Deerfield, IL) under the membrane.
- Cut an additional amniotic membrane the size of the total defect.
- With the amniotic membrane stromal side down, affix the newly cut membrane over the previous placed membrane as well as the bare sclera with Fibrin glue.
- If remaining corneal or epithelial defect is present, the above procedure can be repeated with amniotic membrane until no bare sclera or corneal epithelial defect remains.
- Inject ~0.3 cc of a preservative-free mixture of bupivacaine, cefazolin and dexamethasone as well as 0.1 cc of 40 mg/cc triamcinolone (kenalog) into the subconjunctival space of the inferior fornix.
- Instill a steroid/antibiotic ointment in the operative eye and pressure patch overnight.

If the lesion extends into deeper structures of the cornea or sclera, complete removal should not be attempted as the risk of perforation increases significantly.

Due to the characteristic clinical appearance of limbal dermoids, biopsy is rarely necessary. Nevertheless, all excised tissue should be submitted for pathologic examination after routine excision.

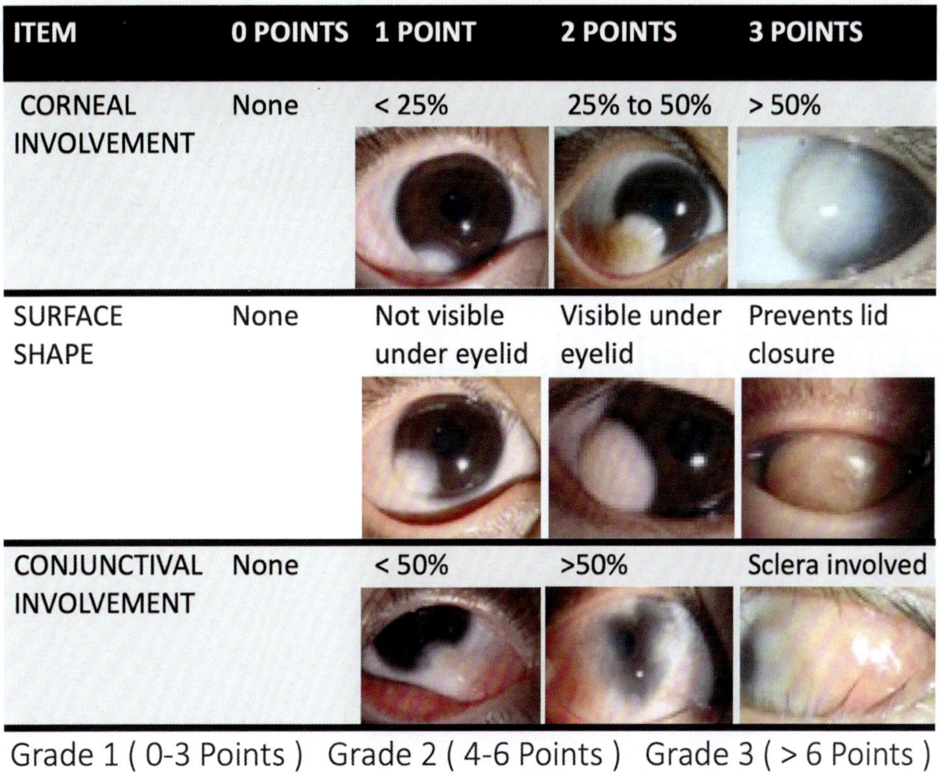

FIGURE 16.2. Limbal dermoid grading scheme and associated visual acuity. (Modified from Zhong J, Deng Y, Zhang P, et al. New grading system for limbal dermoid: a retrospective analysis of 261 cases over a 10-year period. *Cornea*. 2018;37:66-71. doi: 10.1097/ICO.0000000000001429.)

POSTOPERATIVE CONSIDERATIONS

Postoperative visual acuity is quite variable in the case of limbal dermoid excision. A new grading scheme from Zhong et al.[1] is helpful in providing a guideline to patients and their families based on the degree of corneal involvement, surface shape, and conjunctival involvement (Fig. 16.2). For grade 1, average best corrected visual acuity (BCVA) is 20/50, for grade 2 average BCVA is 20/80, and for grade 3 average BCVA is 20/200.

Reference

1. Zhong J, Deng Y, Zhang P, et al. New grading system for limbal dermoid: a retrospective analysis of 261 cases over a 10-year period. *Cornea*. 2018;37:66-71. doi: 10.1097/ICO.0000000000001429.

Suggested Readings

Pirouzian A, Ly H, Holz H, Sudesh RS, Chuck RS. Fibrin-glue assisted multilayered amniotic membrane transplantation in surgical management of pediatric corneal limbal dermoid: a novel approach. *Graefes Arch Clin Exp Ophthalmol*. 2011;249:261-265. doi: 10.1007/s00417-010-1499-2.

Ward M. Limbal Dermoid Removal. https://www.youtube.com/watch?v=TBfPJOFHLEw

CHAPTER 17

EDTA Chelation for Band Keratopathy

Andrew R. Lee, MD

PREOPERATIVE CONSIDERATIONS

- Etiology of band keratopathy[1–4]:
  - Chronic inflammatory ocular disease (uveitis, keratitis, phthisis bulbi).
  - Topical medications containing mercury or phosphates (eg, some steroid preparations, pilocarpine).
  - Hypercalcemia.
  - Silicone oil.
  - Hereditary (primary hereditary band keratopathy, Norrie disease, CHED).
- Indications for ethylenediaminetetraacetic acid (EDTA) chelation for band keratopathy:
  - Visually significant band keratopathy.
  - Pain not controlled with more conservative measures such as lubrication.
- Mechanism of action:
  - EDTA is a metal ion chelator that can help dissolve the calcium present at the level of Bowman membrane in band keratopathy.

If the etiology of the band keratopathy is unknown, serum electrolytes and urinalysis may be performed to assess for metabolic or renal disease. Parathyroid hormone, angiotensin converting enzyme, and assessment for lytic bone lesions can also be considered.[4]

- Surgical planning:
  - Preoperative examination:
    - Assess for any ocular surface disease that may impair epithelial healing postoperatively (dry eye, limbal stem cell deficiency, neurotrophic keratopathy).[2]
    - If performing surgery to improve vision, assess for any other ocular pathology that may limit visual potential (retinal disease, optic neuropathy, glaucoma).
  - Preoperative discussion with patient and parent and/or guardian:
    - Risk of recurrence (reported in literature from 17.8%[3] to 28.1%[1]).
    - Limitations in visual potential.

Alternatives to EDTA chelation include mechanical debridement (superficial keratectomy), peeling with forceps, diamond burr, Nd:YAG laser, lamellar keratoplasty, and excimer laser phototherapeutic keratectomy.[3]

SURGICAL PROCEDURE:[1–5]

- Obtain EDTA (start with 0.5% dilution, can increase up to 3.75% if not dissolving well)—not commercially available, needs to be compounded.
- For children, perform this procedure under general anesthesia given the prolonged time that chelation may require.
- Administer topical anesthetic and/or retrobulbar anesthetic (see Chapter 1).
- Debride the corneal epithelium over desired area of treatment with ethanol in a LASIK well, and/or mechanically.
- Soak a cotton tip applicator or cellulose spear in disodium EDTA (concentration can range from 0.5% to 3.75%) and apply to the areas of band keratopathy for 3 minutes. Attempt to debride mechanically with the applicator or spear; repeat as needed to clear the band keratopathy. A well can be used to confine the chelating solution. Chelation can take 5-45 minutes.
- Gentle scraping can be performed with care to not damage Bowman layer.
- Irrigate with normal saline.

POSTOPERATIVE CONSIDERATIONS

- Apply a bandage contact lens.
  - For cases with concern for poor epithelial healing, consider amniotic membrane transplantation (see Chapter 20).[6]
- Prescribe topical antibiotic and cycloplegic for the immediate perioperative period.
- Possible complications:
  - Nonhealing epithelial defect: mean time to healing reported to be 8 days, possibly longer than a typical corneal epithelial defect due to underlying ocular diseases.[3]
  - Infectious keratitis.
  - Recurrence.
  - Corneal haze.

References

1. Al-Hity A, Ramaesh K, Lockington D. EDTA chelation for symptomatic band keratopathy: results and recurrence. *Eye (Lond)*. 2018;32:26-31.
2. Jhanji V, Rapuano CJ, Vajpayee RB. Corneal calcific band keratopathy. *Curr Opin Ophthalmol*. 2011;22:283-289.
3. Najjar DM, Cohen EJ, Rapuano CJ, et al. EDTA chelation for calcific band keratopathy: results and long-term follow-up. *Am J Ophthalmol*. 2004;137:1056-1064.
4. Roy FH, Fraunfelder FW, Fraunfelder FT. *Corneal and Conjunctival Calcifications. Roy and Fraunfelder's Current Ocular Therapy*. Elsevier Saunders; 2008.
5. Nagra PK, Hammersmith KM. EDTA chelation. In: Dunn JP, Langer PD, eds. *Basic Techniques of Ophthalmic Surgery*. San Francisco, USA: American Academy of Ophthalmology; 2009.
6. Anderson DF, Prabhasawat P, Alfonso E, et al. Amniotic membrane transplantation after the primary surgical management of band keratopathy. *Cornea*. 2001;20:354-361.

CHAPTER 18

Corneal Collagen Cross-Linking

Sonali Talsania, MD

Collagen cross-linking (CXL) was first described in 2003 for the treatment of progressive keratoconus in adults and received FDA approval in 2016 for treatment of patients over 14 years of age with progressive keratoconus. CXL uses reactive oxygen species generated when riboflavin 5′-phosphate is activated by ultraviolet A (UVA) light to create covalent bonds between collagen fibrils in the corneal stroma, thereby cross-linking them to strengthen the cornea.[1] The goal of CXL is to achieve disease stabilization; improvement in visual acuity has been described but is not the primary goal. CXL is performed in patients younger than 14 years of age, but is not covered by most insurance plans as it is not currently FDA approved for this age group.

PREOPERATIVE CONSIDERATIONS

Patients who demonstrate progressive keratoconus are candidates for CXL (see below for adult guidelines from CXL studies; currently, there are no strict guidelines for patients ≤14 years old). The age of the patient should be considered when assessing a patient's fitness for CXL. Children with keratoconus progress more quickly and may be considered for CXL at the time of their diagnosis. Many still opt to monitor closely given the risks of CXL and lack of insurance coverage for the procedure.[2,3] Adults can be monitored for progression every 3 months and considered for CXL if meeting criteria for progression as listed below.

- Preoperative testing:
  - Tomography (Pentacam most commonly used) to diagnose keratoconus and monitor for progression (Fig. 18.1).
  - Corneal pachymetry to monitor for progression and also determine if patient is candidate for CXL; current standards require a corneal thickness of at least 400 μm due to concerns for endothelial damage in thinner corneas.
  - Refraction to monitor for progression.
- Criteria for progression (these may differ from insurance approval guidelines, which should be reviewed for each patient):
  - Steepest keratometry (Kmax) 1 D increase from baseline.
  - Flattest keratometry (Kmin) 1 D increase from baseline.
  - Mean keratometry (Kmean) 0.75 D increase from baseline.
  - Corneal apex power 1 D increase from baseline.
  - Manifest spherical equivalent 0.5 D difference from baseline.
  - Central corneal thickness 2% decrease from baseline.

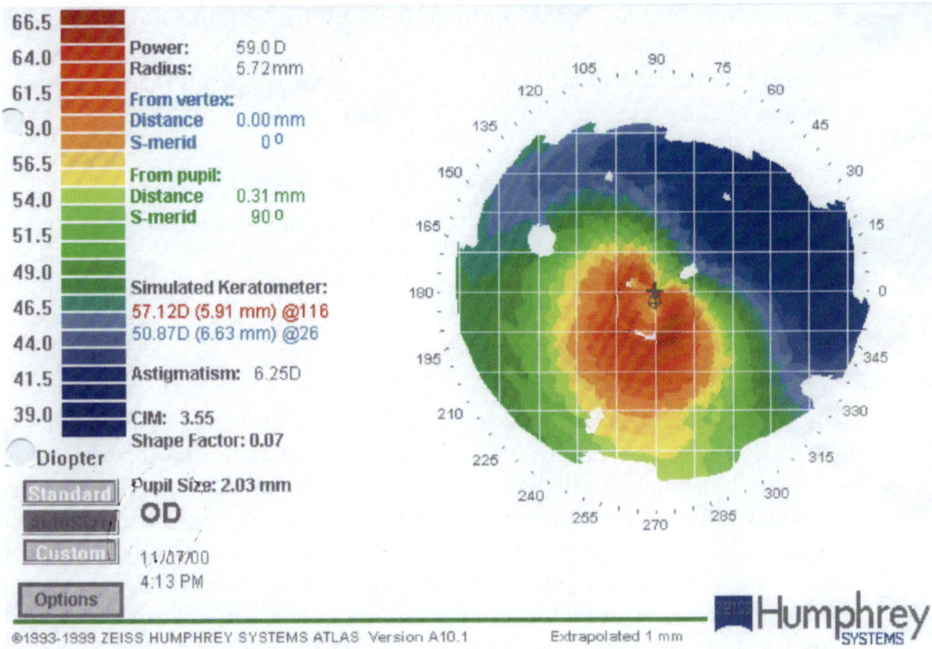

FIGURE 18.1. Representative topography of keratoconus demonstrating inferior corneal steepening. (Image courtesy of David Jones, MD.)

- Preoperative medications:
  - In patients with a history of HSV infection, CXL can cause recurrence.[2]
  - Consider placing these patients on a prophylactic oral acyclovir prior to treatment.
- Anesthesia considerations:
  - CXL can be performed under topical or general anesthesia depending on the patient's age and developmental level (see Chapter 1).

Patients with Down syndrome have an increased risk of developing keratoconus. In addition, eye rubbing is a risk factor for keratoconus and is commonly seen in children with developmental delay. Diagnosis in these high-risk patient populations is often difficult due to issues obtaining a reliable clinical examination and corneal topography.

SURGICAL PROCEDURE

Standard Corneal Cross-Linking: Dresden Protocol

- Apply topical anesthetic drops.
- Remove the corneal epithelium using one of the following techniques:
  - Manual removal with a beaver blade using long strokes to remove epithelium.
  - Alcohol-assisted epithelium removal: Use a 8- to 9-mm corneal marker on surface to create a well. Apply 20% alcohol solution to surface for 20 seconds (this loosens the epithelium). Use a Weck-Cel sponge (Beaver Visitec International, Inc., Waltham, MA) or beaver blade to remove epithelium.
  - Laser-assisted removal using phototherapeutic keratectomy.
- Apply 0.1% riboflavin formulation drops every 1-2 minutes for 30 minutes.
- Evaluate for riboflavin diffusion to anterior chamber by identifying flare under blue light (more important with transepithelial CXL, described below); this step is important to ensure good uptake of riboflavin throughout the corneal stroma prior to irradiation.
- Irradiate cornea for 30 minutes with UVA of 370 nm, 3 mW/cm^2 for total energy 5.4 J/cm^2 using Avedro system (Avedro Inc., Waltham, MA; currently only

FDA-approved machine). Continue to instill 0.1% riboflavin 2 drops every 2 minutes during the irradiation process.

- Consider placing bandage contact lens or occlusive patch for comfort at the termination of the procedure.

Standard Corneal Cross-Linking: Alternative Protocol (A-CXL)

- A-CXL uses higher fluence (up to 30 mW/cm^2) allowing for shorter treatment times.
- Mixed evidence from current studies on the efficacy as compared to standard CXL.
- Concerns regarding effects of higher UVA fluence on the lens, retina, and endothelial cells.[2]

Transepiethelial Corneal Cross-Linking

Transepithelial CXL is currently in clinical trials and pending FDA approval.[2] Transepithelial CXL does not require the removal of the epithelium prior to riboflavin administration; riboflavin is applied directly to the epithelium. There are certain formulations of riboflavin used for transepithelial CXL; the FDA-approved formulation is not considered as effective as formulations that are currently under study. Advantages include easier surgical procedure (most children can tolerate procedure under topical anesthesia since no need for epithelium removal), and reduced risk of infectious keratitis/pain/haze. There are still questions about the efficacy and long-term results, as it can be more difficult to achieve full corneal loading of riboflavin with transepithelial delivery compared to epithelium-off procedures.[2]

POSTOPERATIVE CONSIDERATIONS

- Follow-up on post-operative day 1 and post-operative week 1 to monitor for epithelial healing. Some practitioners follow daily until epithelium has healed in order to titrate steroid.
- Patients who have undergone corneal epithelial removal are prescribed a topical antibiotic during bandage contact lens use and until epithelium has healed, as well as a higher potency steroid taper (prednisolone acetate 1%). Some practitioners add a low-potency topical steroid like fluorometholone for several months subsequently to reduce risk of corneal haze, but this practice varies.[4]
- Plan for Pentacam evaluation 3-6 months post-operatively to establish new baseline.
- Regression has been reported in pediatric patients, and they should be followed to monitor for regression every 4-6 months.
- Treat underlying allergic conjunctivitis/vernal keratoconjunctivitis aggressively to prevent regression.

References

1. Rubinfeld R, Caruso C, Ostacolo C. Corneal cross-linking: the science beyond the myths and misconceptions. *Cornea*. 2019;38(6):780-790.
2. Mohammadpour M, Masoumi A, Mirghorbani M, Shahraki K. Updates on corneal collagen cross-linking: indications, techniques and clinical outcomes. *J Curr Ophthalmol*. 2017;29(4):235-247. doi: 10.1016/j.joco.2017.07.003.
3. Kankariya VP, Kymionis GD, Diakonis VF, Yoo SH. Management of pediatric keratoconus—evolving role of corneal collagen cross-linking: an update. *Indian J Ophthalmol*. 2013;61(8):435-440.
4. Hatch K, Stahl E. MD Roundtable, Part 1: corneal cross-linking for pediatric keratoconus. *Eyenet Magazine*. 2019:29-31.

Suggested Reading

Andreanos K, Hashemi K, Petrelli M, Droutsas K, Georgalas I, Kymionis G. Keratoconus treatment algorithm. *Ophthalmol Ther*. 2017;6(2):245-262.

CHAPTER 19

Corneal Transplantation in Children

Melissa B. Daluvoy, MD

PREOPERATIVE DECISION-MAKING

- When evaluating a pediatric patient for corneal transplantation (CT), one must consider the entire clinical picture, including:
  - Visual status of the fellow eye.
  - Overall health of the child, who will require multiple exposures to anesthesia for surgery and postoperative management.
  - Social support of the child, who will require complex postoperative care and frequent follow-up appointments.
- Once the decision is made to proceed with CT, the surgeon must balance the risk of amblyopia with the risk of transplant rejection and anesthesia risk in deciding when to perform the surgery.
  - Younger patients have robust immune systems making immune rejection much more common than in adults. However, deprivation can lead to dense irreversible amblyopia.
  - Manage expectations for visual prognosis as refractive issues and amblyopia can limit acuity even with successful surgery.
  - Prepare the family for the demanding postoperative care required, and necessity for long-term ophthalmology follow-up and treatment (amblyopia management, glaucoma risk, monitoring for rejection, etc.).

ENDOTHELIAL KERATOPLASTY

Preoperative Considerations

- Endothelial keratoplasty (EK) carries a higher success rate than full-thickness penetrating keratoplasty (PKP) in children because of its faster visual recovery, stronger structural stability, and decreased risk of immunologic rejection.[1]
  - For conditions involving only the endothelium (ie, CHED 1 & 2), performing EK should be strongly considered.

- Descemet's stripping endothelial keratoplasty (DSEK) and Descemet's membrane endothelial keratoplasty (DMEK) can achieve similar results, and the surgeon should choose the procedure with which he or she is most comfortable.

Surgical Procedure

- Use the EK technique you are most comfortable with; most techniques can be adapted to pediatric cases taking into account the smaller anterior chamber, floppy iris, and likely phakic status. Also plan to stay in the operating suite longer under sedation to allow time for the graft to attach as sustained positioning in young children is difficult once they are awake.
- If the patient is phakic, consider pilocarpine preoperatively to protect the lens during graft insertion.
- General anesthesia is recommended for all pediatric patients.
- Position patient and yourself as you feel most comfortable taking into account any synechiae or glaucoma devices; EK can be performed sitting temporally or superiorly.
- Measure the cornea and decide on the size of the graft. Mark the size of the graft on the epithelium.
  Note: The epithelium can be removed for better visualization if needed. Some centers may have access to MIOCT (microscope-integrated OCT) that can be of great assistance in cases with poor visibility.
- Make two paracentesis wounds aimed slightly posteriorly.
- Instill cohesive viscoelastic agent into the anterior chamber (AC).
- Make a triplanar main wound.
- Prior to removing endothelium, it is best to ensure the readiness of your graft. We prefer precut thin DSEK tissue, which we trephine to our desired size (~8 mm) prior to removing endothelium, then store safely in BSS
  Note: Err on the side of smaller graft for your first few cases. This will make it easier to unfold in a small AC.
- Score the endothelium 360 degrees using your predetermined epithelial markings. There are several methods for scoring Descemet membrane (DM); our preferred method is the use of a reverse Sinskey hook (a bent 27G needle can also be used) to apply gentle but consistent pressure to the DM. The correct pressure will produce a light "snail track" behind your instrument but should not encounter any resistance against stroma. Once 360 degrees have been scored, remove DM with a stripping instrument (Gorovoy stripper) pulling centrally and trying to remove endothelium and DM in one sheet.
  Note: Pediatric patients have a stronger adhesion of DM to stroma; if the endothelium and DM does not remove easily (or at all), you can still proceed and place the graft over their existing DM.
- Remove all viscoelastic agent, fill AC with air to ensure smooth surface, and visualize any remaining tags of DM. Again, irrigate the AC to remove the air bubble and any possible remaining viscoelastic agent.
- Insert the graft.
  Note: Our preferred method of insertion is using a single-use inserting device that provides irrigation which helps maintain the AC depth and prevent iris prolapse and lenticular touch. Other methods of insertion include Sheets glide, suture pull through, or Busin glide, etc.
- In pediatric patients, it is advisable to suture the wound closed with 10-0 nylon.
  Note: Iris prolapse can be a challenge in pediatric eyes, and the paracentesis wounds may also need to be sutured to maintain AC depth and air fill.
- Inject air into the AC. Be sure the cannula is behind the graft prior to injecting air. Inject slowly and steadily. Iris tissue is floppy and can be unpredictable in pediatric cases.
- Center the graft and be sure to remove any interface fluid.

- The goal is to center the graft and achieve an IOP above 30 mm Hg at this point (assuming a healthy optic nerve and adjusted for severe glaucoma). Leave a full air fill in the OR for ~30 minutes while the patient is under sedation. Instill cycloplegic drops every 5-10 minutes to dilate the pupil.
- Prior to leaving the OR exchange air for BSS until the air bubble is approximately the size of the graft and well above the dilated pupil when the patient is upright. The IOP is ideally between 15 and 25 mm Hg.
  Note: It is also reasonable to perform an inferior peripheral iridotomy prior to graft insertion, which allows for a larger air bubble and negates the need for intraoperative pupil dilation.

Postoperative Management

- Check the position of the graft, air bubble, and IOP 1-hour after surgery, prior to the patient being discharged; this can be done in the recovery area with a Tono-Pen and handheld slit lamp.
- Depending on the age and cooperation of the patient, an EUA may be necessary post-op day 1 to ensure graft attachment. Additional EUAs may be needed for examination, suture removal, and measuring refractive error.
- Postoperative drop regimen should include:
  - Broad spectrum antibiotics (fluoroquinolone) qid for at least 1 week or until all epithelial defects have closed.
  - Steroid drops Q 1 hour for the first week (alter as necessary for epithelial defects and elevated intraocular pressure) then Q 2 hours for 4 weeks and tapered slowly every 4 weeks, keeping bid for at least 1 year post surgery.

PENETRATING KERATOPLASTY

Preoperative Considerations

- Have a clear understanding of the AC anatomy prior to surgery; this often requires an EUA with hand-held slit lamp examination, ultrasound biomicroscopy, B-scan ultrasonography, and anterior segment OCT. It is important to know if there are any lens-corneal adhesions prior to beginning surgery so you can be prepared to remove the lens if necessary.
- Ideally, other ocular conditions such as glaucoma should be treated prior to transplantation.
- Consider pilocarpine at the time of surgery to constrict the pupil and protect the lens.
- General anesthesia should be used; retrobulbar anesthesia is avoided because it can increase posterior pressure (a peribulbar block can be given later in the case for postoperative pain control).
- Mannitol can be given (0.25-1.0 mg/kg iv) in the OR and the eye can be massaged to help reduce posterior pressure prior to starting the case.
- Future EUAs should be planned before the initial surgery, especially if the patient is difficult to examine in the clinic. At minimum plan for OR visits to remove sutures at ~6-8 weeks and another OR visit to remove the remaining sutures 2-4 weeks after that.

VIDEO

Surgical Procedure (Video 19.1)

- Take time to achieve good positioning and exposure without undue pressure on the globe; when possible use a slight reverse Trendelenburg position.
- Place a Flieringa ring with ~8 interrupted sutures or a running suture using 7-0 Vicryl suture. This is important due to decreased scleral rigidity; take care not to perforate the thin sclera or apply uneven tension which will cause irregular astigmatism during corneal suturing.[2]

- Mark the center of the cornea, measure the diameter, and choose the trephination size.
  Note: Use the trephination blade to place a light mark on the surface of the eye to check the size and centration of the graft prior to trephination.
- Choose the donor size: for children under 2 years old, oversize the graft by 1 mm, and for those over 2 years old oversize by 0.5 mm.
- Prepare the donor tissue–trephine to determine size and keep in sterile solution.
- Return your attention to the recipient and use a suction trephine to penetrate the cornea ~75% but do not enter the AC.
- Use a blade to enter the AC at an area you know is free of iris tissue.
- Fill the AC with a cohesive viscoelastic agent.
- Using the curved scissors, begin to remove the corneal button, taking care to visualize the tips of the scissors to ensure you are not engaging iris.
  Note: If at this time you encounter severe posterior pressure, place a suture in each quadrant as you cut to maintain equal pressure. Now with the host tissue fully cut but held in place with four (or more if needed) sutures; cover with a cohesive viscoelastic agent and place the donor tissue on top. Secure this in place using four interrupted sutures. Once secure, cut the sutures holding the original cornea and pull it out from under the donor tissue (see Fig. 19.1). This technique cannot be used if there is lenticular-corneal adhesions, as in some cases of anterior segment dysgenesis.

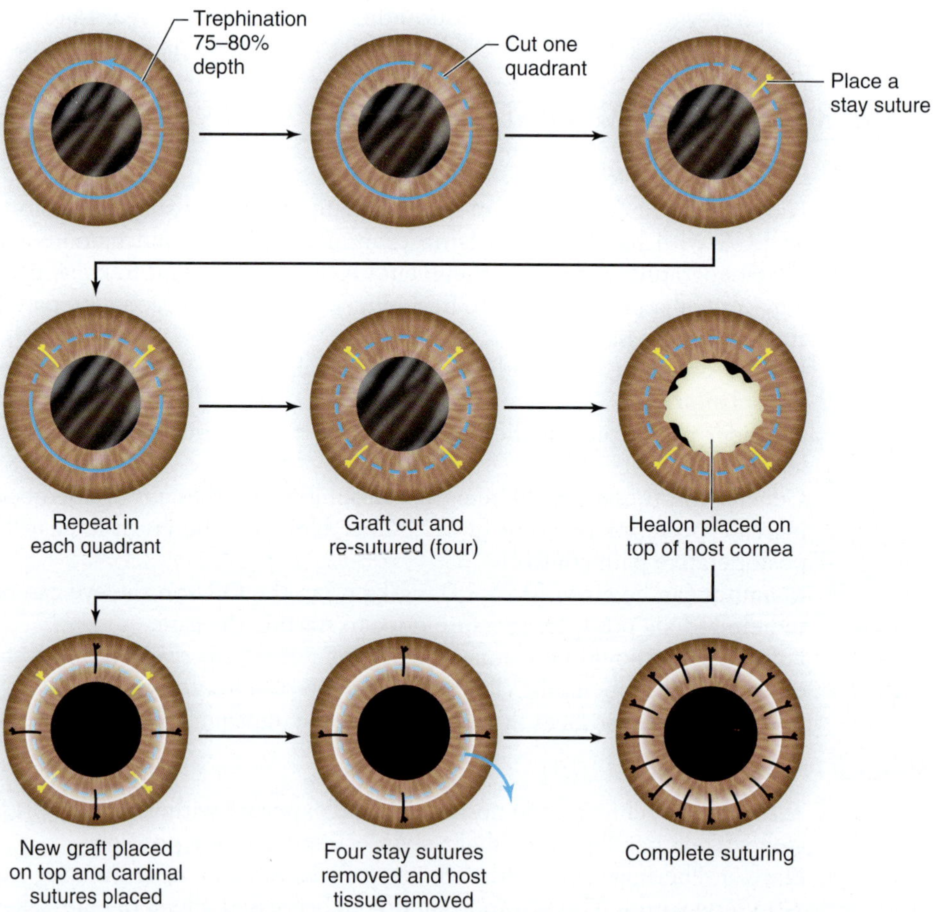

FIGURE 19.1. Technique of securing donor tissue to recipient rim in the setting of posterior pressure: Place four cardinal sutures in corneal button to be removed. Then place the donor tissue on top and secure to recipient rim using four cardinal sutures. Once donor tissue is secure, remove the sutures from the original corneal button and remove.

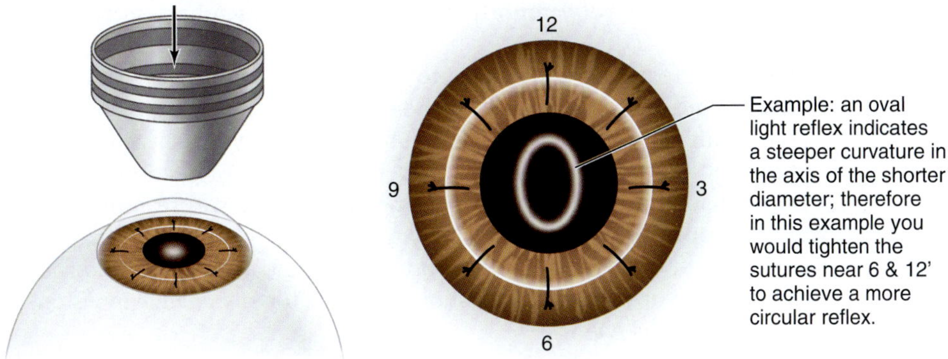

FIGURE 19.2. A Maloney ring can be used to assess astigmatism during a penetrating keratoplasty. By observing the light reflex on the cornea, it is possible to adjust suture tension to reduce the induced astigmatism.

- If there is known lenticular cornea touch or uncontrolled posterior pressure that causes loss of the crystalline lens, an efficient and effective anterior vitrectomy should be performed to clear any prolapsed vitreous from the AC.

Loss of the crystalline lens decreases graft survival and visual outcomes in pediatric patients. Great care should be taken to reduce posterior pressure and preserve the lens if possible.

- If there is concern for shallow AC, inflammation, or synechiae, consider making small peripheral iridectomies at this time.
- Secure the graft using 16 interrupted 10-0 nylon sutures. The cardinal sutures may be placed with locking 3-1-1 style sutures and the rest placed with slip knots so that tension can be adjusted to reduce astigmatism prior to locking the knot

A Maloney ring is an effective tool to assess astigmatism during the case. By observing the light reflex on the cornea it is possible to adjust suture tension to reduce astigmatism (see Fig. 19.2).

- After 6-8 sutures have been placed, remove the viscoelastic agent by irrigating the AC with BSS.
- Tie knots, and bury all sutures.
- Remove the Flieringa ring.
- Subconjunctival antibiotics and steroids should be injected at the conclusion of the case as well as a peribulbar block for post-op pain control.

Postoperative Management

- Multiple EUAs may be necessary to provide adequate visualization of the graft and to ensure epithelialization of the graft (by ~1 week), that all sutures are intact, and that there are no signs of rejection or infection. Additional EUAs will be needed for full evaluations, refraction, and suture removal.
- Postoperative drop regimen should include the following:
  - Broad spectrum antibiotics (fluoroquinolone) qid for at least 1 month and after suture removal procedures.
  - Steroid drops should be used Q 1 hour for the first month (augment as necessary for epithelial defects), then Q 2 hours for 4 weeks, then qid. Frequent dosing of topical steroids for the first 6 months may help prevent rejection. One must balance threat of rejection with risk of infection, epithelial defects, and increased pressure.

- Suture removal is very important due to children's robust scarring. EUA may be necessary.
  - For young patients, the goal is to remove all sutures by ~3 months postoperatively. One may remove half of the sutures at 4-8 weeks postoperatively and the remaining sutures at 8-12 weeks. Any loose or vascularized sutures should be removed as soon as possible to prevent infection or rejection.
- Visual rehabilitation should start immediately after suture removal is completed, and amblyopia should be aggressively treated.
- Parents must be aware that rejection is a lifelong risk and the child should maintain regular follow-ups with low threshold for visits for any change in vision, behavior, or appearance of the eye.

References

1. Trief D, Marquezan MC, Rapuano CJ, et al. Pediatric corneal transplants. *Curr Opin Ophthalmol.* 2017;28:477-483.
2. Zazzo AD, Bonini S, Crugliano S, et al. The challenging management of pediatric corneal transplantation: an overview of surgical and clinical experiences. *Jpn J Ophthalmol.* 2017;61:207-217.

Section V

Other Pediatric Anterior Segment Surgeries

CHAPTER 20

Conjunctival Lesions and Conjunctivoplasty

Derek W. DelMonte, MD

PREOPERATIVE CONSIDERATIONS

- Children rarely have cancerous ocular surface and epibulbar growths; however, lesions can arise from many tissues in and around the ocular surface, and can be characterized as:
  - Epithelial
  - Melanocytic
  - Vascular
  - Fibrous
  - Lymphoid
- The most common lesions in children are conjunctival nevi, which can range in pigmentation from nonpigmented to dark[1,2] (Fig. 20.1).
- Malignancies can include melanoma and lymphoma, although both are rare.[1,2]

In a retrospective case series of pediatric conjunctival tumors, Shields et al. reported that melanoma, compared with nevus, was associated with older age (>10-15 years), larger tumor, hemorrhage, and lack of cyst. The series showed lymphoma, compared with benign reactive lymphoid hyperplasia, was associated with larger size and diffuse involvement.

- Preoperative documentation of conjunctival lesions is critical, and should include:
  - Size.
  - Shape.
  - Vascularity.
  - Growth pattern.
  - Involved tissues.
  - Color.
  - Solid vs cystic.
- Perform a full conjunctival examination under the eyelids and into the fornix either intraoperatively or preoperatively to avoid missing satellite or second lesions.

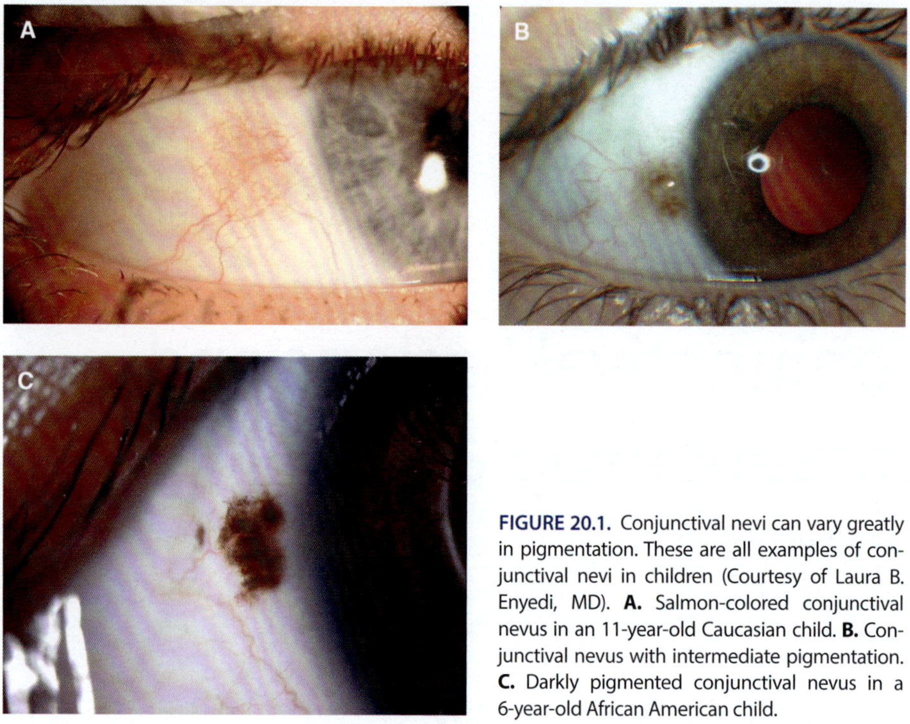

FIGURE 20.1. Conjunctival nevi can vary greatly in pigmentation. These are all examples of conjunctival nevi in children (Courtesy of Laura B. Enyedi, MD). **A.** Salmon-colored conjunctival nevus in an 11-year-old Caucasian child. **B.** Conjunctival nevus with intermediate pigmentation. **C.** Darkly pigmented conjunctival nevus in a 6-year-old African American child.

Slit lamp photographs are most helpful and aid in following suspicious lesions and directing postoperative care.

SURGICAL PROCEDURE: INCISIONAL BIOPSY

- Incisional biopsies are performed to diagnose conjunctival lesions or to determine response to topical treatment.

Incisional biopsy should be avoided when concerned about solid malignant tumors—an excisional biopsy with a no-touch technique is preferred in these cases.

  - In children, the procedure is generally done in an operating room under general anesthesia.
  - In cooperative teenagers or adults, this can be performed in a minor procedure room with topical anesthesia alone.
- A lid speculum is placed.
- Specimens are obtained with tiny non-toothed forceps and scissors, avoiding crushing of the tissue.
- Multiple specimens can be taken from different parts of the lesion if necessary.
- Sutures to close conjunctiva are not required unless the biopsy is large (>5 × 5 mm); then, dissolvable sutures (8-0 Vicryl) are preferred.
- Antibiotic ointment or drops are administered.
- An eye patch can be placed, which can be removed in 2-3 hours.

If concern for lymphoma, fresh tissue should be placed in saline-soaked gauze and sent for flow cytometry and gene rearrangement studies in addition to formalin-fixed tissue.

SURGICAL PROCEDURE: EXCISIONAL BIOPSY (VIDEO 20.1)

Although rare, malignant conjunctival lesions can arise in the pediatric population. If there is a high suspicion for malignancy, an excisional biopsy is preferred over incisional biopsy to avoid tumor spread.

- General anesthesia or monitored anesthesia with a peri/retrobulbar block is administered.
- The extent of the tumor should be outlined in ink prior to manipulation of the tissue.
- Greater than 3-mm margins around the lesion are preferred, although 1-2 mm is acceptable when unable to get more due to anatomy. Wide margins are not necessary if the lesion is not suspicious for malignancy and is being removed for comfort and/or cosmesis.
- Subconjunctival lidocaine with or without epinephrine can help elevate and create a cleavage plane between the lesion and the underlying tissue.
- Care should be taken to avoid manipulation of the lesion itself, instead touching only the unaffected margins (a "no-touch" technique).
- If there is an associated corneal component, it can be removed with absolute alcohol (epithelial) or en bloc removal with a spatulated blade (stromal).
- For scleral involvement, a spatulated blade is used to find a lamellar plane below the depth of the lesion and carried under the entirety of the lesion.
- It is helpful to place the specimen on paper with orientation markings to aid in pathology margin determination. Alternatively, different length or colored sutures may be passed through the cardinal meridians of the tissue (eg, a long nylon suture in the superior boarder, short Vicryl suture at the limbal margin, etc.).
- Double freeze-thaw cryotherapy should be applied at the conjunctival margins and scleral base. This is not necessary for lesions that are not suspicious for malignancy.
- The surgical site can be closed primarily with 8-0 Vicryl if small or may be reconstructed with amniotic membrane (see below for details).
- Subconjunctival injections of an antibiotic and steroid (eg, cefazolin and dexamethasone) can be applied opposite the surgical site or a combination antibiotic/steroid ointment can be applied.
- The eye is patched and shielded overnight and checked the next day.
- Oral acetaminophen can be used for pain control.

SURGICAL PROCEDURE: TRAUMATIC CONJUNCTIVAL LACERATION REPAIR

Ocular trauma can include isolated conjunctival abrasions or lacerations, or more serious underlying injury.

- Any traumatic ocular injury must be fully evaluated, under sedation if necessary, to rule out deeper ocular trauma such as scleral perforation (see Chapters 22 and 25).
- Gentle probing with a cotton-tip applicator or cellulose spear can help determine the extent of the injury (if you suspect scleral involvement, do this in the operating room).
- Small isolated conjunctival lacerations can often be observed with topical antibiotics.
- Larger lacerations may require suture closure with 8-0 Vicryl in the operating room under general anesthesia.
- If there is a loss of significant tissue in the trauma, reconstruction with amniotic membrane grafts can help reduce healing time and prevent significant scarring (see below).

SURGICAL PROCEDURE: OCULAR SURFACE REPAIR WITH AMNIOTIC MEMBRANE (VIDEOS 16.1 AND 20.1)

- Small conjunctival defects will heal well without intervention; however, larger defects left untreated may result in conjunctival scarring, infection, and/or symblepharon. In these cases reconstruction with amniotic membrane may be indicated.
- General anesthesia or monitored anesthesia with a peri/retrobulbar block is administered.
- The defect should be measured in all dimensions.
- Amniotic membrane should be trimmed to 1-2 mm larger than the measured defect.
- Large bleeding vessels may be gently cauterized to avoid hematomas under the graft; however, some vascularity should be left to aid in healing.
- The graft is tucked under the conjunctival margins and fastened into place with fibrin tissue glue or 8-0 Vicryl sutures.
- Excess glue is trimmed from margins.

Tips for orienting amniotic membrane: Fresh frozen tissue is attached to a cardboard backing. The side that was attached to the cardboard should be oriented against the sclera. This can be confirmed by gently touching the surface with a cellulose spear, and if it appears sticky, this should be placed down. Freeze dried tissue will often have markings to help with orientation.

References

1. Shields CL, Shields JA. Conjunctival tumors in children. *Curr Opin Ophthalmol.* 2007;18(5):351-360.
2. Shields CL, Sioufi K, Alset AE, et al. Clinical features differentiating benign from malignant conjunctival tumors in children. *JAMA Ophthalmol.* 2017;135(3):215-224.

CHAPTER 21

Iridectomy and Sphincterotomy

Sharon F. Freedman, MD • Maria Gomez-Caraballo, BA

SURGICAL IRIDECTOMY AND SPHINCTEROTOMY

Surgical procedures on the iris in children fall into three main categories:

- Peripheral iridectomy to treat or prevent pupillary block glaucoma.
- Optical iridectomy to make a visual axis, usually in settings where a central opacity of the cornea prevents the central visual axis from being adequate and where one wishes to avoid penetrating keratoplasty (See Chapter 19).
- Manipulations of the iris in the course of other surgery. Discussion of the topic here is limited to sphincterotomy.

PERIPHERAL IRIDECTOMY

One or more openings are made in the peripheral iris, specifically avoiding involvement of the pupillary sphincter, to treat or to prevent angle-closure glaucoma from pupillary block mechanism. Note that, in some instances, a laser iridotomy may be effective in older and cooperative children, but caution is recommended in using laser iridotomy in cases where cooperation is in question or likelihood of reclosure is high (eg, uveitis, see others below).

- Indications:
  - Acute closed-angle glaucoma with or without elevated IOP: Acute closed-angle glaucoma usually occurs secondary to iris bombe with uveitis, after surgery (aphakic or occasionally pseudophakic eye after childhood cataract removal), in eyes with a history of severe retinopathy of prematurity, and less often with spherophakia or lens subluxation.
  - Narrow closeable angles (eyes in which there is a higher risk for acute close-angle glaucoma and pupillary block): Narrow closeable angles can present in patients noted above before the angle is completely closed and in addition may be noted in eyes with microphthalmia, spherophakia, and selected other developmental abnormalities.

    - Prophylactically in high-risk situations for angle-closure despite a deep anterior chamber angle and open angle. Examples include high-risk cataract cases (ie, eyes with a history of retinopathy of prematurity), eyes with silicone oil after retinal detachment surgery (iridectomy must be placed inferiorly), rarely in cases of iris cyst, and other nonmalignant space-occupying lesions of the anterior segment.
- Comparing laser iridotomy and peripheral iridectomy:
    - Consider laser iridotomy in select cases. This technique can be difficult in the pediatric population as some children are not able to remain still during the laser iridotomy procedure.
    - There are some cases when a more definitive treatment, such a peripheral iridectomy, is required as laser iridotomy may prove inadequate to remove significant synechiae[1] or to definitively treat recurrent pupillary block.[2]
- Nonsurgical management (temporizing and preoperative preparations):
    - The goals of preoperative medications are to decrease intraocular pressure pending more definitive iridectomy, to decrease inflammation in cases of uveitis or where the angle closure has caused inflammation, and to help clear the view in cases of corneal edema to improve technical ease of surgery. Useful medications include aqueous suppressants such as timolol and dorzolamide, and apraclonidine 0.5% for pressure reduction (with oral acetazolamide in severe cases), prednisolone acetate 1% topically (and systemic steroid in cases of severe inflammation or known uveitis); sodium chloride 5% topically in cases of corneal edema (see Chapter 9).
    - Pilocarpine can be used in cases where the pupil is able to react, but caution is recommended in cases where there may be a component of "posterior pushing" from a relatively anteriorly positioned crystalline lens or uveitis, which may be made worse with pilocarpine.
- Procedure:
    - Equipment needed:
        - Number 64 microsurgical blade with a handle.
        - A 15-degree Super Sharp blade or equivalent for paracentesis.
        - Forceps.
        - Colibri or very fine toothed forceps.
        - Utrata forceps in special cases.
        - Westcott (or micro Westcott) scissors.
        - Iris or Vannas scissors.
    - Surgical steps:
        - Choose a limbal site: Superotemporal and superonasal sites are usually preferred in order to conceal the iridectomy underneath the superior lid; although in adult cases with laser iridotomy, the current recommendation is in the horizontal meridian to reduce diplopia risk.
        - Placement of a traction suture under the superior rectus is recommended, but not mandatory.
        - Make a small conjunctival peritomy (~2-2.5 mm) at the intended site of iridectomy.
        - Make a groove with a Super Sharp blade (~2 mm long) in the anterior surgical limbus and very vertically oriented (to at least ~ 2/3-3/4 depth).
        - Consider performing another paracentesis at another convenient location (eg, temporal) with a Super Sharp blade and inserting a small amount of viscoelastic if there is a shallow anterior chamber.
        - Enter the anterior chamber at the base of the groove with a Super Sharp blade. If needed, add more viscoelastic to allow safe enlargement of the entry site to the full 2 mm. CAUTION—watch carefully to avoid iris injury.
        - Grasp peripheral iris with Colibri forceps. Use Utrata forceps if friable iris is suspected.

- Carefully lift peripheral iris through the wound; cut flush with iris or Vannas scissors. CAUTION—watch to be sure that the iris sphincter muscle is still inside the eye.
- Ensure that enough iris is in forceps to include iris pigment epithelium (this ensures it is a full-thickness iridectomy).
- Inspect the specimen to ensure that the removed iris contains iris pigment epithelium.

It is helpful to rub the specimen on the surgeon's surgical glove and look for pigment unless the specimen needs to be sent to pathology.

- Reposition the iris if necessary and look for red reflex and confirmation of iridectomy patency. CAUTION—avoid adding too much viscoelastic, which may expel more iris out the limbal opening; use a small amount of Miochol or Miostat if needed to pull iris back in and constrict pupil.
- Irrigate the wound with balanced salt solution if there is some pigment remaining.
- Deepen the anterior chamber through the previously performed paracentesis if necessary, to avoid iris entrapment in the wound.
- Irrigate viscoelastic from the eye through the paracentesis.
- Place a small filtered air bubble if desired.
- Close the primary opening with 10-0 polyglactin (Vicryl) suture (use two interrupted or one figure-of-8-style suture).
- Close the conjunctiva with the same suture.
- Close the side paracentesis if needed (often can hydrate this closed).
- Standard subconjunctival antibiotics and steroid therapy (see Chapter 3).
- Place standard patch and eye shield.
- Additional procedures like lysis of posterior synechiae may be needed in eyes with uveitis or in postcataract eyes.
  - Lysis of posterior synechiae in some cases of iris bombé patients: Sometimes these cases may require anterior vitrectomy in addition to iridectomy (eg, in cases of aphakic, postcataract eyes with synechial pupillary block).
  - In these cases, consider performing the surgery with a 23G vitrectomy device through two standard ports in a closed chamber. The vitrector is used port down to engage and cut the iris making a small peripheral iridotomy.

- Postoperative care:
  - Treat patient with a course of topical antibiotic and steroids (See Chapter 3).
  - Consider addition of glaucoma medications to avoid spikes in IOP.

OPTICAL IRIDECTOMY: SECTOR OR COMPLETE IRIDECTOMY

Surgical removal of portions of the iris sphincter in children with congenital or acquired central corneal defects. This helps create a clear, noncentral visual axis and may improve visual development[3,4] while avoiding penetrating keratoplasty.

- Indications:
  - Visual axis obstruction (seen in children with corneal opacities such as in Peters anomaly, postinfectious scars, among others).
  - Consider only if there is potential for creating a visual axis through the native cornea (Fig. 21.1).
- Advantages:
  - There is often improvement in visual acuity, especially in bilateral cases.[5]

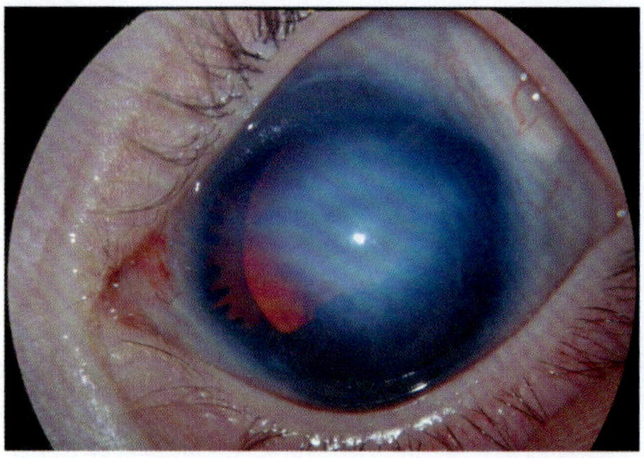

FIGURE 21.1. Child with bilateral Peters anomaly and bilateral glaucoma. This eye had an Ahmed placed superotemporal, and then, once the IOP was controlled, had an optical iridectomy, which helped the child to see. The other eye had a penetrating keratoplasty and eventually was lost to multiple complications, and this became the better seeing eye.

- As an alternative to pediatric penetrating keratoplasty without incurring the risks of graft failure, rejection, or suture-related complications (See Chapter 19).[5] Optical iridectomy also allows for faster recovery and initiation of amblyopia treatment immediately postoperatively.[6]
- Does not require prolonged use of dilating drops to ensure clear visual axis (which may add the complication of cycloplegia in phakic eyes with large corneal opacity).

- Nonsurgical management and preoperative considerations:
  - Consider pharmacological pupillary dilation as the first option if the opacity is restricted to the central cornea and the native pupil is not adherent and easily dilated to well outside the opacity.
  - Agents used include phenylephrine, which is given multiple times per day and may have systemic side effects such as increased blood pressure[5]; cycloplegic agents, such as cyclopentolate and atropine, are stronger but result in blurred vision in phakic patients.

Phakic patients maintained on cycloplegics long-term need bifocal glasses for optimal visual results.

  - Administer maximal dilation (eg, cyclopentolate and phenylephrine) prior to surgery to make it easier to remove the more central iris, which includes the pupil sphincter.

VIDEO

- Procedure (Video 21.1):
  - Equipment needed:
    - Number 64 microsurgical blade with a handle.
    - A 15-degree Super Sharp blade or equivalent for paracentesis.
    - Forceps.
    - Colibri or very fine toothed forceps.
    - Utrata forceps.
    - Angled Kelman-McPherson forceps.
    - Westcott (or micro Westcott) scissors.
    - Iris or Vannas scissors.
  - Surgical steps:
    - Choose a limbal site: Superotemporal or superonasal sites are usually preferred.
    - Place 7-0 Vicryl traction suture at the limbus above and below the intended incision site.
    - Make small conjunctival peritomy (~2-2.5 mm) at intended site of iridectomy.
    - Make groove with a Super Sharp blade (~2 mm long) in the anterior surgical limbus and very vertically oriented (to at least ~2/3-3/4 depth).
    - Consider performing another paracentesis at another convenient location (eg, temporal) with a Super Sharp blade and inserting a small amount of viscoelastic if there is a shallow anterior chamber.

- Enter the anterior chamber at the base of the groove with a Super Sharp blade. May place more viscoelastic to allow safe enlargement of the entry into a shallow anterior chamber. CAUTION—watch carefully to avoid iris injury.
- Grasp iris as far centrally as possible with nontoothed Utrata or angled Kelman-McPherson forceps.
- Carefully remove additional iris through the surgical opening using a hand-over-hand technique with great care not to allow the iris to tear and retract back into the anterior chamber before an adequate portion of the iris, and especially the pupillary sphincter, has been removed.

It is much easier to keep removing the iris hand over hand than it is to try to reach back into the eye once the iris has shredded so move gently, firmly, and deliberately and contact as much iris as possible with the nontoothed grasping forceps.

- Once enough iris has been removed, cut flush to get "extra" iris with the iris or Vannas scissors. The first cut will be the best one.
- At times, the iris may "keep coming," and in selected cases, especially anterior segment dysgenesis, the iris root may be intentionally disinserted, resulting in a total iridectomy, which maximizes the visual axis through all available clear cornea.
- Inspect the specimen to ensure that the removed iris contains iris epithelium.
- Reposition the iris if necessary; proceed with caution to prevent lens damage in phakic patients.
- Look for red reflex and confirmation of iridectomy patency.
- Irrigate the wound with balanced salt solution if there is some pigment remaining.
- Deepen the anterior chamber through the previously performed paracentesis if necessary, to avoid iris entrapment in the wound.
- Irrigate viscoelastic from the eye through the paracentesis.
- Place small filtered air bubble if desired.
- Close the primary opening with 10-0 polyglactin (Vicryl) suture (use two interrupted or one figure-of-8-style suture).
- Close the conjunctiva with the same suture.
- Close the side paracentesis if needed (often can hydrate this closed).
- Standard subconjunctival antibiotics and steroid therapy (See chapter 3).
- Place standard patch and eye shield.

- Postoperative care:
  - Treat patient with a course of topical antibiotic and steroids (See chapter 3).
  - Consider addition of glaucoma medications to avoid spikes in IOP.

SPHINCTEROTOMY

There are times that the pupil does not enlarge adequately to allow performance of concurrent necessary cataract removal. Less often, there may be a form of anterior segment dysgenesis, in which the pupil is totally occluded and does not provide an adequate visual axis. In these cases, manipulation of the iris is needed (eg, iris stretching, iris hooks, etc.), which is not covered in the following more general discussion of sphincterotomy.

- Indications include surgical pupillary enlargement when cataract surgery is also being performed and iris stretching with hooks is not practical or ill advised.
  - Most common cases include microcornea and congenital cataract with abnormal or poorly dilating pupil, uveitis, or trauma in which tight synechiae to lens or damage/scarring/membranes make the pupil unable to dilate even after attachments to the lens are broken (hooks will often cause tearing and excess technical

difficulty in these cases, resulting in a pupil that does not become round again after their release).

- Consider after truly heroic attempts to dilate in cases where there are not synechiae or scars on the iris.
  - Pharmacologic dilation techniques include placing a small cotton pledget of phenylephrine/cyclopentolate into the fornix prior to surgery. Alert the anesthesia staff as this may result in elevations in blood pressure and/or bradycardia requiring removal of the pledget (see Chapter 3).
- VIDEO Procedure (Fig. 21.2) (Video 21.2):
  - Equipment needed:
    - Same as for infant cataract surgery (see Chapter 5).
    - Cyclodialysis spatula and Sinskey hook.
    - 23G curved (retina) scissors.
    - 23G vitrector, which will be used for the cataract removal to follow.
    - Viscoelastic and 23G infusion (anterior chamber maintainer, same as for the cataract surgery to follow).
- Surgical steps:
  - Begin as for infant/pediatric cataract surgery (traction suture, two entries into anterior chamber, either limbal or clear cornea).
  - May begin with infusion in place, but often better to fill anterior chamber with viscoelastic (see Chapter 3) to maintain chamber and protect corneal endothelium; once it is clear, sphincterotomy will be needed.
  - Use careful blunt dissection with cyclodialysis spatula or Sinskey hook to separate iris adhesions from lens capsule, if present.

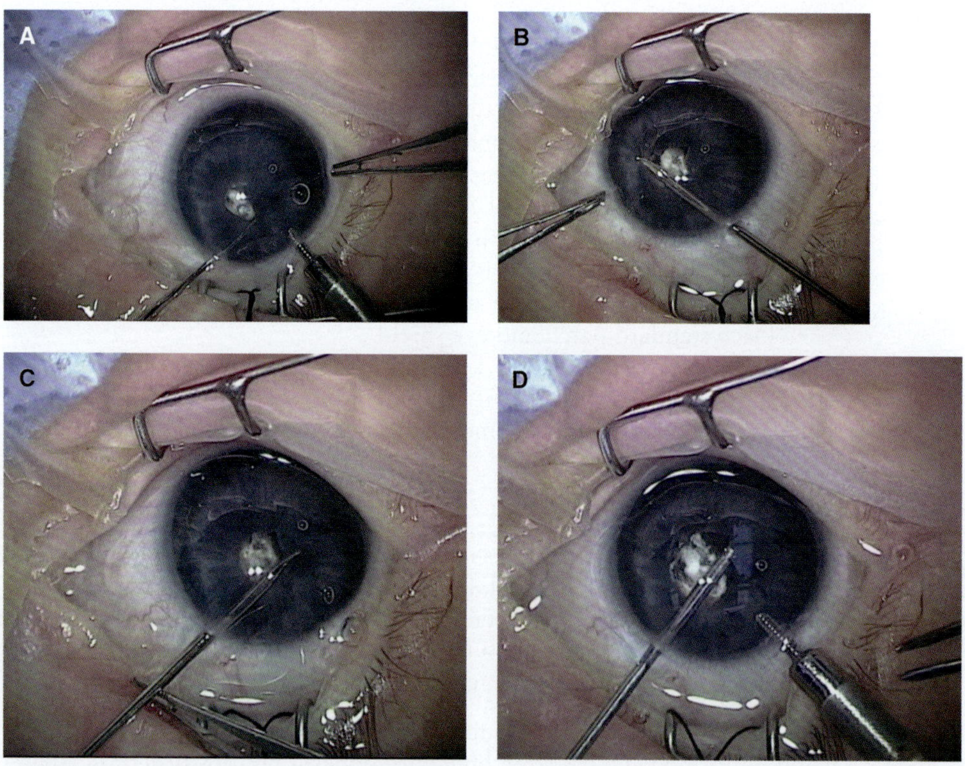

FIGURE 21.2. 2-month old otherwise healthy infant born with microcornea, poorly dilating pupils, and calcified cataracts in both eyes. When the pupil did not dilate, it was first stretched to break any iridolenticular adhesions **(A)**, then sphincterotomies were created with a 23G curved scissor **(B and C)**. When the resultant pupil remains inadequate for cataract removal, the 23G vitrector was used to additionally round and enlarge the now-surgically-enlarged pupil **(D)**.

- Once it has been confirmed that the pupil size is inadequate for safe cataract removal (the pupil should typically be at least as large as the anterior capsulotomy—eg, ~5 mm minimum diameter), remove infusion and fill anterior chamber with viscoelastic (see also above).
- Use 23G curved scissors from one wound to make at least three separate incisions in the pupillary sphincter to full depth of the scissors (about 1.5 mm), separated equally by about 2 clock hours.
- Switch the scissor to the other wound to allow at least three more incisions to be made from the opposite side.
- Replace the infusion line, and when the Healon has escaped, place the vitrector and "nibble" the "ragged" iris between the scissor incisions, rounding the pupil gradually and enlarging it.

Surprisingly, there is usually not much bleeding with these maneuvers. If iris bleeding does occur, use the blunt tip cautery on a very low setting (eg, 8-10 rather than the customary setting of 20 on the Constellation machine).

- Proceed with the cataract surgery as usual.
- Standard subconjunctival antibiotics and steroid therapy (see Chapter 3).
- Place standard patch and eye shield.

- Postoperative care:
  - Treat patient with a course of topical antibiotic and steroids (see Chapter 3).
  - Consider addition of glaucoma medications to avoid spikes in IOP.
  - Strongly consider oral steroid (see Chapter 3) in cases where the iris has required sphincterotomy, especially in cases where the cataract and abnormal pupil are the result of anterior uveitis (see Chapter 7).

References

1. Romano JH, Hitchings RA, Pooinasawmy D. Role of Nd:YAG peripheral iridectomy in the management of ocular hypertension with a narrow angle. *Ophthalmic Surg.* 1988;19(11):814-816.
2. Wand M, Clark JA, Hill DA. Nd: YAG laser iridectomies: 100 consecutive cases. *Ophthalmic Surg.* 1988;19(6):399-402.
3. Zaidman GW, Rabinowitz Y, Forstot SL. Optical iridectomy for corneal opacities in Peter's anomaly. *J Cataract Refract Surg.* 1998;24(5):719-722.
4. Jünemann A, Gusek GC, Naumann G. Optical sector iridectomy: an alternative to perforating keratoplasty in Peters' anomaly. *Klin Monbl Augenheilkd.* 1996;209(2-3):117-124.
5. Spierer O, et al. Outcome of optical iridectomy in Peters anomaly. *Graefes Arch Clin Exp Ophthalmol.* 2018;256(9):1679-1683.
6. Sundaresh K, Jethani J, Vijayalakshmi P. Optical iridectomy in children with corneal opacities. *J AAPOS.* 2008;12(2):163-165.

Section VI

Pediatric Trauma

CHAPTER 22

Pediatric Trauma: Preoperative Considerations

Erin O. Schotthoefer, MD

OCULAR TRAUMA

- Pediatric ocular trauma occurs at a rate of 3.3-5.7 million children annually.[1]
- Boys are more likely to injure their eyes than girls, and different mechanisms of injury occur more commonly in different age groups.[1]
- High-risk activities include those that involve projectiles such as air-powered guns or sharp projectiles such as darts. Injuries can also occur at a higher rate during sporting events, related to bungee cord use or secondary to airbag deployment.[1] However, the majority of pediatric open globe injuries occur at home.[2]
- Determine the mechanism of injury by history, if possible, to guide examination and treatment considerations. Pediatric trauma is unique because children may not be reliable historians and the injury may be unwitnessed.

In addition to the accidental mechanisms of injury listed above, children are also at risk for nonaccidental trauma inflicted by another person.

EXAMINATION

- Check recognition visual acuity if possible or fixation behavior in preverbal children.
- Defer measurement of intraocular pressure until globe rupture has been ruled out.
- Evaluate with slit lamp (portable slit lamp, if needed) for conjunctival and corneal injury, traumatic iritis, hyphema, and traumatic cataract.
  - Hemorrhagic chemosis can be a sign of a full-thickness scleral injury.
  - A flat anterior chamber or a peaked pupil is concerning for a corneal or scleral laceration.
- Perform Seidel testing on suspected penetrating injuries if possible.
- Consider CT scan if intraocular foreign body is suspected.
- B scan should be performed with caution if there is concern for open globe injury.

- Concussive injuries: evaluate for orbital fractures. Evaluate sensory testing of the fifth cranial nerve. Perform full motility testing to evaluate for entrapment. Be suspicious if there is vomiting or vasovagal response with eye movements in children. Even in the absence of globe trauma or significant ecchymosis, pediatric patients' orbital bones are more flexible and a small fracture of the orbital floor can entrap the inferior rectus or surrounding tissues (the "white-eyed blow out fracture").[3]
- Non-accidental Trauma: Suspect in cases wherein:
  - The child is under the age of 1 year
  - Examination findings do not match history.
  - There is evidence of multiple ocular injuries having occurred over different periods of time.
  - There is evidence of injury of multiple organ systems without an appropriate history.
  - Report any suspicion of abuse to the proper state authorities for investigation. It is often helpful to communicate with the patient's primary care physician during this process.

Preoperative preparation: If the child is determined to have a ruptured globe, the patient should be taken to the OR for repair as soon as possible.

- Make patient NPO (nothing by mouth).
- Shield the eye.
- Consider IV antiemetics if the patient is nauseated to prevent emesis that can exacerbate a rupture.
- A single dose of IV antibiotics perioperatively followed by an oral course of antibiotics can be considered.[5]
  - Levofloxacin has broad organism coverage (except for *Pseudomonas aeruginosa*) and good vitreous penetration.[5] (The American Academy of Pediatrics warns of possible arthrotoxicity in pediatric patients based on studies of animals and complications in adults. Physicians may weigh the risks and benefits for use in pediatric patients and discuss this with the patient and their parents).[4] Alternatively, cefazolin, a first-generation cephalosporin, can be used as a first-line antibiotic.
- If IOFB is suspected, the patient should be admitted for a course of intravenous vancomycin and ceftazidime.[2]
- Antifungal medication is not generally recommended unless patient has evidence of fungal infection on culture.[5]
- Determine if tetanus shot is up-to-date and give if it is not.
- Obtain informed consent from the patient's guardian/caretaker. Discuss the risks, benefits, and alternatives to ruptured globe repair. Provide prognostic information and educate on the likely need for long-term follow-up after surgical repair.

The rate of successful treatment after pediatric open globe injury, defined as having a final VA of 20/40 or better, is between 54% and 56.5% in industrialized countries.[2]

ORBITAL FRACTURES

Pediatric orbital fractures with entrapment should be taken to the operating room as soon as possible for repair due to the risk of scarring and resulting strabismus and diplopia.

The most common muscles affected by entrapment are the inferior rectus and inferior oblique.

References

1. Abbot J, Shah P. The epidemiology and etiology of pediatric ocular trauma. *Surv Ophthal.* 2013;58(5):476-485.
2. Li X, Zarbin MA, Bhagat N. Pediatric open globe injury: a review of the literature. *J Emerg Trauma Shock.* 2015;8(4):216-223.
3. Nerad JA, Carter KD, Alford M. *Oculoplastic and Reconstructive Surgery*. St. Louis, MO: Mosby Elsevier; 2008. Print.
4. Jackson MA, Schutze GE, AAP Committee on Infections Diseases. The use of systemic and topical Fluoroquinolones. *Pediatrics*. 2016;138(5):e20162706
5. Ahmed Y, Schimel AM, Pathengay A, Colyer MH, Flynn HW. Endophthalmitis following open-globe injuries. *Eye*. 2012;26(2):212-217.

CHAPTER 23

Lid and Canalicular Laceration Repairs

R. Kevin Winkle, MD

PREOPERATIVE CONSIDERATIONS

- Perform a complete exam to rule out open globe.
  - Repair globe if necessary, before repairing eyelid lacerations.
- Assess tetanus status and order vaccination if indicated.
- Always explore for canalicular lacerations when lid lacerations are present as trauma to the lid is often associated with canalicular avulsion injuries as well. This is particularly true in dog bite injuries and blunt lid trauma.
  - Lacerations medial to the punctum should be explored for canalicular injury.
  - Pass a probe through the upper or lower punctum and along the canaliculus.
  - If the probe is visible in the laceration, the canaliculus has been lacerated and requires repair (Fig. 23.1).
- Repair canalicular and lid margin lacerations first, and then close additional lid wounds.

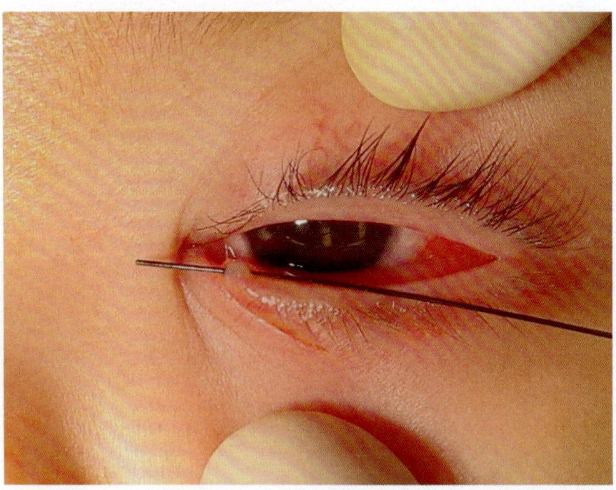

FIGURE 23.1. A probe placed through the punctum is visible in the eyelid laceration, indicating a laceration of the canaliculus.

CANALICULAR LACERATIONS

- Equipment needed:
  - Canalicular stent of choice. Ritleng canalicular stents are excellent in trauma involving the lacrimal drainage system. Bicanalicular and monocanalicular stents are available.
  - High magnification loupes and an operating microscope.
- Procedure:
  - Depending upon where the laceration is located, the nylon suture attached to the Ritleng stent may be passed through the punctum first without the introducer, or an introducer may be used. If there is a large separation between the cut ends of the canaliculus, then pass the suture and stent through the puncta into the lateral portion of the wound first, and then use the introducer to pass the stent through the proximal canaliculus into the nose (Fig. 23.2). This prevents inadvertent tearing of the often fragile tissue of the distal canaliculus when the introducer is rotated to pass downward into the nose.
  - Identify the cut end of the canaliculus.
    - The canaliculus typically has a whitish coloration compared to the background red and pink of the surrounding tissue, and inspecting for an apparent lumen is beneficial (Fig. 23.3). This color difference can help to identify the proximal canaliculus. Often the proximal canaliculus retracts, especially when the medial canthal tendon is ruptured.
    - An operating microscope and the use of cotton-tipped applicators or a low-powered suction catheter help to facilitate the view.
    - 0.3 and 0.5 Castroviejo forceps can be used to gently pull the tissue into view when the canaliculus has retracted, and often this is when the lumen can be seen in conjunction with its characteristic white coloration.
    - If the proximal end is not identified, perform the following steps:
      - Inject air or fluorescein via a 27G cannula into the opposite punctum. Observe for dye or bubbles emanating from the nasal portion of the canaliculus.
    - Use topical phenylephrine to cause construction of the vascular and muscular tissues surrounding the canaliculus.

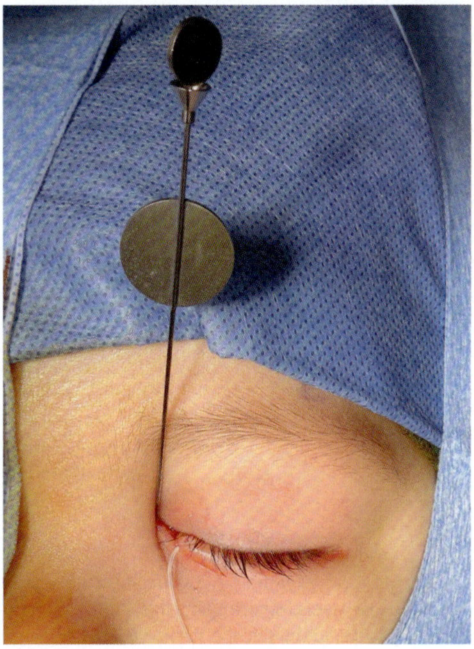

FIGURE 23.2. Placement of stent through the punctum, and localization of the proximal canaliculus with metal introducer.

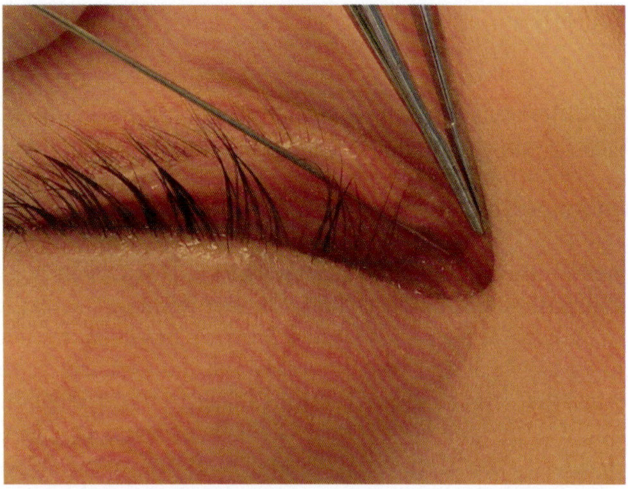

FIGURE 23.3. Visualization of the cut end of the canaliculus. Forceps can be used to pull tissue into view when canaliculus has retracted.

- The metal introducer is then passed through the proximal canaliculus and into the nose followed by passage of the suture into the introducer and removal of the suture and stent from the nose.
- Alternatively, a pigtail probe can be passed through the intact canaliculus and retrieved through the cut canalicular end.
- 8-0 Vicryl is used to reapproximate the canaliculus on two or three sides of the canaliculus.
- If the medial canthal tendon is ruptured (Fig. 23.4), resuspend the anterior and posterior portion of the tendon to the proximal stumps of the tendon or to the periosteum using 5-0 Vicryl sutures on a P-2 needle but do not tie the sutures yet. Pass two to three 8-0 Vicryl sutures on multiple sides of the canaliculus but do not tie them since there is often significant tension present. Tighten the 5-0 Vicryl to bring both sides of the canaliculus together, and then tie the 8-0 Vicryl. Secure the 5-0 Vicryl.
- If using a monocanalicular stent, secure the stent end in the nose with a 4-0 or 5-0 silk suture.
- If using a bicanalicular stent, pass the other end of the stent through the unaffected punctum and out the nose. Tie a knot in the bicanalicular stent, and suture it in the nose with 4-0 or 5-0 silk suture.

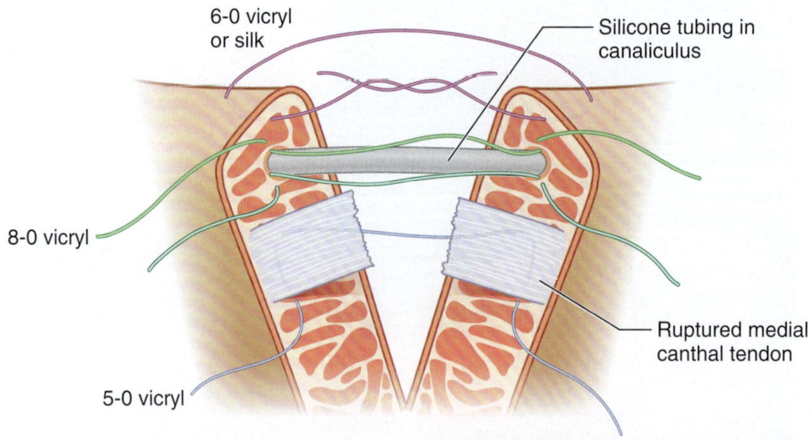

FIGURE 23.4. Repair of canalicular and medial canthal tendon laceration. A 5-0 Vicryl suture is placed to reapproximate the medial canthal tendon and deep orbicularis layers. Before tying this suture, multiple 8-0 Vicryl sutures are placed to repair the cut ends of the canaliculus around the silicone stent. A 6-0 silk or Vicryl suture may be placed in the lid margin, and the skin is closed.

- Use topical antibiotic/steroid combination drops in the eye for 1-2 weeks and antibiotic ointment to the lid wounds for 7-10 days.
- Remove the Ritleng tube in 6 weeks to 3 months. This can usually be done in the office especially when monocanalicular stents are used. It is also possible to remove bicanalicular stents in the office by pulling the knotted portion of the stent through the unaffected canalicular system to prevent trauma to the previously injured area. Stents may also be removed in the operating room.

EYELID LACERATIONS NOT INVOLVING THE CANALICULUS

- Reapproximate lid margin lacerations first.
  - Use 6-0 Vicryl on an S-28 needle for children too young for suture removal. Use 6-0 silk on a TG-140 needle for older children.
  - Pass the suture into the tarsus and reapproximate the lid margin with sutures passed through the mucocutaneous junction, the gray line, and the lash margin. Ensure that the exit depth on one side of the laceration matches the entrance depth on the opposite side to minimize potential lid notching postoperatively (Fig. 23.5).
  - Leave the tails of the 6-0 silk suture long, and following any other lid repairs, suture them away from the lid margin using 6-0 Prolene or nylon sutures. This prevents corneal erosions from the knots touching the cornea.
  - Remove lid margin sutures in 2-3 weeks.
  - In younger children, use 6-0 Vicryl as described. Secure the mucocutaneous junction and gray line sutures, and leave the tails long. Tie the lash margin suture, and then drape the tails of the two sutures closer to the globe under slight tension over the lash margin knot and secure them (Fig. 23.6). Trim short. This keeps the knots of the mucocutaneous border and gray line sutures adequately away from the globe in most situations. Buried 6-0 Vicryl along the lid margin is an alternative. Suture removal is typically not required.
  - Reapproximate tarsal injuries with buried 6-0 Vicryl S-28 sutures passed partial thickness into the tarsus.
- Close the remaining lid laceration with interrupted or running locking 6-0 fast absorbing suture in young children or 6-0 Prolene in children who can tolerate suture removal in 1 week.

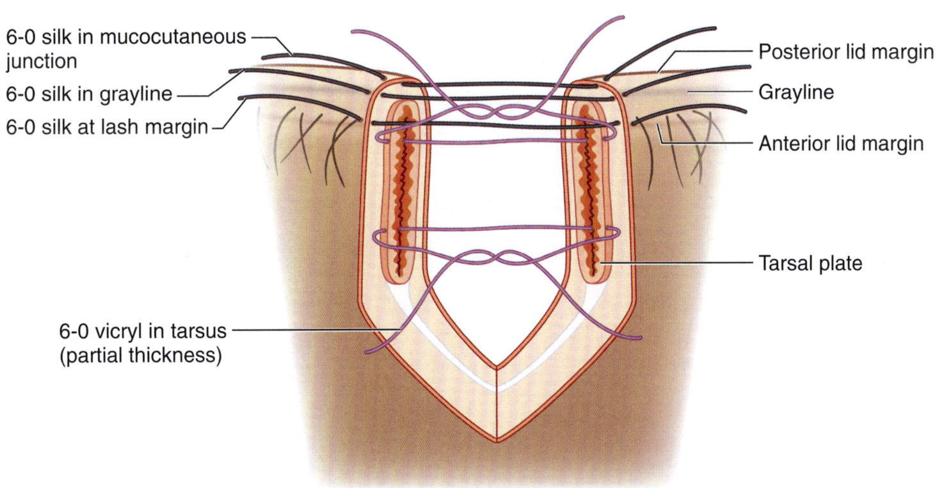

FIGURE 23.5. Reapproximation of lid margin lacerations with sutures through the mucocutaneous junction, the gray line, and the lash margin.

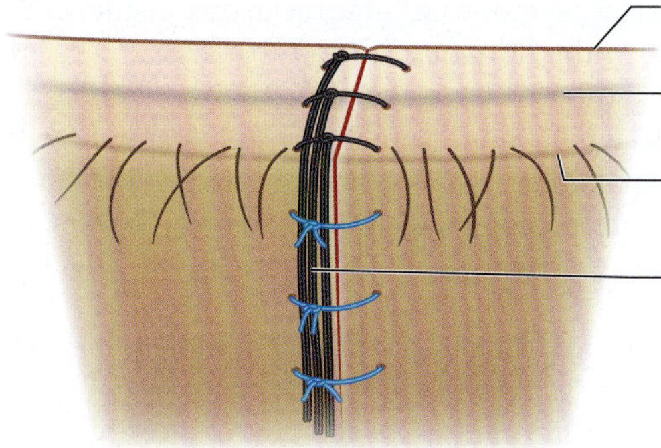

FIGURE 23.6. Tie the lash margin suture, and drape the tails of the two sutures closer to the globe under slight tension over the lash margin knot. This keeps the suture tails away from the globe during the healing process.

COMPLEX EYELID LACERATIONS

- Find the apex of stellate or multi-angulated lid and facial lacerations and reapproximate the apices first using 5-0 or 6-0 fast absorbing gut suture.
  - If significant tension is present, instead of fast absorbing gut, use subcutaneous 5-0 or 6-0 Vicryl with buried knots at the apices.
- The remaining laceration may be closed with interrupted or running locking 6-0 fast-absorbing gut in young children or 6-0 Prolene in older children.
- Postauricular skin grafts may be used if lid skin is absent.
- A Tenzel semicircular flap arising from the lateral canthal region may be utilized if part of the lid is missing.
- Apply bacitracin ointment to the wounds for 7-10 days.

Suggesting Readings/Videos

https://www.aao.org/basic-skills/surgical-repair-of-eyelid-canalicular-laceration
https://eyewiki.org/Eyelid_Laceration
Reifler DM. Management of canalicular laceration. *Surv of Ophthalmol.* 1991;36(2):113-132. doi.org/10.1016/0039-6257(91)90125-Y.

CHAPTER 24

Traumatic Hyphema

Evan Silverstein, MD

Traumatic hyphemas in children require both close immediate follow-up and long-term monitoring for secondary glaucoma.[1]

ETIOLOGY

- Obtain a good history of etiology. If not known, keep a broad differential. Have a high suspicion for open globe injuries.
- Without known trauma, consider nonaccidental trauma, retinoblastoma, leukemia (or other bleeding diathesis), and juvenile xanthogranuloma.

INITIAL EVALUATION

- Examine entire globe and surrounding adnexa. Be on high alert for other injuries including:
  - Retrobulbar hemorrhage (tight lids, very high IOP, resistance to retropulsion).
  - Orbital fractures (consider CT scan based on etiology and motility examination to evaluate for muscle entrapment).
  - Open globe (associated diffuse hemorrhagic chemosis or peaked pupil).
- Obtain complete eye examination including visual acuity, IOP, pupil examination (looking specifically for a relative afferent pupillary defect, traumatic mydriasis, and iridodialysis), motility, and anterior and posterior examination.
- Measure hyphema in millimeters (if possible). This allows objective tracking of the resolution or worsening of the hyphema.
- If no view to the fundus, obtain B-scan to evaluate for retinal detachment.
- Additional history: Sickle cell trait or disease (obtain sickle cell prep to screen for sickle cell disease in African American patients of unknown status), hemophilia, von Willebrand disease.

Children with sickle cell disease or trait are at higher risk of elevation of intraocular pressure as a result of obstruction of trabecular meshwork with sickled red blood cells. Oral carbonic anhydrase inhibitors (eg acetazolamide) are contraindicated in these patients.

MEDICAL MANAGEMENT

- Protect eye with clear shield at all times until hyphema resolves.
  - Using a clear shield allows the child to see through the shield, which decreases the risk of amblyopia and also enables the child to report vision changes and the parents to visualize if the hyphema significantly worsens.
- Strict bed/chair rest.
  - Limit physical activity to decrease the risk of rebleed and allow blood to settle out of the visual axis.
  - Elevate the head and/or head of the bed while sleeping.
- Prednisolone acetate 1% topical drops.
  - Often prescribed four times daily.
  - Be aware that topical steroids can cause steroid-induced ocular hypertension.
  - Stop steroids when hyphema is resolved.
- Atropine 1% topical drops.
  - Prescribed daily until hyphema resolves to treat discomfort from ciliary spasm.
- Hold all oral blood thinners, if possible. Consult primary care physician and/or cardiologist prior to discontinuing medically necessary blood thinners.
- If IOP is elevated, start aqueous suppressants:
  - Timolol 0.5% (avoid in asthmatics), apraclonidine 0.5% (avoid in patients younger than 2 years of age), dorzolamide (avoid in sickle cell disease/trait patients).
  - Consider acetazolamide 5 mg/kg up to four times daily (can crush and mix in apple sauce) if IOP still elevated. Oral carbonic anhydrase inhibitors are contraindicated in sickle cell disease/trait patients.
  - Antifibrinolytics like aminocaproic acid or tranexamic acid are not routinely used in the management of hyphema, but can be considered for higher-risk patients.

SURGICAL MANAGEMENT

- Consider anterior chamber washout if:
  - IOP > 50 mm Hg for 2 days or >50 mm Hg and large hyphema.
  - IOP > 30 mm Hg for 5 days.
  - New relative afferent pupillary defect.
  - Corneal blood staining (Fig. 24.1).
  - Have a lower threshold to intervene for patients with sickle cell disease/trait and uncontrolled intraocular pressure. In patients with sickle cell trait or sickle cell disease who have hyphemas of any size that are associated with intraocular pressures of >35 mm Hg for more than 24 hours, consider AC washout.

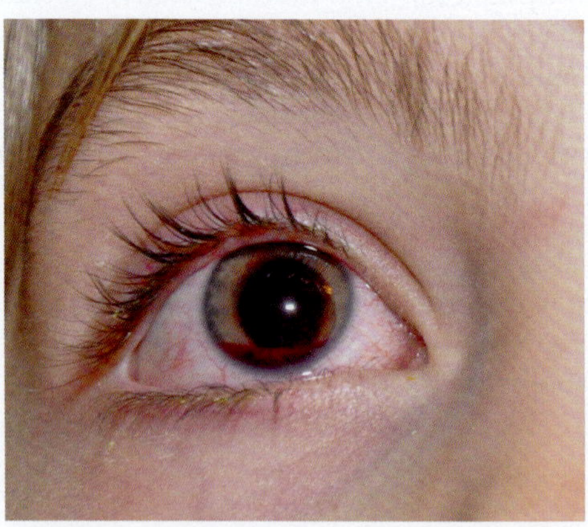

FIGURE 24.1. Hyphema with corneal blood staining and conjunctival injection. (Courtesy of Laura B. Enyedi, MD.)

- Anterior chamber washout technique:
  - Goal: To reduce IOP.
  - Make 2 paracenteses with Super Sharp blade—large enough to allow cannula into anterior chamber. Allow first paracentesis to decompress the eye before making second paracentesis. Flush anterior chamber with BSS through first paracentesis while depressing second paracentesis to allow flow of blood out of the eye until blood is cleared.
  - Gentle anterior vitrectomy may assist with evacuation of hyphema.
    - Maintain normal IOP, and use gentle suction and a relatively low cut rate.
    - Take care to avoid injuring the iris or lens, which may be difficult to visualize.
  - Inject a large air bubble into the anterior chamber. This will help clear out additional blood. Air can also be helpful to quickly pressurize the eye and tamponade rebleeding intraoperatively.
  - Do not try to remove blood clots, as this may cause a rebleed.
  - Inject BSS until IOP is about 15 mm Hg.
  - Close paracenteses with dissolvable suture if leaking.
  - Place shield over eye.
  - If intraocular pressure remains uncontrolled, further glaucoma surgical management (see Section III) and repeat washout may be indicated.

FOLLOW-UP

- When treating nonsurgically, follow daily for the first 5 days watching for decreased vision, afferent pupillary defect, increased IOP, and rebleeds (increased size of hyphema, new layering of hyphema).
  - Rebleeds are most likely to occur in the first 5 days following the initial trauma, so care should be taken to monitor for this.
- Return precautions: increased pain, decreased vision, nausea, increased size of hyphema.
- Then, follow weekly until hyphema resolved. Other injuries to the iris or lens may become apparent with resolution of hyphema (Fig. 24.2).
- Try gonioscopy after 1 month to look for angle recession.
- Follow every 3 months watching for secondary ocular hypertension for first year. Then, every 6 months for the next 3 years.

Sequelae of Traumatic Hyphema

- Traumatic optic neuropathy from the initial injury.
- Optic neuropathy from increased IOP.
- Traumatic mydriasis.

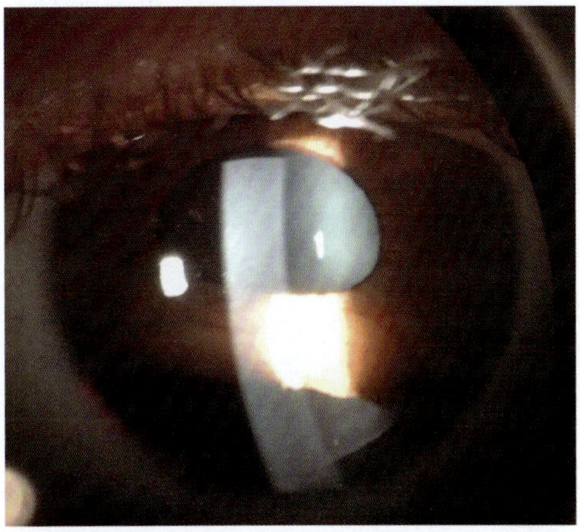

FIGURE 24.2. Iridodialysis that became apparent after resolution of large hyphema. (Courtesy of Laura B. Enyedi, MD.)

- Traumatic cataract.
- Angle recession and glaucoma.
- Amblyopia.

Reference

1. Gharaibeh A, Savage HI, Scherer RW, Goldberg MF, Lindsley K. Medical interventions for traumatic hyphema. *Cochrane Database Syst Rev.* 2019;(1):CD005431. doi: 10.1002/14651858.CD005431.pub4.

CHAPTER 25

Pediatric Open Globe Repair

Marina Roizenblatt, MD • Kim Jiramongkolchai, MD

PREOPERATIVE CONSIDERATIONS

Open Globe Injury Classification[1,2]

- Type:
  - *Rupture:* full-thickness wound of the eye, usually caused by a blunt object.
  - *Penetrating:* presence of a single entrance wound, usually caused by a sharp object.
  - *Perforating:* presence of both entrance and exit wounds, usually caused by a sharp object.
  - *Intraocular foreign body (IOFB)*: a retained foreign object, responsible for the entrance laceration, found within the eye cavity.
- Grade:
  - Defined by the VA at the presentation exam.
  - Baseline VA is a significant prognostic indicator for visual outcome.
- Pupils:
  - *Positive* (presence of an afferent pupil defect).
  - *Negative* (absence of an afferent pupil defect).
- Zones:
  - *Zone I:* cornea and limbus.
  - *Zone II:* 0-5 mm posterior to the limbus (excludes the retina).
  - *Zone III:* >5 mm posterior to limbus.
  - In cases involving a perforating injury, the most posterior defect, (usually the exit site) is used to classify the zone.

Examination

- Signs that may indicate an occult open globe (see Chapter 22):
  - Significantly reduced vision (out of proportion to findings).
  - Afferent pupillary defect.
  - Blood at multiple layers: hemorrhagic chemosis, hyphema, and/or vitreous hemorrhage.
  - Corectopia.
  - Hypotony (intraocular pressure of 5 mm Hg or less).
  - An abnormally deep or shallow anterior chamber.

- Avoid manipulating or applying pressure to the open globe.
  - Avoid intraocular pressure measurement, gonioscopy, forced duction testing, or scleral depression.
  - B-scan ultrasonography, if absolutely necessary, should be performed gently over a closed eyelid.
- Children frequently need sedation or anesthesia for adequate examination.

Ketamine is typically avoided in patients with suspected ruptured globe injury as it has been reported to increase intraocular pressure.

- If open globe is suspected, make the patient NPO, provide pain control and antiemetics if needed, and place an eye shield to protect the eye
- Preoperative CT scanning indications:
  - Suspected occult open globe, IOFB, or facial fractures.
  - Lack of visualization of the posterior segment with funduscopic exam.
- Assess for child abuse:
  - Consider consultation with child abuse specialist if there are inconsistencies in the caregiver's history of the event, multiple associated and unexplained injuries, repeated trauma, or delay in presentation to the hospital. In most states, physicians are legally obligated to report any suspected abuse.
- Check for tetanus immunization status, and update if necessary.
- Consider the administration of IV antibiotics preoperatively and intravitreal antibiotics intraoperatively. While these decisions are based on surgeon's discretion, below are some general guidelines:
  - Adults: cefazolin 1 g IV q8h or vancomycin 1 g IV q12h and moxifloxacin 400 mg IV daily.
  - Children <12 years old: cefazolin 25-50 mg/kg/d IV in 3 divided doses and gentamicin 2 mg/kg IV q8h.
  - Consider 48 hours of intravenous antibiotics to reduce the risk of posttraumatic endophthalmitis.
  - If IOFB is suspected, intravenous vancomycin and ceftazidime should be started on admission.[3,4]
  - Intravitreal vancomycin (1 mg/0.1 mL) and ceftazidime (2.25 mg/0.1 mL) after globe repair or IOFB removal.[5]

SURGICAL MANAGEMENT[1,6-8]

Open globe repair should be performed as soon as reasonably possible under general anesthesia. Do not put any pressure on the globe when prepping and try not to instill any iodine directly into the eye. Use an eyelid speculum that puts minimal pressure on the globe (*ie*, Jaffe eyelid retractor).

Anterior Segment Surgical Reconstruction

Corneal Laceration

- Create an incision at the limbus with a keratome or a sideport blade.
- Gently irrigate the anterior chamber with a blunt infusion cannula (avoid this if there is extensive prolapse of intraocular tissue).
- Inject viscoelastic to reform the anterior chamber.
- If lens fragments, necrotic iris, or vitreous are noted to prolapse through the corneal defect, they should be carefully excised so as not to cause traction on the vitreous body or zonular fibers. Gently sweep viable iris tissue back into the anterior chamber using a separate limbal incision.

- Suture the corneal wound using interrupted 10-0 nylon sutures.
  Tips:
  - If the laceration involves the limbus, start suturing from this point with 9-0 or 10-0 nylon.
  - Suture passes should be partial thickness through the cornea.
  - Knots are buried within corneal stroma, not in the wound.
  - In case of difficulty in closing a complex corneal laceration, consider X-shaped sutures or even cyanoacrylate glue and a therapeutic bandage contact lens.
  - Sutures should be longer with increased interval spaces between sutures in the peripheral cornea, but shorter, and closer to adjacent sutures in the central cornea. This pattern of suture placement will help restore the normal cornea curvature.
  - In cases where the corneal wound edges are irregular, the sutures may need to be longer in order to incorporate healthy tissue.
- Clot removal from the anterior chamber can be performed with a vitreous cutter or with an irrigation and aspiration unit after the corneal wound is closed. This should be done with care, as dislodging a clot can occasionally precipitate worse bleeding.

Lens Injuries

- Penetrating or blunt trauma may result in traumatic cataract formation (see Chapter 7).
  - Cataract extraction is usually postponed until after repair of the primary rupture, thereby allowing for the resolution of intraocular inflammation prior to cataract surgery.
  - This also allows for intraocular lens calculations (see Chapter 4) to be performed in a controlled setting either in the clinic or under a subsequent anesthesia.
  - Intraocular lens placement may be deferred because of capsular instability or persistent intraocular inflammation (see Chapter 26).

Traumatic Iris Defect

- McCannel suture technique is a safe option to repair iris lacerations (Fig. 25.1).
- First, a limbal paracentesis is created at the clock hour of the iris discontinuity. A double armed 10-0 polypropylene suture on a long, curved needle is then passed through the peripheral cornea, the edges of the iris defects, and finally the opposite peripheral cornea. A Sinskey hook is then inserted through the paracentesis to grasp the suture loop and draw it back out of the anterior chamber. The needles are then cut and the suture tied in a 3-1-1-1-1 fashion.[9]

IOFB Removal from the Anterior Segment

- Make sure to explore the entire entry site.
- Create a limbal corneoscleral incision as large as the material to be removed. Avoid removing the IOFB through the traumatic wound.
- Fill the anterior chamber with viscoelastic to maintain chamber depth and protect adjacent tissues.
- Intraocular forceps are usually the tool of choice for IOFB extraction. When removing metallic IOFB, magnets may be used.
- Remove the viscoelastic and close the extraction incision.

If the lens capsule is violated, the lens may be removed at the time of IOFB removal.

An inert IOFB may be left in place if it is small and not obstructing the visual axis; this is especially relevant when the material is found several days after injury. Electroretinography is helpful in the follow-up of these cases. Examples of inert IOFB: metallic (gold, silver, and platinum) and nonmetallic (stone, sand, glass, porcelain, plastic, and cilia).

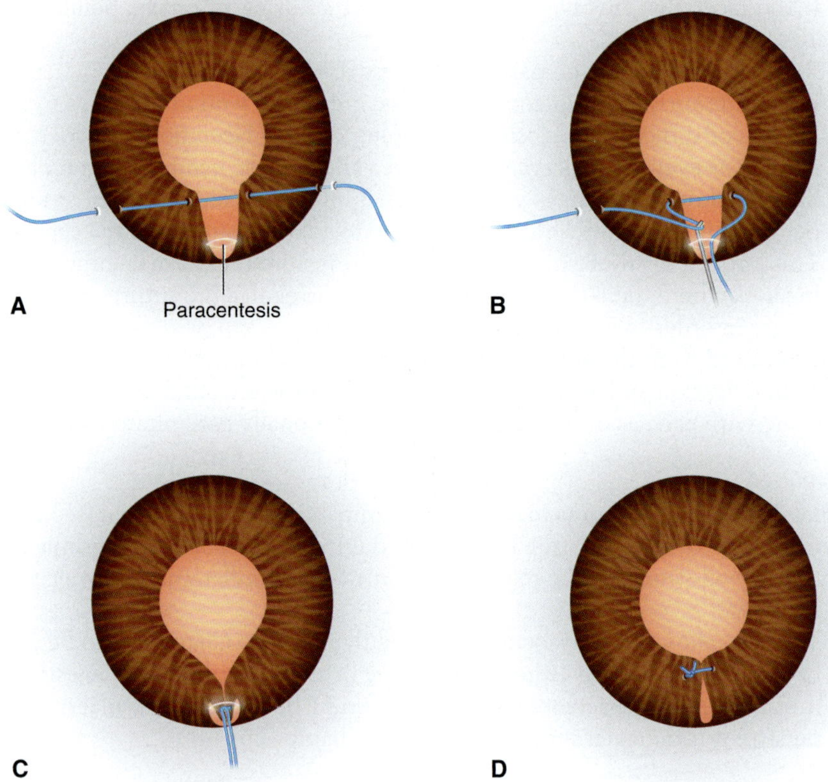

FIGURE 25.1. **A.** A limbal paracentesis is made over the iris defect. A 10-0 polypropylene suture is passed through the peripheral cornea, the edges of the iris, and the opposite peripheral cornea. The suture is then cut. **B.** A Sinskey hook is inserted through the paracentesis, and each end of the suture is drawn out through the paracentesis. **C.** The suture is tied in 3-1-1-1 surgeon's knot. **D.** The excess suture is cut and iris allowed to retract. Image from: https://www.aao.org/image/mccannel-technique

Posterior Segment Surgical Reconstruction

Consultation with a vitreoretinal specialist is recommended for posterior injuries.

Posterior Scleral Laceration

- Make a peritomy that is large enough to expose the entire scleral wound. If an occult open globe is suspected, perform a wide exploration by doing a 360-degree peritomy.
- Prolapsed vitreous should be amputated at the scleral surface. Retina and non-necrotic uvea should be gently reposited to avoid incarceration of the tissue in the wound.
- Scleral lacerations are generally sutured with 8-0 or 9-0 silk or nylon.
- When closing very posterior scleral lacerations, a muscle hook can aid in the exposure of the wound. When the wound extends under the rectus muscle, the involved muscle may need to be temporarily disinserted (isolate with a double armed 6-0 Vicryl) and then reattached after the scleral defect closure (see Chapter 44).
- Avoid excessive traction with the muscle hook as this may cause additional tissue prolapse. It may not be possible to close very posterior lacerations as a result of limited exposure.

Choroidal Detachment

- Accurate preoperative B-scan ultrasonography is impractical in open globe injuries due to the risk of further intraocular tissue extrusion and additional risk of infection.[10]
- If there is hemorrhagic choroidal detachment, drainage is usually not performed prior to clot liquefaction, which occurs 7-14 days after trauma.[11]
- If there are appositional choroidals, surgical drainage should be considered.
- To drain a choroidal detachment, insert an anterior chamber maintainer at the limbus, create a posterior drainage sclerotomy to access the suprachoroidal space at the maximal fluid accumulation site, and gently massage the eye to allow for drainage of the choroidals.

Retinal Detachment (see Chapter 31)

- Scleral buckling indications: clear media, anterior retinal break, retinal dialysis, and absence of proliferative vitreoretinopathy (PVR).
- Pars plana vitrectomy indications: media opacities, multiple and complex retinal breaks, posterior retinal breaks, giant retinal tear, PVR, retinal, or vitreous incarceration.
    - Follow age-based guidelines for sclerotomy placement in pediatric pars plana vitrectomy (see Chapter 31).[12]
    - The incidence of PVR is higher in children than adults, probably due to the greater fibroblast activity in this age group, as well as the intrinsic difficulty of the exam, which may delay surgical intervention.[13]
    - At the end of surgery, silicone oil should be considered for children, as this vitreous substitute stabilizes the retina during the critical period of active PVR, provides a relatively clear view, and requires no postoperative positioning.[4,14]

IOFB Removal from the Posterior Segment

- A standard 3-port pars plana vitrectomy is the ideal approach (see Chapter 31).
- The entry wound should be avoided when creating the sclerotomy to prevent further damage to intraocular tissues, especially when retinal incarceration is suspected.
- In order to avoid retinal traction while removing the IOFB, the material must first be completely isolated from potential adhesions to the vitreous body. This is accomplished with a thorough vitrectomy, removal of posterior hyaloid, and shaving of the vitreous base.
- When removing a magnetic foreign body, intraocular electromagnetic adherent instruments with intraocular forceps are recommended. Nonmagnetic IOFB's can be removed using retinal forceps alone.
- Remove the IOFB from the posterior segment through the conventional sclerotomy site, through a circumferentially enlarged sclerotomy or, if the IOFB is very large, through a limbal corneoscleral incision after a lensectomy.
- Perform endolaser around retinal breaks that can be caused either directly by the IOFB or by surgical manipulation.
- Intravitreal vancomycin (1 mg/0.1 mL) and ceftazidime (2.25 mg/0.1 mL) should also be given after the open globe injury is repaired and the IOFB has been removed.[5]

POSTOPERATIVE CONSIDERATIONS (SEE CHAPTER 27)

- There are no "gold standard" guidelines for endophthalmitis prophylaxis, and oral antibiotics are used at the individual surgeons' discretion.[15]
- Postoperative medications should include steroid and antibiotic eye drops.
- Corneal sutures may be removed starting at postoperative week 6, either at the slit lamp or in the operating room, depending on the child's age and cooperation.

- Follow-up should focus on the treatment of amblyopia, especially in young children. Polycarbonate spectacle correction and optical penalization is typically required. If there is irregular or high astigmatism, a scleral lens might be helpful.
- The incidence of sympathetic ophthalmia following open globe injury is between 0.14% and 0.5%. Patients should be monitored for this in the postoperative period as well.[16-18]

References

1. Kuhn F, Pieramici DJ. *Ocular Trauma: Principles and Practice*. New York, Stuttgart: Thieme; 2002.
2. Kuhn F, Morris R, Witherspoon CD, Heimann K, Jeffers JB, Treister G. A standardized classification of ocular trauma. *Ophthalmology*. 1996;103(2):240-243.
3. Andreoli CM, Andreoli MT, Kloek CE, Ahuero AE, Vavvas D, Durand ML. Low rate of endophthalmitis in a large series of open globe injuries. *Am J Ophthalmol*. 2009;147(4):601-608.e2.
4. Li X, Zarbin MA, Bhagat N. Pediatric open globe injury: a review of the literature. *J Emerg Trauma Shock*. 2015;8(4):216-223.
5. Bhagat N, Nagori S, Zarbin M. Post-traumatic infectious endophthalmitis. *Surv Ophthalmol*. 2011;56(3):214-251.
6. Grob S, Kloek C. *Management of Open Globe Injuries*. Cham, Switzerland: Springer; 2018.
7. MacCumber MW. *Management of Ocular Injuries and Emergencies*. Philadelphia, PA: Lippincott-Raven; 1998.
8. American Academy of Ophthalmology. *Basic and Clinical Science Course 2007–2008: Section 8: External Disease and Cornea*. San Francisco, CA: American Academy of Ophthalmology; 2019-2020.
9. McCannel MA. A retrievable suture idea for anterior uveal problems. *Ophthalmic Surg*. 1976;7(2):98-103.
10. Shiraki N, Wakabayashi T, Sato T, Sakaguchi H, Nishida K. Intraoperative B-scan ultrasonography and pars plana vitrectomy for severe open globe injury with hemorrhagic retinal and choroidal detachment. *Graefes Arch Clin Exp Ophthalmol*. 2017;255(11):2287-2291.
11. Agrawal R, Shah M, Mireskandari K, Yong GK. Controversies in ocular trauma classification and management: review. *Int Ophthalmol*. 2013;33(4):435-445.
12. Wright LM, Harper CA III, Chang EY. Management of infantile and childhood retinopathies: optimized pediatric pars plana vitrectomy sclerotomy nomogram. *Ophthalmol Retina*. 2018;2(12):1227-1234.
13. Wang NK, Chen YP, Yeung L, et al. Traumatic pediatric retinal detachment following open globe injury. *Ophthalmologica*. 2007;221(4):255-263.
14. Szurman P, Roters S, Grisanti S, et al. Primary silicone oil tamponade in the management of severe intraocular foreign body injuries: an 8-year follow-up. *Retina*. 2007;27(3):304-311.
15. Ahmed Y, Schimel AM, Pathengay A, Colyer MH, Flynn HW Jr. Endophthalmitis following open-globe injuries. *Eye (Lond)*. 2012;26(2):212-217.
16. du Toit N, Motala MI, Richards J, Murray AD, Maitra S. The risk of sympathetic ophthalmia following evisceration for penetrating eye injuries at Groote Schuur Hospital. *Br J Ophthalmol*. 2008;92(1):61-63.
17. Savar A, Andreoli MT, Kloek CE, Andreoli CM. Enucleation for open globe injury. *Am J Ophthalmol*. 2009;147(4):595-600.e1.
18. Gurdal C, Erdener U, Irkec M, Orhan M. Incidence of sympathetic ophthalmia after penetrating eye injury and choice of treatment. *Ocul Immunol inflamm*. 2002;10(3):223-227.

CHAPTER 26

Pediatric Traumatic Cataract

Dinah Chen, MD • Fatema Ghasia, MD

PREOPERATIVE CONSIDERATIONS

Examination

- Have a high suspicion for nonaccidental trauma. Look for other associated ocular or periocular injuries, and ensure the child has had a complete physical examination to evaluate for other signs of trauma.
- Assess child's visual acuity using age-appropriate methods.
- Assess the red reflex in the undilated state to determine whether the opacity is visually significant in infants and toddlers.
  - Absence of view of the fundus or a dull retinoscopic reflex preventing refraction suggests a visually significant cataract.
- Assess ocular motility and look for the presence of strabismus or nystagmus.
  - If either are present, this could suggest cataract is long standing, causing dense deprivation amblyopia.
- Assess for other signs of ocular trauma, including corneal scar, iridodonesis, or phacodonesis.
- Assess for lens dislocation and depth of anterior chamber.
- Assess the morphology and location of cataracts.
  - More central and posterior location is more visually significant than more peripheral and anterior.
  - Bilateral posterior subcapsular cataracts and/or lens dislocation can be seen in nonaccidental trauma.
- Assess anterior and posterior capsule integrity.
- Note the extent of pupillary dilation.
- If there is a history of hyphema, assess for angle recession, and monitor intraocular pressure.
- Perform B-scan ultrasonography to evaluate for vitreous hemorrhage or retinal detachment if the view to the fundus is not clear.
- Assess the cooperation of the child at slit lamp.
  - If the child is able to sit for a YAG capsulotomy, the posterior capsule may be left intact.
- Obtain intraocular lens implant calculations in the outpatient setting if possible.
  - If the child cannot cooperate with awake lens calculations, perform lens calculation under anesthesia (see Chapter 4).

- Discuss postoperative care and considerations.
  - Refractive correction including aphakic contact lenses and the need for spectacles with bifocals for all children (see Chapter 4).
  - Importance of compliance with follow-up and post-op medications.
  - Importance of amblyopia treatment.
  - Risk of visual axis opacification after surgery.
  - Risk of glaucoma and retinal detachment.

Timing of Surgery

Visually significant cataracts acquired in a child <6 years old should be removed within weeks. In children >6 years, it is acceptable to wait for inflammation to resolve prior to surgery.[1]

In children with penetrating trauma and subsequent cataract, primary repair of the anterior segment wound is generally performed initially (see Chapter 25). Cataract surgery with IOL can be performed 1-4 weeks following.

When to Consider IOL Implantation (see Chapter 4)

- Most children <6 months are left aphakic.
- IOL implantation in children between 6 months and 2 years is controversial, and the pros and cons should be considered for each patient individually.
- In children >2 years of age, an IOL may be implanted in the capsular bag. If compromised, consider capsular tension ring, sulcus IOL, or leaving patient aphakic.
- The IOL target is usually mild to moderate hyperopia in children <6 years and emmetropia at 7 years or older.
- If IOL calculations cannot be performed awake, ultrasound biometry and IOL calculations can be obtained under anesthesia.
  - Holladay (axial length [AL] 21.00-21.49 mm) and Hoffer Q (AL 20.00-21.99 mm) may be used for short eyes.[2]

SURGICAL PROCEDURE

Surgical Planning

- Anesthesia: general
- Dilate patient using drops q5min ×3 (see Chapter 3).
- Examination under anesthesia should include the following elements:
  - Measurement of intraocular pressure.
  - Slit lamp examination.
  - Gonioscopy.
  - Fundus examination.
  - Keratometry measurements.
  - IOL calculations.
  - Complete examination of the fellow eye including refraction (if not done previously).

General intraoperative considerations for pediatric cataract surgery include:

- **Children have thin sclera with decreased rigidity compared to adults, placing them at higher risk for posterior pressure, vitreous prolapse, and anterior chamber collapse.**
- **Corneal incisions generally require closure with suture. Corneal vascularization is less common using absorbable (Vicryl) vs nonabsorbable suture.**
- **A superior wound with scleral/corneal tunnel is generally preferred in young children as this location is more protected (brow and Bell phenomenon). One can consider a clear cornea incision in older children.**
- **The anterior capsule is very elastic; capsulorrhexis is generally performed with a vitrector in very young children.**

Surgical Approach: IOL and Anterior Vitrectomy (see Chapter 6)

- Place a 4-0 silk traction suture into the superior rectus muscle, cut off the needle and clamp to the drape superiorly to infraduct the eye.
- Perform 6 mm superior conjunctival peritomy.
- Cauterize the sclera for hemostasis.
- Make a partial thickness scleral groove of ~4 mm length with a #64 blade and extend to clear cornea with a #66 Beaver blade. Be careful to keep the blade in the same plane as the wound is carried forward. Make sure both sides/corners are opened well.
- Using an MVR blade, make 2 sideport incisions adjacent to the groove in the anterior surgical limbus (11 and 1 o'clock).
- Consider using iris hooks, Malyugin ring, or manual expansion for small pupils (see Chapter 7).
- Use trypan blue if necessary for adequate capsular visualization (see Chapter 3).
  - This can be helpful to delineate the capsule in white cataracts or situations in which the capsule has been traumatically ruptured.
- Place irrigating cannula into one of the sideport incisions (usually side of the non-dominant hand) and the vitrector into the other (usually side of dominant hand).
- Using the vitrector, make a flap tear in the anterior capsule and create a 5-mm capsulorrhexis (by aiming for a smaller 4-mm rhexis).
  - If performing a continuous curvilinear capsulorrhexis, be aware that the capsule in children's eyes is very elastic and at risk for running outward. Pull toward the center of the pupil to prevent radialization.
  - The vitrector can be used for a vitrectorhexis instead of tearing the anterior capsule.
- Remove the lens using aspiration mode.
- Remove vitrector and turn off irrigation.
- Reform the anterior chamber and inflate capsular bag with ophthalmic viscosurgical device (OVD) (see Chapter 3).
- Enlarge scleral wound with a keratome to insert the IOL into the capsular bag.
- Close the scleral tunnel with interrupted buried 9-0 Vicryl or 10-0 nylon sutures.
- Remove OVD from AC with the vitrectomy handpiece.
- Close the vitrector limbal wound with 9-0 Vicryl.
- Make incision perpendicular to sclera posterior to limbus and preplace 8-0 absorbable suture across sclerotomy site (see Chapter 6).
  - Distance of sclerotomy site from limbus differs by age (see Chapter 31).
  - For children aged 1.5-3 years and 3-6 years, the sclerotomy should be placed 2.5 mm and 3.0 mm posterior to the limbus, respectively.[3]
- Restart the irrigation and insert the vitrector into the anterior vitreous cavity.
- Cut a posterior capsulotomy of ~4 mm and perform limited anterior vitrectomy.
- Close scleral wound with 9-0 Vicryl and check for leaks.
- Remove irrigating cannula and close the limbal incision with 9-0 Vicryl suture. Check wounds for leakage.
- Consider injecting Miochol, intracameral antibiotics, and/or filtered air (see Chapter 3).
- Confirm IOL position and close conjunctiva with 9-0 buried Vicryl sutures.
- Consider subconjunctival antibiotics and/or steroids. Consider IV steroids and/or acetazolamide (see Chapter 3).

Surgical Approach: No IOL Placement (see Chapter 5)

- After aspiration of the lens, perform posterior capsulotomy and limited anterior vitrectomy from an anterior approach.
- Inject Miochol to look for peaked pupil and assess presence of vitreous at the surgical incision sites.

- Close the limbal incisions with 9-0 Vicryl sutures and check for wound leakage.
- Consider injecting Miochol, intracameral antibiotics, and/or filtered air (see Chapter 3).
- Close the conjunctiva with 9-0 interrupted Vicryl sutures.
- Consider subconjunctival antibiotics and/or steroids. Consider IV steroids and/or acetazolamide (see Chapter 3).

POSTOPERATIVE CONSIDERATIONS

- Prescribe frequent topical steroids for 1 month, oral steroids (½-1 mg/kg/d) for 1-2 weeks, topical antibiotic for 2 weeks, and a cycloplegic for 2-4 weeks (see Chapter 3). Note: avoid putting a cycloplegic eye drop immediately postop in the operating room in patients undergoing IOL placement.
- Assess vision and look for inflammation, visual axis opacification, IOL position, and any posterior segment pathology.
- Monitor intraocular pressure.
- For patients left aphakic, schedule contact lens fitting after surgery. For patients with IOL, plan to prescribe glasses ~1 month after surgery (see Chapter 4).
- Treat amblyopia as soon as possible.

References

1. Wilson ME, Trivedi R, Pandey S. *Traumatic Cataracts in Children. Pediatric Cataract Surgery Techniques*. Philadelphia, PA: Lippincott Williams & Wilkins; 2005.
2. Aristodemou P, Knox Cartwright NE, et al. Formula choice: Hoffer Q, Holladay 1, or SRK/T and refractive outcomes in 8108 eyes after cataract surgery with biometry by partial coherence interferometry. *J Cataract Refract Surg*. 2011;37(1):63-71. doi: 10.1016/j.jcrs.2010.07.032.
3. Liu X, Zheng T, Zhou X, et al. Comparison between limbal and pars plana approaches using microincision vitrectomy for removal of congenital cataracts with primary intraocular lens implantation. *J Ophthalmol*. 2016;2016. doi: 10.1155/2016/8951053.

CHAPTER 27

Pediatric Trauma: Postoperative Management

Irene T. Tung, MD

TIMING OF SUTURE REMOVAL

- 10-0 nylon corneal sutures can be removed as soon as 4-6 weeks after surgery, but may need to stay in longer in order to allow the corneal wounds to heal. Consider removing in stages.
- If left in place, corneal sutures may cause induced astigmatism, keratitis, corneal vascularization, or conjunctivitis.[1]
- Sutures may need to be removed during an examination under anesthesia (EUA).

OPTICAL REHABILITATION

- When able, the patient should be given the appropriate spectacle correction. The cycloplegic refraction can be checked at the time of EUA for suture removal.
  - If there are concerns about cylinder induced by sutures, consider performing refraction in the clinic 2-4 weeks after suture removal.
- Pediatric patients are at risk for amblyopia due to either deprivation/occlusion from media opacities such as corneal haze or traumatic cataract, and/or refractive amblyopia due to induced astigmatism. Amblyopia should be treated as soon as possible after initial surgery.[2]

MEDICATIONS

- Systemic antibiotics should be considered based on the method of injury as well as the timing of the injury. In cases of penetrating eye trauma, the incidence of endophthalmitis is 2%-30%.[3] Cultures taken at the time of surgery can help target antibiotic use. Broad-spectrum antibiotics with good ocular penetration should be used prophylactically.
  - Consider cefazolin (first-generation cephalosporin) for less complex injuries.[4]
  - Consider admission for intravenous vancomycin and ceftazidime for suspected intraocular foreign body or more complex injuries.[4]

  - Unless no other option exists, oral fluoroquinolones should not be the first line of treatment due to concerns for musculoskeletal adverse events, as well as peripheral neuropathy in adults.[5]
- Topical antibiotic drops should also be utilized after surgery and targeted as needed based on culture results.
- Topical corticosteroid drops after surgery are critical in the management of postoperative inflammation. The use of steroids should be balanced against the risk of infection.
  - Steroids can also help prevent neovascularization around sutures prior to suture removal.
- Topical cycloplegic drops after surgery are useful to help manage discomfort from ciliary spasm. The patient may need full cycloplegic refraction and bifocal if cycloplegia is used long-term.

EYE PROTECTION

- Prescribe full-time protective spectacles for children after ocular trauma.
- Counsel family on risk reduction and activities to avoid (ie, contact sports, non-powder gun use, etc).

PROGNOSIS

- Risk of sympathetic ophthalmia is low but should be discussed with the family.
- Prognosis is guarded especially in the presence of retinal detachment, endophthalmitis, corneal injury in the visual axis, and amblyogenic age at time of injury.
- Approximately ½ of pediatric patients will achieve a final VA of 20/40 or better.[4]
- Corneal opacity and amblyopia are common causes of persistently low final VA.[4]
- Families should be counseled on the need for long-term follow up to monitor for the development of traumatic cataract, glaucoma, refractive issues, and amblyopia.

References

1. Acheson JF, Lyons CJ. Ocular morbidity due to monofilament nylon corneal sutures. *Eye*. 1991;5:106-112.
2. Vora GK, Haddadin R, Chodosh J. Management of corneal lacerations and perforations. *Int Ophthamol Clin*. 2013;53(4):1-10.
3. Macsai MS. The management of corneal trauma: advances in the past twenty-five years. *Cornea*. 2000;19(5):617-624.
4. Li X, Zarbin MA, Bhagat N. Pediatric open globe injury: a review of the literature. *J Emerg Trauma Shock*. 2015;8(4):216-223. doi:10.4103/0974-2700.166663.
5. Jackson MA, Schutze GE; AAP Committee on Infectious Diseases. The use of systemic and topical fluoroquinolones. *Pediatrics*. 2016;138(5):e1-e13.

Section VII

Pediatric Posterior Segment

CHAPTER 28

Retinopathy of Prematurity

Xi Chen, MD, PhD • Lejla Vajzovic, MD • Cynthia A. Toth, MD

Preterm infants are at risk for retinopathy of prematurity (ROP), a disease caused by delayed or pathological retinal vascular growth. Left untreated, ROP could lead to fibrosis, retinal detachment, and blindness. With improvement in neonatal medicine and increased survival of very preterm infants, ROP severity has increased and become more prevalent.

ROP SCREENING

Screening guidelines (United States): Infants with a birth weight of 1500 g or less or a gestational age of 30 weeks or less, and selected infants with a gestational age of more than 30 weeks or a birth weight between 1500 and 2000 g who are believed to be at risk for ROP. Screening is performed starting at 4 weeks after birth or at 31 weeks postmenstrual age (whichever is later). Standard screening is performed by an ophthalmologist using eyelid speculum, topical anesthesia, scleral depressor, and indirect ophthalmoscopy with a 28-diopter lens.

ROP classification (defined by International Classification of Retinopathy of Prematurity [ICROP][1]): ROP is described as zone, stage, and vascular activity (plus disease) (Fig. 28.1).

Zone I: circle with radius of twice the distance between fovea and optic nerve centered at the optic nerve.

Zone II: radius of the distance between the nasal ora in the horizontal meridian centered at the optic nerve.

Zone III: the remaining retina.

Stage 1: narrow white line at the vascular-avascular junction.

Stage 2: ridge of thickening at the vascular-avascular junction.

Stage 3: neovascularization with growth of vessels toward the vitreous cavity.

Stage 4: partial retinal detachment not involving (4A) or involving the fovea (4B).

Stage 5: total retinal detachment.

Plus disease: two or more quadrants of dilated and tortuous vessels at the posterior pole.

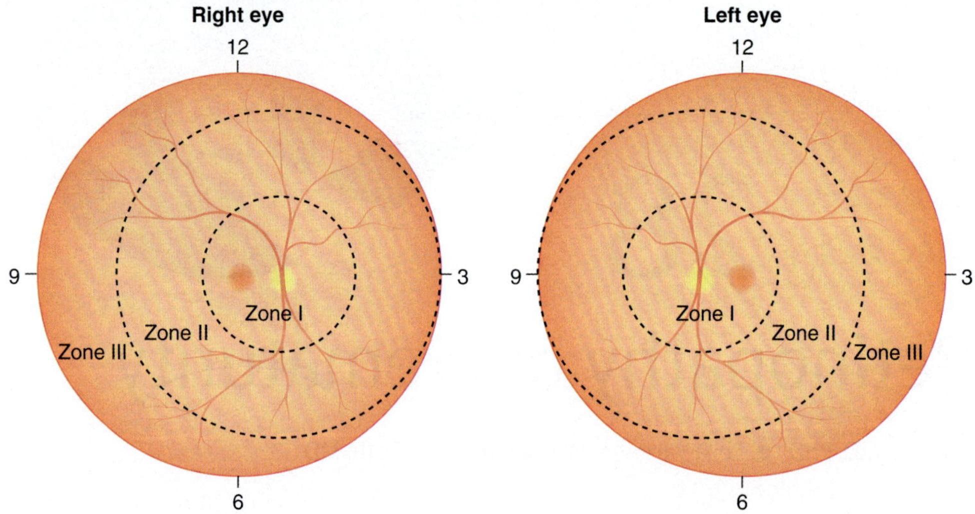

FIGURE 28.1. Schematic diagram illustrating the zones of disease in retinopathy of prematurity.

Aggressive posterior ROP: Posterior severe plus disease, with the absence of obvious neovascular elevations but marked circumferential shunt vessels and flat neovascularization (sometimes presumed). These eyes have a high degree of vascular activity and therefore carry a higher risk of progression to retinal detachment.

Isolated neovascular tufts ("popcorn")[2]: Small isolated tufts of neovascular tissue, often observed posterior to stage 2 ridge, are believed to increase the risk of progression to stage 3 disease.

IMAGING IN ROP

Indirect ophthalmoscopy is the gold standard for ROP diagnosis. The goal of telemedical screening for ROP is to identify referral-warranted ROP[3] (defined as any ROP in zone I, plus disease, or stage 3 ROP). Imaging in infants at risk for ROP helps to document and evaluate ROP and serves as a vehicle for telemedical screening.

Fundus photography: Fundus photography with commercially available fundus cameras (such as RetCam, Neo, etc.) has been used by trained neonatal nurses. These methods have been shown to have high sensitivity and specificity in detecting referral-warranted ROP.

Fluorescein angiography: Fluorescein angiography, necessitating intravenous fluorescein injection, has been helpful in elucidating vascular structure and processes seen in eyes with ROP. Pediatric ophthalmologists and retina specialists use this method at their discretion in evaluating ROP.

Optical coherence tomography: Optical coherence tomography has been adapted to handheld use and is used as an adjunct for evaluation of ROP. It has been shown to be helpful to detect macular edema and retinal neovascular elevations, as well as to differentiate retinoschisis and retinal detachment.

TREATMENT OF ROP

Indication for treatment: Recommendations are based on outcomes of the Early Treatment Retinopathy of Prematurity (ETROP) study.[4] Treatment is indicated for type 1 ROP.

Type 1:

Zone 1 with any stage of ROP with plus disease.

Zone 1 stage 3 with or without plus disease.

Zone 2 stage 2 or 3 with plus disease.

Type 2:

Zone 1 stage 1 or 2 without plus disease.

Zone 2 stage 2 or 3 without plus disease.

Laser treatment: Indirect laser confluent photocoagulation of the avascular retina.

Laser can be done at the bedside with sedation (per neonatology team in neonatal intensive care unit [NICU]) or in the operating room under anesthesia.

- An eyelid speculum is placed between the eyelids.
- Using indirect diode laser, laser application is placed in the avascular retina anterior to the vascularized retina to the ora serrata in multiple interlocking rows for 360 degrees in a semiconfluent pattern. Care is taken to avoid treating the vascular retina, iris, and lens. Typical settings are power: 100-200 mW; duration: 300 ms.
- Following treatment, retinal examination is performed to detect and treat skip areas.

Intravitreal anti-VEGF injections: Intravitreal bevacizumab and ranibizumab have been used off-label to treat ROP since 2007 following the same indications as described above. Some practitioners reserve intravitreal anti-VEGF for posterior disease. The benefits of intravitreal anti-VEGF injections include ease of use and less peripheral retinal ablation. Disadvantages of this treatment include delayed or incomplete vascularization, possibly higher recurrence rate, and need for longer-term follow-up (Table 28.1). Ongoing studies are investigating the effect of various doses of bevacizumab and potential ocular and systemic effects.

- Under sedation, the treatment eye is marked with a sticker on infant's forehead.

Permanent markers can tattoo the skin in very young infants.

- Topical proparacaine is applied.
- Betadine is used to clean the periorbital skin, lids, and lashes.
- A sterile lid speculum is placed between the eyelids.
- Another Betadine swab is used between the eyelids and on the conjunctiva at the planned injection site.
- The correct drug and concentration is confirmed and witnessed, and excess drug expelled through the tip of the 30G needle until 0.02 mL remains in the syringe.
- A scleral depressor is used to rotate the eye to better expose the injection site.
- The injection needle tip is placed 2 mm from the limbus, aiming back toward the optic nerve and enter through the eyewall into the vitreous cavity, with advancement of the needle ~3 mm.
- An assistant injects the drug while the surgeon holds the eye and the syringe.
- A cotton tipped applicator is applied to the injection site as soon as the needle is withdrawn.
- Sterile saline is used to irrigate the eye and fornices and two drops of antibiotic eye drop is placed on the eye.

TABLE 28.1. Comparison of laser photocoagulation and anti-VEGF injection for treatment of type 1 retinopathy of prematurity

Laser treatment	Anti-VEGF injection
Can be performed at bedside or OR	Usually given at bedside and requires less time to administer treatment
Con: Potential ablation of fovea in severe posterior diseases	Pro: Less destruction of the peripheral retina
Con: Likely more refractive changes	Pro: Likely less refractive changes
Pro: Decreased concern for incomplete vascularization and reactivation	Con: Delayed vascularization or incomplete vascularization
Pro: Less requirement of frequent long-term follow-up	Con: Recurrence rate may be higher and occurs at a later age necessitating longer follow-up period
Pro: Less concern for systemic effects	Con: Controversial concern for neurodevelopment and systemic effects

From VanderVeen DK, Melia M, Yang MB, Hutchinson AK, Wilson LB, Lambert SR. Anti-vascular endothelial growth factor therapy for primary treatment of type 1 retinopathy of prematurity: a report by the American Academy of Ophthalmology. *Ophthalmology.* 2017;124(5):619-633.

- The indirect ophthalmoscopy is performed to confirm clear cornea, clear lens, clear vitreous, and attached retina as preinjection.
- The eyelid speculum is removed.

Referral for surgical evaluation: Timely referral for surgical evaluation is important to improve ROP outcomes. Pay close attention to vitreous hemorrhage and consider early referral if retinal status is uncertain.

ROP surgery: Vitreoretinal surgery (see Chapter 31) is required for treatment of advanced stage 4 or 5 ROP. Lens-sparing vitrectomy is usually performed for stage 4 ROP. Lensectomy and vitrectomy is sometimes performed for more advanced stage 4 or stage 5 ROP. Some pediatric retina specialists have also used endoscopic vitrectomy with great success.

LONG-TERM FOLLOW-UP AND COMPLICATIONS

Post-discharge clinic appointments are critical to follow the infants with ROP until full vascularization. This is especially important in infants who received anti-VEGF injections alone for ROP treatment. Despite treatments to prevent progression to retinal detachments, infants who develop ROP are at increased risk of decreased visual acuity, refractive errors, strabismus, and amblyopia. Active research is currently under way to provide more effective screening methods and improve treatment of ROP.

References

1. International Committee for the Classification of Retinopathy of Prematurity. The International Classification of Retinopathy of Prematurity revisited. *Arch Ophthalmol.* 2005;123(7):991-999.
2. Wallace DK, Kylstra JA, Greenman DB, Freedman SF. Significance of isolated neovascular tufts ("popcorn") in retinopathy of prematurity. *J AAPOS.* 1998;2(1):52-56.
3. Quinn GE, Ying GS, Daniel E, et al. Validity of a telemedicine system for the evaluation of acute-phase retinopathy of prematurity. *JAMA Ophthalmol.* 2014;132(10):1178-1184.
4. Good WV, Hardy RJ. The multicenter study of Early Treatment for Retinopathy of Prematurity (ETROP). *Ophthalmology.* 2001;108(6):1013-1014.
5. VanderVeen DK, Melia M, Yang MB, Hutchinson AK, Wilson LB, Lambert SR. Anti-vascular endothelial growth factor therapy for primary treatment of type 1 retinopathy of prematurity: a report by the American Academy of Ophthalmology. *Ophthalmology.* 2017;124(5):619-633.

CHAPTER 29

Nonaccidental Trauma (Shaken Baby Syndrome)

Martha A. Howard, MD

The diagnosis of nonaccidental trauma cannot be made upon isolated physical examination findings. It requires the careful synthesis of information from physical and ophthalmic examinations and radiologic and laboratory studies.

Shaken baby syndrome is a subset of abusive head trauma that occurs when a baby is forcefully shaken, causing bleeding in the brain and eyes secondary to acceleration-deceleration forces.

EPIDEMIOLOGY

- Majority <12 months of age, almost always <5 years of age.
- Risk factors:
  - Prematurity.
  - Multiple medical problems/disabilities.
  - Male gender.

HISTORY

- Out of proportion with extent of injuries.
- May be vague and/or inconsistent.
- Mental status deterioration, seizures, respiratory depression.

SIGNS AND SYMPTOMS (TYPICALLY NONSPECIFIC)

- Poor feeding.
- Vomiting.
- Apnea.
- Irritability.
- Seizures.
- Decreased tone.
- Decreased consciousness.

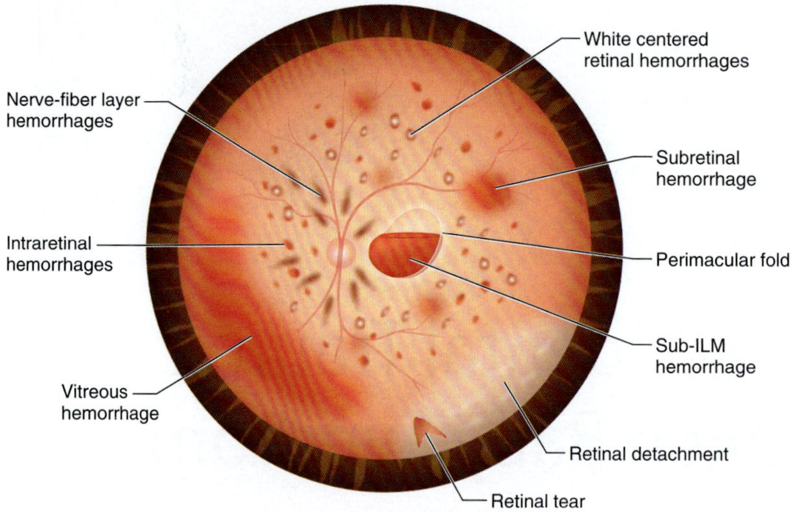

FIGURE 29.1. Diagram showing various types of hemorrhage seen in nonaccidental trauma patients.

OPHTHALMOLOGIC FINDINGS

- Common (Fig. 29.1):
  - Retinal hemorrhages (85% of cases) (Fig. 29.2).
    - Location:
      - Preretinal or vitreous.
      - Intraretinal (flame and dot blot).
      - Subretinal.
      - Tend to cluster in posterior pole but may extend throughout fundus.
    - Can be too numerous to count.
    - Usually bilateral but may be unilateral or asymmetric.
    - Last days to months, depending on location and severity, and it is impossible to date the hemorrhages by their appearance.
  - Circumferential macular folds.
  - Retinoschisis.
- Other:
  - Periorbital hematoma.
  - Eyelid laceration.

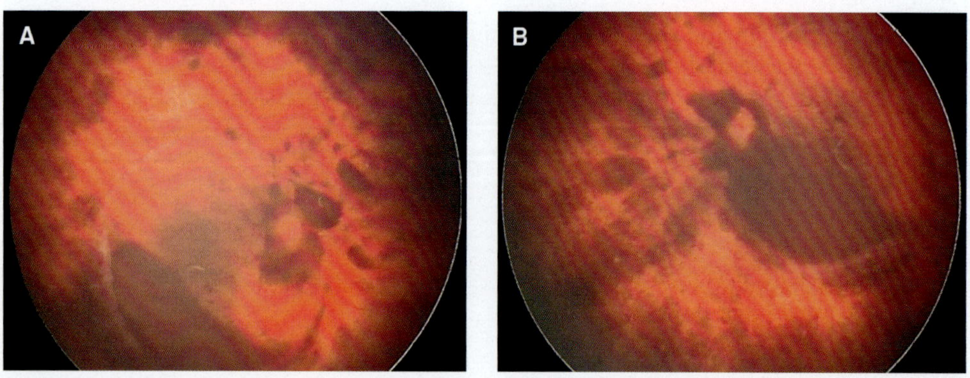

FIGURE 29.2. **A** (right eye) and **B** (left eye): Multiple and confluent retinal hemorrhages of different layers centered on the posterior pole in a 5-month-old child hospitalized for nonaccidental trauma. Note that many of the hemorrhages are white centered. There is also preretinal hemorrhage and a macular posterior vitreous detachment with perimacular folds OU. (Courtesy of Janine Collinge, MD.)

- Subconjunctival hemorrhage.
- Subluxed or dislocated lens.
- Cataracts.
- Glaucoma.
- Anterior chamber regression.
- Iridodialysis.
- Macular hole.
- Retinal breaks.
- Retinal detachment.
- Optic atrophy.
- Papilledema.

MANAGEMENT

- Check visual and pupillary responses
- Perform dilated (if permitted) fundus examination ideally within 24-48 hours.
- Carefully document examination findings.
  - Describe retinal hemorrhages:
    - Type.
    - Number.
    - Distribution/location.
    - Severity.
  - Make schematic drawings and/or obtain photographs.
  - Perform B-scan ultrasonography if there is no view posteriorly.
  - Provide differential diagnosis of retinal hemorrhages in assessment.
    - Nonaccidental trauma.
    - Perinatal (newborn retinal hemorrhages typically resolve by 4-6 weeks).
    - Fulminant meningitis.
    - Leukemia.
    - Coagulopathies.
    - Ruptured aneurysm.
- Communicate with pediatrician and abuse team and report suspicions to child protective services, if not already done. Be prepared to admit the child to the hospital to ensure safety.
- Monitor for resolution of hemorrhage.
- Consider vitrectomy for nonclearing vitreous hemorrhage, which may be amblyogenic.

LABORATORY TESTING AND RADIOLOGIC STUDIES

- Usually ordered by pediatrician or child abuse team.
- CBC.
- Liver function tests.
- Amylase.
- Coagulation studies:
  - PT: Prothrombin time
  - PTT: Partial thromboplastin time
  - INR: International normalized ratio
  - PFA: Platelet function assay
  - von Willebrand factor.
- Noncontrast head CT or MRI.
- Skeletal survey.

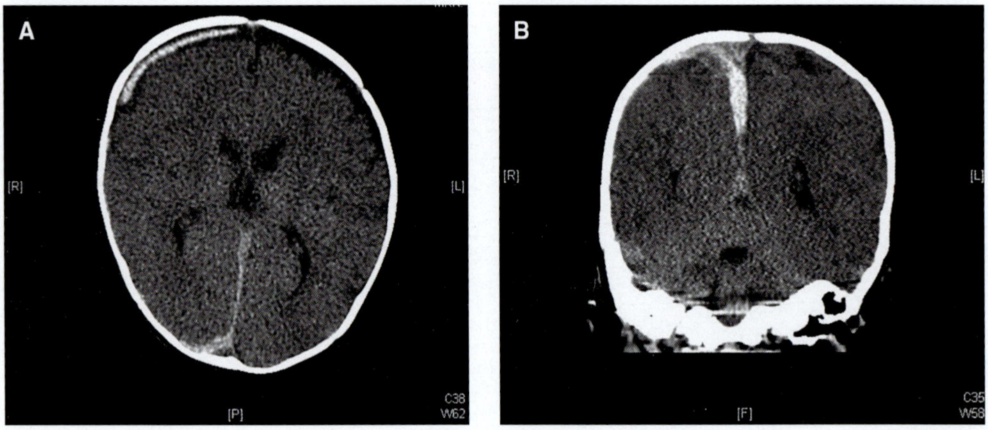

FIGURE 29.3. **A** (transverse) and **B** (coronal): CT images of the same infant presented in Figure 29.2 showing an acute subdural hematoma along the right aspect of the interhemispheric falx and along the right frontotemporal convexity.

X-ray findings such as long bone spiral fractures, skull fractures, and multiple rib fractures suggest abuse.

The most common finding on the head CT is subdural hematoma (Fig. 29.3A and B), but findings of cerebral edema, subarachnoid hemorrhage, and vascular infarction can also be seen.

Episodes of abuse are often repeated, and injuries of various ages are common and suggestive of abuse.

PROGNOSIS

- Thirty percent mortality; most survivors are left with permanent disability, including blindness, seizures, and cerebral palsy.
- Greater than 50% of survivors suffer visual impairment. The most common cause of decreased visual function in survivors is cortical injury, and second most common cause is optic atrophy.

Poor initial visual and pupillary responses strongly correlate with death.

Suggested Readings

Kempe CH, Silverman FN, Steele BF, et al. The battered-child syndrome. *JAMA*. 1962;181(1):17-24.

Sturmm V, Kecht PB, Landau K, Menke MN. Rare retinal haemorrhages in translational accidental head trauma in children. *Eye*. 2009;23(7):1535-1541.

Kaur B, Taylor D. Fundus hemorrhages in infancy. *Surv Ophthalmol*. 1992;37(1):1-17.

Morgan LA, Fouzdar Jain S, Svec A, et al. Clinical comparison of ocular and systemic findings in diagnosed cases of abusive and non-abusive head trauma. *Clin Ophthalmol*. 2018;22(12):1505-1510.

Chong CF, Misra SL, Escardo-Paton JA, et al. Predictors of long-term neurological outcomes in non-accidental head injury. *Eye*. 2018;32:608-614.

Levin AV, Alexander R, Binenbaum G, et al. Abusive Head Trauma/Shaken Baby Syndrome, AAO ONE Network, American Academy of Ophthalmology, Quality of Care Secretariat, Hoskins Center for Quality Eye Care, March 2015.

CHAPTER 30

Retinoblastoma

Miguel A. Materin, MD

BACKGROUND

Retinoblastoma is the most common intraocular primary malignancy in children with an estimated incidence of 1/15 000 live births. If untreated, it is a fatal condition.[1] Survival is about 95% in developed countries. Incidence of death is still high in Asia and Africa (up to 50%).[2] Retinoblastoma has no predilection for gender or race. Most patients are diagnosed before 5 years of age, typically in the first 3 years of life.

The most common sign on presentation is leukocoria; however, patients can also present with strabismus, red eye, glaucoma, orbital cellulitis, pseudohypopyon, and others.

Whenever retinoblastoma is suspected, the patient should be referred immediately to a specialized ophthalmologic cancer treatment center.

CLASSIFICATION

- Germline mutation: Usually represents the hereditary form; about 30%-40% of patients with retinoblastoma are affected with this type. They present at an early age, mostly in the first year of life. It can be bilateral (more common) or unilateral. These patients will be at higher risk to develop second, third, and even fourth cancers later in life. There is a 50% of chance patients with germline mutation will pass it to their offspring.[2]

The most common types of second, nonocular malignant neoplasm include osteosarcoma, soft tissue sarcoma, and cutaneous melanoma.

- Somatic mutation: 60%-70% of children with retinoblastoma have this type. It is unilateral and usually presents later compared to patients with germline mutations.

DIAGNOSIS

- Detailed family and personal history—specifically focusing on a history of retinoblastoma and other cancers.

> **All children with a family history of retinoblastoma should be screened soon after birth; screening should be repeated every 4-6 weeks until 1 year of age and then every 2-3 months until 3 years of age.**

- Complete ophthalmological examination (examination under general anesthesia).
- Indirect ophthalmoscopy (Figs. 30.1-30.3).
- B-scan ultrasonography (Fig. 30.2B).
  - Irregular mass.
  - Increased echogenicity compared to vitreous.
  - Fine calcifications (highly reflective foci with characteristic acoustic shadowing).

> **Calcifications are key in differentiating retinoblastoma from other mass lesions in young children.**

- Color fundus photography (wide angle).
- Fluorescein angiography.
- MRI scan.
- Genetic testing (on ALL patients with retinoblastoma).
- Do **not** perform biopsy or diagnostic vitrectomy because of risk of seeding.
- Differential diagnosis (most common):
  - Cataract.
  - Coats disease.

> **The major features of Coats disease include retinal telangiectasias, massive yellow exudates underlying an edematous retina, and exudative retinal detachment.**

  - Retinopathy of prematurity.
  - Ocular toxocariasis.
  - Persistent fetal vascular syndrome (PFV).

> **PFV is often unilateral and typically presents with moderate microphthalmia and other ocular malformations such as uveal coloboma.**

  - Astrocytic hamartoma.
  - Medulloepithelioma.
  - Retinal detachment.

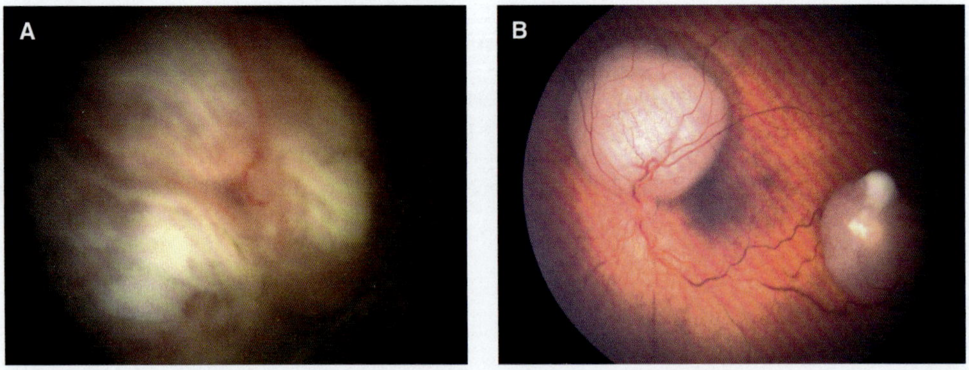

FIGURE 30.1. A 10-month-old boy with bilateral retinoblastoma. **A.** Right eye. **B.** Left eye.

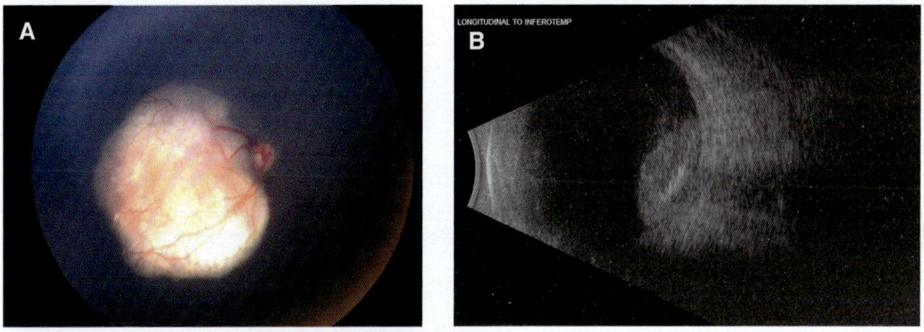

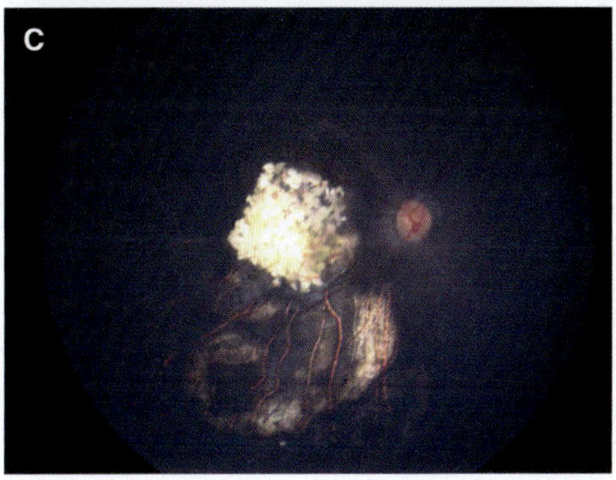

FIGURE 30.2 An 8-month-old girl with unilateral sporadic retinoblastoma. **A.** Fundus photograph of macular lesion. **B.** Ultrasound lesion demonstrates calcifications. **C.** Same patient after intra-arterial chemotherapy and transpupillary thermotherapy.

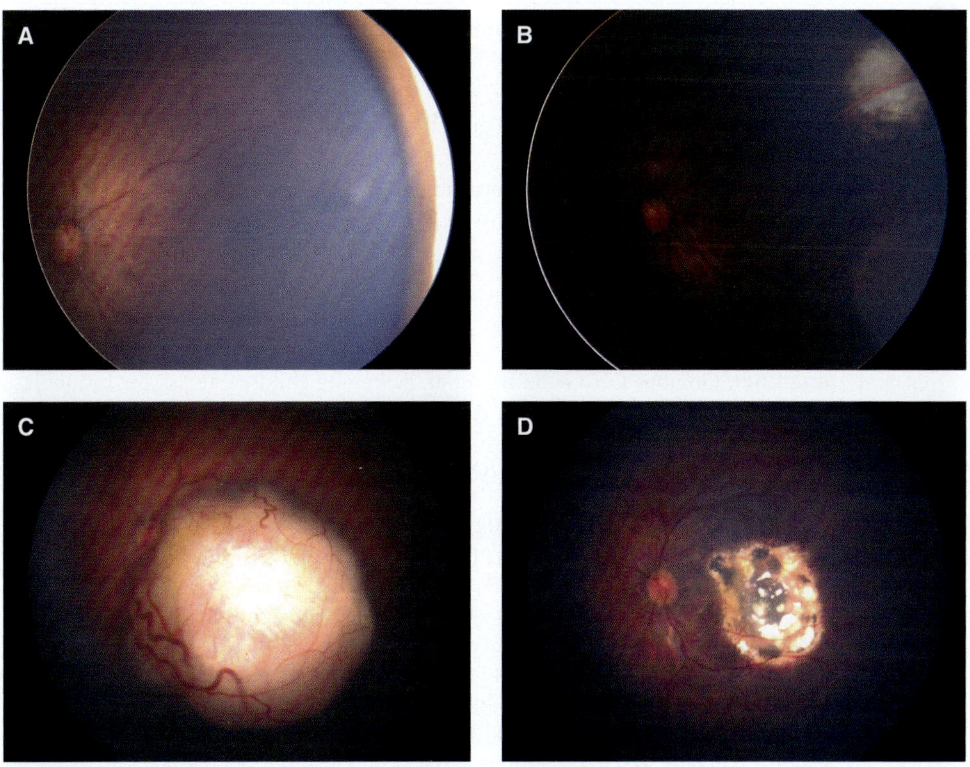

FIGURE 30.3. **A.** Right eye before treatment with small retinoblastoma. **B.** Right eye after systemic chemotherapy and cryotherapy. **C.** Left eye before treatment with large macular retinoblastoma. **D.** Left eye after systemic chemotherapy and transpupillary thermotherapy.

MANAGEMENT

- Multidisciplinary approach including ocular oncology, pediatric ophthalmology, pediatric oncology, neurosurgery or interventional neuroradiology, social workers, and nurses.
- Brain and orbit MRI before treatment—high resolution, contrast-enhanced.

It is important to avoid CT scans in these patients as the radiation exposure can increase the child's risk for other cancers in the future.

- Individualized treatment options based on patient presentation:
  - Chemotherapy:
    - Systemic (mainly for bilateral cases or post-enucleation in high-risk retinoblastoma or metastatic disease) (Fig. 30.3B).
    - Intra-arterial (for unilateral or bilateral cases)[3] (Fig. 30.2C).
    - Intravitreal (for vitreous seeds).[4]
  - Enucleation (see Chapter 37): mostly unilateral (for advanced intraocular retinoblastoma, neovascular glaucoma, failure of other treatments).
  - Radiation:
    - Brachytherapy.
    - External beam radiation (very last option due to increased risk to develop other cancers and orbit deformation).
  - Localized treatment:
    - Transpupillary thermotherapy (Figs. 30.2C and 30.3D).
    - Cryotherapy (Fig. 30.3B).
    - Laser photocoagulation.

Overall, over 9 out of 10 children with retinoblastoma in the United States are cured.

  - Late effects of treatment:
    - Children with retinoblastoma have an increased risk of developing subsequent neoplasms (see above).
    - Other late effects after retinoblastoma treatment:
      - Diminished orbital growth
      - Visual field defects
      - Hearing loss

References

1. Skalet AH, Gombos DS, Gallie BL, et al. Screening children at risk for retinoblastoma: consensus report from the American Association of Ophthalmic Oncologists and Pathologists. *Ophthalmology*. 2018;125:453-458.
2. Ramasubramanian A, Shields CL. *Retinoblastoma*. 1st ed. New Delhi, IND: Jaypee-Highlights Medical Publishers, INC; 2012.
3. Abramson DH, Marr BP, Francis JH, et al. Simultaneous bilateral ophthalmic artery chemosurgery for bilateral retinoblastoma (tandem therapy). *PLoS One*. 2016;11(6):e0156806. doi: 10.1371/journal.pone.0156806.
4. Francis JH, Brodie SE, Marr BP, et al. Efficacy and toxicity of intravitreous chemotherapy for retinoblastoma: four-year experience. *Ophthalmology*. 2017;124:488-495.
5. Abramson DH, Friedman DN, Gallie BL, et al. Clinical update. Retinoblastoma: Gentics That Affect Treatment and Lifelong Follow-Up. *EyeNet Magazine*. 2014.
6. PDQ Pediatric Treatment Editorial Board. Retinoblastoma Treatment (PDQ®): Health Professional Version. 2019 December 3. In: *PDQ Cancer Information Summaries* [Internet]. Bethesda, MD: National Cancer Institute (US); 2002. https://www.ncbi.nlm.nih.gov/books/NBK66006/

CHAPTER 31

Retinal Detachments and Vitrectomy

Xinxin Zhang, MD • Lejla Vajzovic, MD

HISTORY

- Onset—often delayed presentation as patient or caregivers may not recognize or report vision loss.[1]
- Birth history—retinopathy of prematurity, TORCH infections (rare cause).
- Medical history—Stickler (Fig. 31.1), Marfan, Wagner, Knobloch, atopic dermatitis, incontinentia pigmenti, hemoglobinopathies.
- Ocular history—previous intraocular surgery, X-linked retinoschisis, choroidal coloboma, retinal vascular disease (persistent fetal vasculature, familial vitreoretinopathy, uveitis).
- Family history.
- Trauma (Fig. 31.2)—most frequent cause; history may be lacking.
- Secondary findings—leukocoria and strabismus.

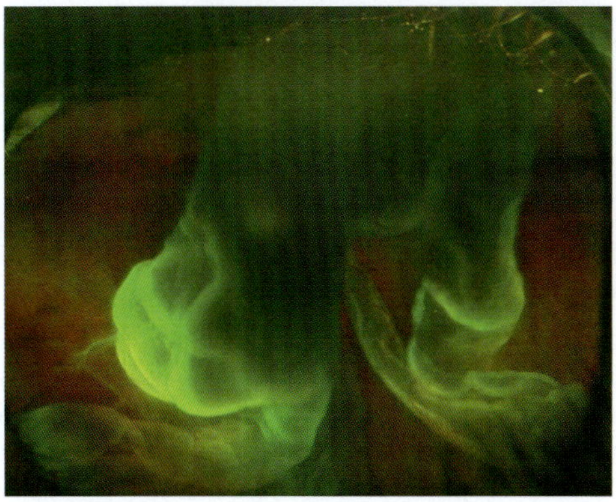

FIGURE 31.1. A 12-year-old male with amblyopia OD and moderate myopia OU presented with new-onset floaters and decreased visual acuity in the right eye. He was found to have retinal detachment of the right eye with giant retinal tears. Initial visual acuity on presentation was LP OD and 20/20 OS. The patient underwent repair with scleral buckle, pars plana vitrectomy, and endolaser. Subsequent repair was needed for PVR and subretinal fluid involving the macula. Visual acuity on follow-up 2 years later is 20/150 OD. Genetic testing showed positive COL2A1 mutation for Stickler syndrome.

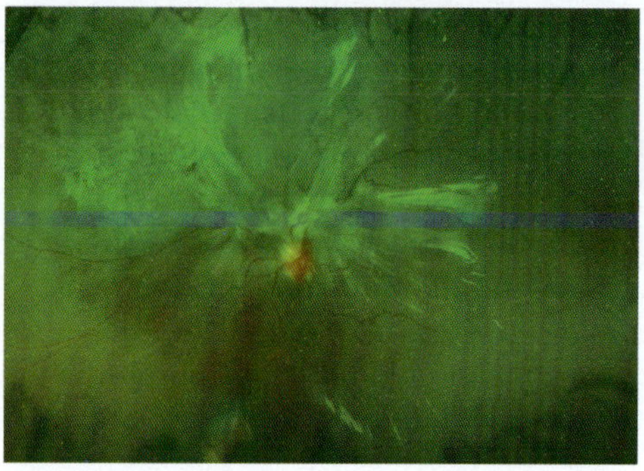

FIGURE 31.2. Macula-off combined tractional and rhegmatogenous retinal detachment of the left eye with grade C vitreoretinal proliferation of an 8-year-old female after BB gun injury to the left eye. The detachment was found at a follow-up appointment ~1 month after initial injury and initial surgery for removal of the BB from the orbit with closure of a conjunctival laceration.

EXAMINATION

Depending on the age and cooperation of the child, an examination under anesthesia may be necessary. Extra attention should be given to the following examination components:

- Best corrected visual acuity.
- Intraocular pressure—check for relative hypotony in the affected eye, which is present in 40% of unilateral uncomplicated retinal detachments.
- Anterior segment—look for pigmented cell in the anterior vitreous as it is strongly predictive of a retinal tear or hole.
- Posterior segment—perform scleral depression, which typically requires an exam under anesthesia. Note the extent of involvement, including the number of quadrants affected and the location of retinal holes, dialyses, and/or proliferative vitreoretinopathy (PVR).

In children, it is particularly important to perform a thorough evaluation of the fellow eye as they have higher incidence of bilateral pathology and bilateral presentation.

DIAGNOSTIC TESTING

Perform a B-scan ultrasonography if the view is inadequate (Fig. 31.3).

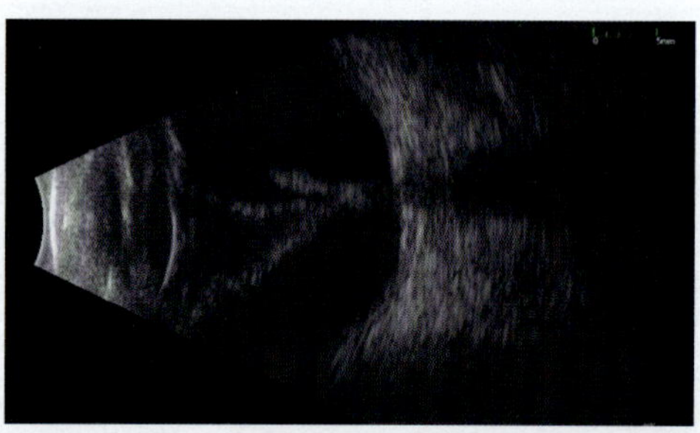

FIGURE 31.3. B-scan ultrasonography (vertical axial view) showing a total retinal detachment in a closed funnel configuration in the right eye of a 9-year-old male. The patient presented with intermittent exotropia and light perception vision in the right eye for likely more than 1-year duration. He was found to have total retinal detachment with giant retinal tear and dense vitreous membranes in the right eye as well as lattice degeneration with atrophic holes, small horseshoe tears, and syneretic vitreous in the left eye. Patient underwent pars plana vitrectomy and lensectomy with scleral buckle, endolaser, retinectomy, PVR peeling and silicone oil fill in the right eye, and 360 prophylactic laser retinopexy in the left eye. Patient is undergoing genetic testing for suspected inherited vitreoretinopathy.

SURGICAL CONSIDERATIONS

Manage patient and caregiver expectations regarding prognosis and possible need for further intervention. Retinal detachments in children tend to present when they are chronic and may require multiple surgeries. Perform prompt refraction and monitor for amblyopia postoperatively in order to achieve the best visual outcome.

Aphakic eyes become less hyperopic when the vitreous cavity is filled with silicone oil (eg, an aphakic eye with 10-12 diopters of hyperopia would have 4-6 diopters of hyperopia when filled with silicone oil). Phakic eyes typically develop 5-7 diopters of hyperopia when the vitreous cavity is filled with silicone oil.[1]

Scleral Buckling with Cryotherapy and Possible Subretinal Fluid Drainage

- Indications:
  - Retinal dialysis.
  - Peripheral tears without traction.[3]
- Contraindications[2]:
  - Opaque media.
  - Significant traction.
  - Breaks posterior to equator.
- Advantages[2]:
  - Minimizes lens injury.
  - Avoids vitreous removal difficulties.
  - Avoids need for a tamponade agent.[2]
- Disadvantages[3]:
  - May cause discomfort, strabismus, and diplopia.
  - May cause possible anterior segment ischemia.
  - May have buckle extrusion and cause secondary infection (rare).

General Vitrectomy Combined with Scleral Buckling Procedure (Fig. 31.4)

- Indications[4]:
  - Severe PVR worse than grade C.
  - Vitreous opacities (such as dense, unresolving vitreous hemorrhage).
  - Traction.

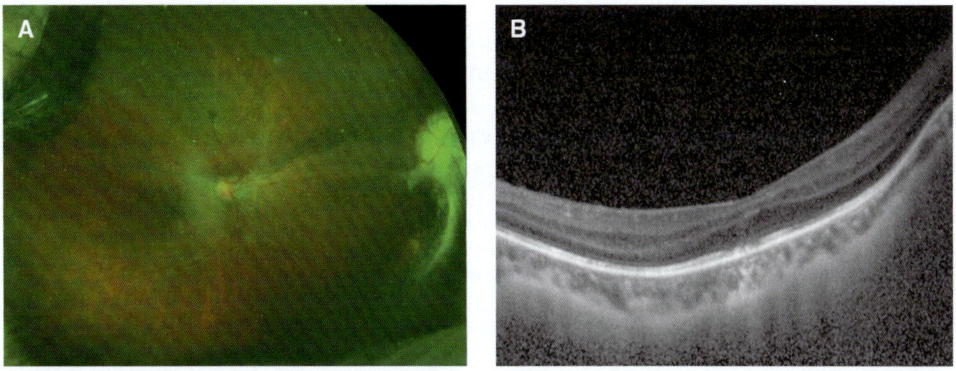

FIGURE 31.4. Postoperative Optos wide-field fundus photography **(A)** and optical coherence tomography **(B)** of the same patient in Figure 31.1 two years after initial presentation. The retina remains attached. The patient was status post combined scleral buckle and pars plana vitrectomy.

- Contraindications[4]:
  - Corneal opacity (inadequate view).
  - Suspected intraocular neoplasm (may seed orbit).
- Advantages[3]:
  - Clears opacities.
  - Enables better visualization of breaks.
- Disdvantages[3]:
  - Requires tamponading agent (typically longer acting gas).
    - If pathology is inferiorly located, silicone oil is required due to positioning difficulties in children.
    - Subsequent procedure required to remove oil.
  - Requires stringent positioning.
  - May result in secondary cataract.

Due to strong vitreoretinal adhesion, attempting complete removal of all vitreous or preretinal tissue may not be possible or desirable (high risk of iatrogenic retinal breaks).[5] However, posterior vitreous detachment induction is very important. Extreme caution should be taken to not create a retinal break in pediatric patients due to aggressive subsequent PVR, which may prompt secondary surgeries.[6]

If a tractional component is present anteriorly, lensectomy with total capsulectomy is needed to remove traction and the capsular scaffold for fibrovascular proliferation and traction.

SURGICAL PROCEDURES

Scleral buckle

- Confirm the size and location of the break.
- Perform a 360-degree conjunctival peritomy.
- Use tenotomy scissors to split Tenon's in four oblique quadrants.
- Using 2-0 silk, loop the rectus muscles.
- Perform 360-degree scleral depressed examination with either an indirect ophthalmoscope or a 25G chandelier.
- Mark retinal tears and perform cryopexy.
- Loop a broad/wide silicone band under the rectus muscles. Secure the band to itself in the superonasal quadrant using a Watzke sleeve.
- Determine band placement by selecting the distance from the limbus or the rectus muscle insertions that allows for the best support of retinal breaks.
- Secure the band in the four oblique quadrants using four mattress sutures (5-0 Mersilene or nylon), and tighten the band to produce sufficient globe indentation.
- Examine the retina again to confirm that the buckle is placed appropriately and that it supports the retinal breaks adequately.
- Consider external fluid drainage in a bullous retina that precludes break support.

Fish-mouthing of retinal breaks can be improved by changing buckle location and using intravitreal gas to flatten the breaks.

Vitrectomy (Video 31.1):

- Using a wide-field viewing system, place the endoilluminator and vitrectomy probe.
- Place trocars to ensure that the retina is drawn anteriorly.

- Typically, a placement of 1 mm posterior to limbus for neonates, 2 mm for 2-year-olds, and 3 mm for 3-year-olds approximates the appropriate location. Ora serrata localization with transillumination should be performed to ensure accurate placement.[7,8]
- If the posterior trans pars plicata lens-sparing technique is not feasible due to advanced and anteriorly displaced detachments with a very narrow operable space between the retina and the lens and high risk for iatrogenic break, use an anterior translimbal approach.[5,9]
- In the anterior translimbal approach, use a high cutting rate to minimize traction. Aspirate the soft lens with a vitrector after ensuring that vitreous has been removed.

- Induce a posterior vitreous detachment over the optic nerve.
- Perform a core pars plana vitrectomy, and shave the vitreous base. Complete removal of vitreous may not be feasible due to strong adhesions; care should be taken to avoid iatrogenic breaks.
- Use perfluorocarbon to flatten the retina, identify all retinal breaks using 360-degree scleral depression, and mark with diathermy.
- Perform a fluid-air exchange.
- Photocoagulate retinal breaks with endolaser.
- Perform air-gas or air-silicone oil exchange.
- Suture all sclerotomies with 7-0 Vicryl suture.

References

1. Stefánsson E, Anderson MM, Landers MB, et al. Refractive changes from use of silicone oil in vitreous surgery. *Retina*. 1988;8(1):20-23. doi: 10.1097/00006982-198808010-00005.
2. Ryan EH, Mittra RA. Scleral buckling vs vitrectomy: the continued role for scleral buckling in the vitrectomy era. *Arch Ophthalmol*. 2010;128(9):1202-1205. doi: 10.1001/archophthalmol.2010.192.
3. Schwartz S, Flynn H. Primary retinal detachment: scleral buckle or pars plana vitrectomy? *Curr Opin Ophthalmol*. 2006;17(3):245-250. doi: 10.1097/01.icu.0000193097.28798.fc.
4. Fine HF, Bhatnagar P, Spaide RF. 23-gauge vitrectomy. In: Bhavsar A, ed. *Retina and Vitreous Surgery: Surgical Techniques*. 1st ed. Surgical techniques in ophthalmology. Philadelphia, PA: Saunders Elsevier; 2009.
5. Ranchod T, Capone A. Tips and tricks in pediatric vitreoretinal surgery. *Int Ophthalmol Clin*. 2011;51(1):173-183. doi: 10.1097/IIO.0b013e3182009b73.
6. Trese MT, Capone A. Surgical approaches to infant and childhood retinal diseases: invasive methods. In: Hartnett ME, ed. *Pediatric Retina*. Philadelphia, PA: Lippincott Williams & Wilkins; 2005.
7. Lemley CA, Han DP. An age-based approach for planning sclerotomy placement during pediatric vitrectomy: a 12-year experience. *Trans Am Ophthalmol Soc*. 2007;105:86-91.
8. Wright LM, Harper CA, Chang EY. Management of infantile and childhood retinopathies: optimized pediatric pars plana vitrectomy sclerotomy nomogram. *Ophthalmol Retina*. 2018;2(12):1227-1234. doi: 10.1016/j.oret.2018.06.008.
9. Gan NY, Lam W-C. Special considerations for pediatric vitreoretinal surgery. *Taiwan J Ophthalmol*. 2018;8(4):237-242. doi: 10.4103/tjo.tjo_83_18.

Section VIII

Pediatric Oculoplastics

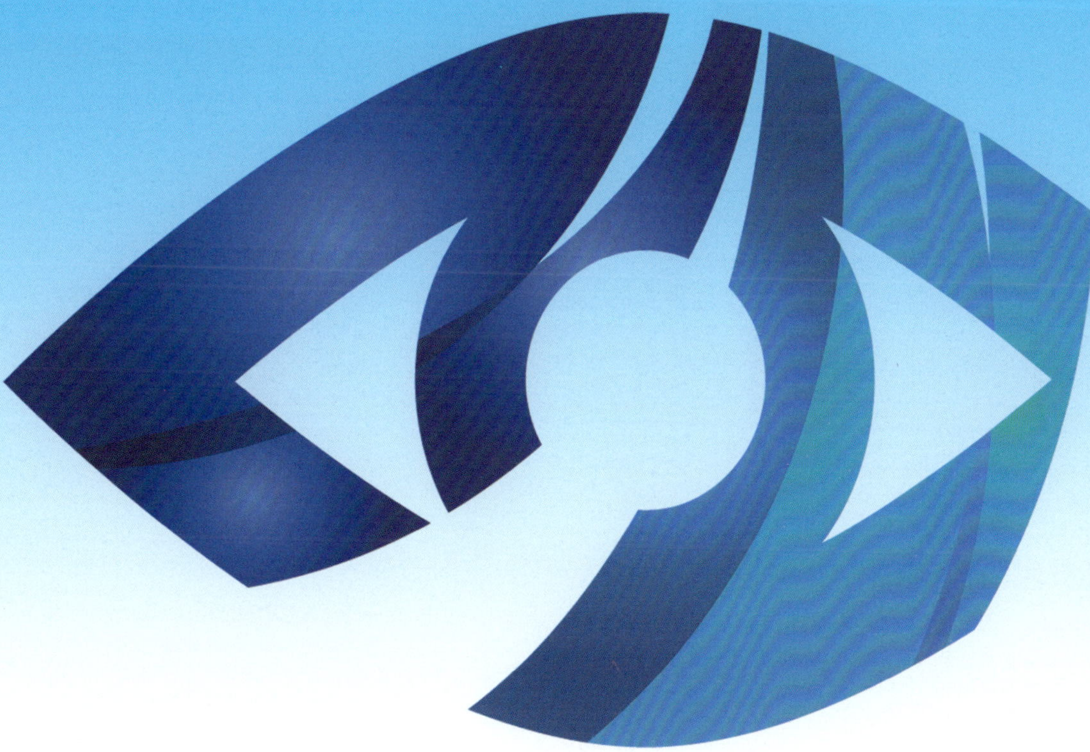

CHAPTER 32

Congenital Nasolacrimal Duct Obstruction

Ryan E. Davis, MD

DISEASE DESCRIPTION/PATHOPHYSIOLOGY

Congenital nasolacrimal duct obstruction (NLDO) is a relatively common problem, occurring in up to 20% of infants in the first year of life.[1] Although most patients are affected in one eye, NLDO is frequently bilateral. Symptoms range from mild epiphora to frank mattering of the eyelids with a mucopurulent discharge. The site of the obstruction is most commonly at the distal end of the nasolacrimal duct (valve of Hasner). Other causes of epiphora/discharge should be ruled out (including primary congenital glaucoma, dacryocystitis, conjunctivitis, or corneal infections) prior to making the diagnosis of NLDO. Clinical findings of NLDO include increased tear lake as well as asymmetric or positive dye disappearance test. The dye disappearance test is performed by placing fluorescein dye in both eyes and waiting for 5 minutes. A positive test is either asymmetric clearing from the suspected involved eye or failure to clear in cases of bilateral NLDO.

Anisometropia occurs at a greater rate in unilateral NLDO patients compared with bilateral NLDO patients and occurs at a greater rate than in the general pediatric population. Due to the increased risk of anisometropic amblyopia in these patients, it is important to perform a cycloplegic refraction and periodically follow patients with NLDO and anisometropia.[2]

MANAGEMENT OPTIONS

Therapeutic interventions for NLDO can be classified according to timing/location of therapy as well as intervention chosen. Infants <6 months are generally observed (unless additional clinical information is available, which favors earlier intervention, ie, dacryocele (Fig. 32.1), recurrent dacryocystitis). The Crigler massage (described below) is a noninvasive treatment option that parents can perform prior to surgical intervention. After 6 months of age, the timing of treatment is provider dependent. Spontaneous resolution is less likely after 9 months of age, and probing efficacy decreases after 15 months of age.[3] Earlier probing may obviate the need for general anesthesia, as younger infants can be safely swaddled and probed in the office. The Pediatric Eye Disease Investigator

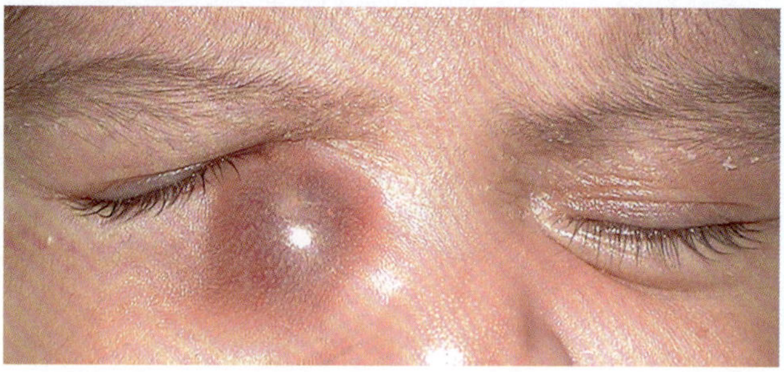

FIGURE 32.1. Dacryocele in a 3-day-old infant. (Courtesy of Laura B. Enyedi, MD.)

Group found that among infants aged 6 to <10 months who were observed for 6 months with Crigler massage, 66% resolved spontaneously. However, in this prospective randomized clinical trial, earlier in-office probing was as successful and less costly than observation/probing under general anesthesia (with the downside that 66% of patients would be probed in-office who would otherwise resolve spontaneously).[4]

NONSURGICAL TREATMENT

Crigler massage: Place the thumb or forefinger in the medial canthus at the level of the nasolacrimal sac and with firm pressure rub the finger down along the path of the nasolacrimal duct. After the massage, upward pressure can be applied to empty the sac and give temporary relief of mucoid discharge.

INDICATIONS FOR SURGERY

Indications for surgical intervention are (1) clinical signs and symptoms consistent with NLDO and (2) failure to spontaneously resolve.

SURGICAL PROCEDURES

Nasolacrimal Duct Probing and Irrigation (Video 32.1)

- Using a nasal speculum, place intranasal oxymetazoline-soaked pledgets into the involved nostril with bayonet forceps.
- Using a punctal dilator or a large safety pin, dilate the superior or inferior punctum. Although either punctum can be used, probing through the superior canaliculus and irrigating through the inferior punctum ensures both are open while avoiding potential iatrogenic trauma to the inferior canaliculus, through which the majority of tear drainage occurs.
- Place a no. 0 or no. 00 Bowman probe into the punctum and pass it through the canaliculus until the hard stop of the bony lacrimal fossa is felt. Following the normal anatomy (holding probe perpendicular to lid while inserting it into punctum, then rotating parallel to the lid to follow the canaliculus) can assist with insertion. Lateral traction of the lid facilitates passing the probe medially, decreasing the risk of trauma to the canaliculus. It is important to ensure that the probe is resting against bone without tissue between the probe and the bony wall, as this tissue may be torn or injured during the next step. Surgeon experience is crucial as proper placement is determined with "feel" as opposed to probe position.
- Once the probe tip abuts the bony wall, discontinue lateral traction on the eyelid and rotate the probe up 90 degrees until it falls inferiorly into the nasolacrimal duct. Keeping the probe on the same plane as the eyelid as it is rotated (bringing the probe over the superior orbital rim/brow) helps the distal tip drop into the nasolacrimal duct. Once in the duct, advance the probe into the nose (Fig. 32.2). If a membranous obstruction is present, the surgeon will frequently feel the release of resistance as the probe clears the obstruction.

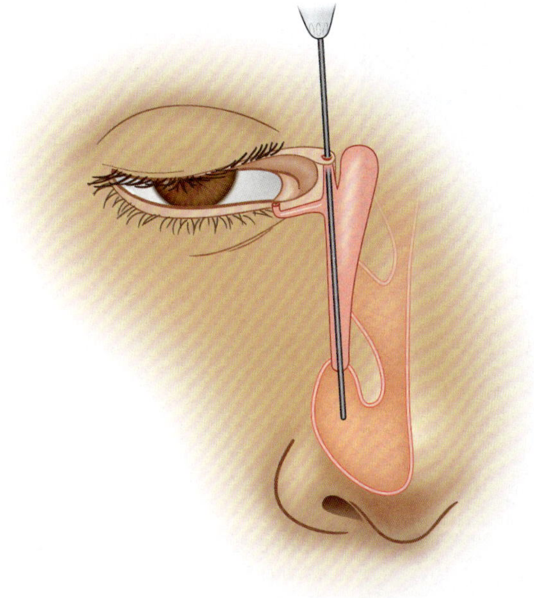

FIGURE 32.2. Probe in nasolacrimal duct. Note the probe exits the nasolacrimal duct at the level of the inferior nasal meatus.

- After removing the pledgets from the nasal cavity, confirm the position of the probe in the nose by placing a second probe behind the inferior turbinate and feeling for "metal-on-metal" contact or by seeing the original probe moving. The second probe should be directed lateral and inferior to the inferior turbinate, which can be visualized when looking into the nostril extending from the lateral wall of the nose. The direction of the second probe will be inferior and lateral pointing in the direction of the earlobe.
- After successful probing, place an irrigating cannula into one of the puncta and irrigate fluorescein-stained balanced salt solution into the nasolacrimal duct while simultaneously suctioning using a French suction catheter through the nose. Successful suctioning of the fluorescein tinted fluid from the nose ensures a patent nasolacrimal system.

Nasolacrimal Duct Balloon Dilation (Fig. 32.3)

- Balloon dilation can be used in both patients who failed simple probing and irrigation as well as primary treatment during a probe where anatomic or intraoperative findings increase the likelihood of probing failure (ie, tight nasolacrimal duct, older patients, patients with Down syndrome).[5]

> **Balloon dacryoplasty has a similar efficacy to monocanalicular stenting in children with congenital NLDO. The major advantage to balloon dacryoplasty is that no silicone tube is left in the lacrimal system.[6]**

- Specific directions can be found on the insert of all commercially available balloons, but the generic technique involves probing with the balloon deflated as you would in a simple probing, advancing the balloon cannula to a specific mark, and then inflating the balloon with the included pump for a specified amount of time at a specific pressure.

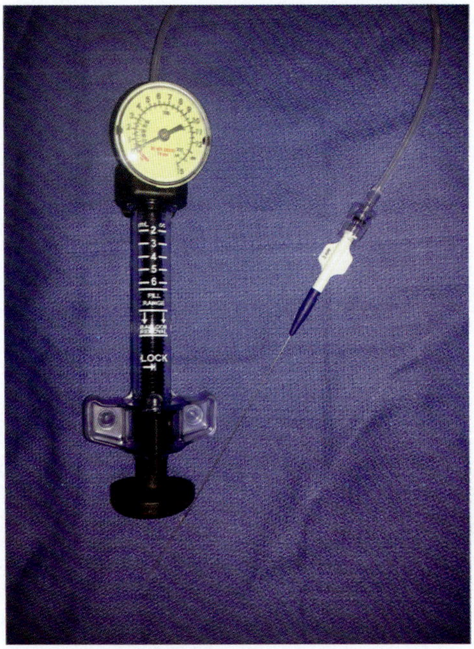

FIGURE 32.3. Balloon dacryoplasty set (Quest Medical, Inc, Allen, TX) includes a probe with a balloon on the end and a device to inflate the balloon in the nasolacrimal system.

For patients ≤30 months of age, the manufacturer recommends the 2-mm balloon diameter. For patients over 30 months of age, the 3-mm diameter balloon is recommended. The 5-mm balloon diameter is used for dacryocystorhinostomy cases.

In order to minimize trauma to the outflow system during removal, maximally deflate the balloon and twist the catheter counterclockwise as you pull it out.

Nasolacrimal Intubation

- Monocanalicular:
  - A variety of monocanalicular stents are commercially available. One common type used for NLDO is composed of a silicone stent that has on one end a self-retaining punctal plug and on the other end a metal probe. The distal end of the metal probe has a round bulbous tip.
  - Insert the metal probe into the punctum (either upper or lower) and pass it down the NLD as described above.
  - Once the rounded tip end of the probe is in the nose, place a special hook under the inferior turbinate in the same manner and direction as the confirmatory probe was placed in the previous step. Slide the hook along the lateral wall of the nose while keeping the opening of the hook oriented toward the septum. This position helps prevent excessive bleeding caused by trauma from the hook.
  - Once the hook is confirmed to be in the correct place as determined by "metal-on-metal" feel of the intranasal probe, hook the shaft of the intranasal probe.
  - Then, slide the hook up the shaft until it engages with the rounded tip. Gently pulling back on the intranasal probe after engagement ensures that the hook stays engaged with the rounded tip as the hook is pulled out of the nose. Once the probe is retrieved through the nose, cut off the metal probe and seat the punctal plug into the punctum.
  - Ritleng type stents (described below) are also available as monocanalicular stents (FCI Ophthalmics, Pembroke, MA).

- Bicanalicular:
  - The two most common bicanalicular stents used for NLDO are the Crawford (Fig. 32.4, FCI Ophthalmics, Pembroke, MA) and the Ritleng.
  - Place the Crawford tubes the same way as the monocanalicular stent described above. However, in bicanalicular stents, the silicone tubing has a separate metal rounded-tipped probe on both ends.
  - Place one probe into the superior canaliculus and retrieve. Then, place the second probe into the inferior canaliculus and retrieve. Then, cut off the probes and tie the silicone ends together. Crawford stents are also available with a Dacron suture within the lumen of the silicone tubing. The silicone ends of these can stripped and the Dacron suture ends tied together. These are less traumatic to remove, as the suture knot is small and easily retrieved through the punctum, but this style takes additional time in the OR to strip the silicone tubing from the suture.
  - Allow the tied ends to retract back into the nose or suture it to the lateral nasal mucosa with a 6-0 silk suture. If sutured, it is important to ensure that there is not excessive traction to avoid cheese-wiring of the punctum.
  - Ritleng probes consist of a hollow introducer probe with stylet. The introducer probe has a narrow slit along the side. Place the introducer probe into position in the nasolacrimal system as described above with the stylet in place, and then, remove the stylet. Feed the stent into the hollow introducer probe and through the nasolacrimal system and retrieve through the nose. Once the guide suture is retrieved through the nose, back the probe out of the nasolacrimal duct to the point where the stent narrows and can be removed from the probe through the narrow groove.
  - Ideally, the stents are left in place for 3-6 months but can be effective if left for shorter time periods. If the stent has been sutured into the nose, check to see if the silk nasal suture is present prior to stent removal. If still present, defer removal another month or two. Removal can be performed by using topical anesthesia and rotating the stent until the knot is visible. The stent is then cut and pulled out of the nasolacrimal system through the puncta.

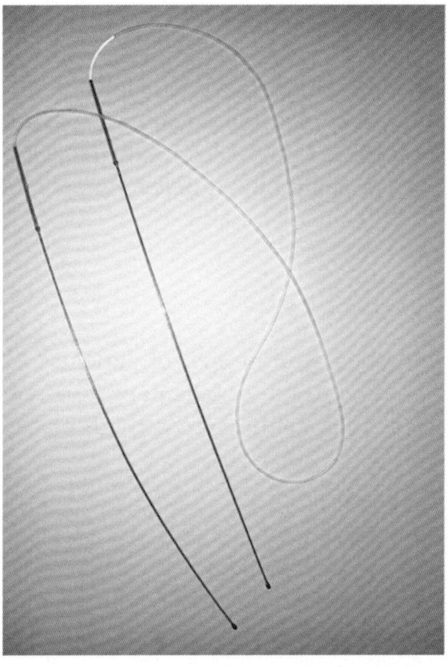

FIGURE 32.4. Crawford bicanalicular stent includes a ball on the end of the stent that is hooked under the inferior turbinate.

Nasal Turbinate Infracture

- Like intubation or balloon dacryoplasty, infracture of the nasal turbinate can be performed at the initial probing or reserved for cases refractive to simple probing. Infracture of the turbinate can be helpful if the tight turbinate impedes retrieval of the canalicular stent.
- To perform infracture, place a periosteal elevator under the inferior turbinate and rotate inward and upward. Alternatively, grasp the inferior turbinate with a hemostat and rotate toward the midline.
- Possible complications of inferior turbinate infracture include nasal bleeding, nasal whistling, or a dry nose.

Dacryocele and Nasal Endoscopy

Dacryocele (Fig. 32.1), also known as dacryocystocele or amniotocele, occurs when both a distal and proximal obstruction prevents any outflow of secretions from the nasolacrimal sac/duct. This usually occurs when an NLDO results in distention of the nasolacrimal sac, which occludes the common canaliculus and prevents retrograde reflux. If not treated with probing, dacryoceles can either resolve spontaneously or become infected/inflamed within a few weeks. If infected, infants are typically admitted for treatment with parenteral antibiotics because of the risk of rapid progression to orbital cellulitis as a result of the fragile infant septum. This is followed by decompression/probing for definitive treatment of the dacryocele. A nasal mucocele (bulging of the nasal mucosa into the nose) can be treated at the time of probing with nasal endoscopy and removal of the nasal cyst.

Dacryoceles can be associated with life-threatening respiratory complications in neonates, who are obligate nasal breathers. Parents should be queried about shortness of breath with feeding in infants with dacryoceles.

POSTOPERATIVE CARE

Symptoms typically resolve immediately following successful probing. Topical antibiotic/steroid can be used for 3-4 days following probing to decrease inflammation. Intranasal oxymetazoline spray can be used for a few days following probing to help with minor bleeding and swelling. Transient bacteremia can occur following any intranasal procedure, so patients at increased risk (ie, congenital heart defects) may require prophylactic systemic antibiotics.[4]

PROGNOSIS

Simple probing and irrigation procedure is successful in 90% of patients.[7] Complications are rare but can include iatrogenic trauma to the canaliculi or false passage into the nose. Other complications with bicanalicular stenting are early displacement and corneal abrasion.

ACKNOWLEDGMENTS

The views expressed are those of the author and do not reflect the official views or policy of the Department of Defense or its Components.

References

1. MacEwen CJ, Young JD. Epiphora during the first year of life. *Eye*. 1991;5:596-600.
2. Kipp MA, Kipp MA Jr, Struthers W. Anisometropia and amblyopia in nasolacrimal duct obstruction. *J AAPOS*. 2013;17(3):235-238.
3. Sathiamoorthi S, Frank RD, Mohney BG. Spontaneous resolution and timing of intervention in congenital nasolacrimal duct obstruction. *JAMA Ophthalmol*. 2018;136:1281-1286.
4. Lee, KA, Chandler, DL, Repka MX, et al. A randomized trial comparing the cost-effectiveness of 2 approaches for treating unilateral nasolacrimal duct obstruction. *Arch Ophthalmol*. 2012;130:1525-1533.
5. Lueder GT. Treatment of nasolacrimal duct obstruction in children with trisomy 21. *J AAPOS*. 2000;4(4):230-232.
6. Wladis EJ, Aakalu VK, Yen MT, et al. Balloon dacryoplasty for congenital nasolacrimal duct obstruction: a report by the American Academy of Ophthalmology. *Ophthalmology*. 2018;125:1654-1657.
7. American Academy of Ophthalmology. *Basic and Clinical Science Course: Pediatric Ophthalmology and Strabismus. 2010–2011*. 2010:208.

Suggested Reading

Valcheva KP, Murgova SV, Krivoshiiska EK. Success rate of probing for congenital nasolacrimal duct obstruction in children. *Folia Med (Plovdiv)*. 2019;61:97-103.

CHAPTER 33

Dermoid Cyst Removal

James W. Weightman, MD

PREOPERATIVE CONSIDERATIONS

On physical examination, determine whether the cystic lesion is a simple superficial dermoid cyst or a complex cyst with orbital or cranial involvement. If orbital or cranial involvement is suspected, imaging is recommended. Removal of a dermoid cyst is performed to prevent slow enlargement over time, remodeling of the underlying bone, and inflammation in the case of rupture. This procedure is often done around the time of the first birthday.

Physical Examination

- Assess for:
  - Cyst mobility (a dermoid should feel rubbery and attached to bone at the base).
  - Location (mobility and location determine incision location).
  - Inflammation (if already ruptured, the cyst may be more difficult to dissect free).
  - Orbital involvement (proptosis or ptosis, assess whether cyst extends into orbit beyond the rim).
- Differential diagnosis includes lipoma, hemangioma, encephalocele, meningocele.
- The location of the cystic lesion guides the differential diagnosis.
  - Lateral orbital rim (frontozygomatic suture)—assess for mobility to rule out a "dumbbell" dermoid with orbital or intracranial extension.
  - Medial orbital rim (frontoethmoid or frontolacrimal sutures).
    - Assess mobility to rule out meningocele or meningoencephalocele and intracranial or intraorbital extension.
    - Determine if the mass expands with Valsalva or is pulsatile as this may indicate a meningocele or encephalocele.
  - Orbit.
    - Assess for proptosis.
    - Assess for ptosis.

Imaging

- CT scan[1]:
  - Dermoid cysts are usually well-circumscribed lesions with a low-density lumen.
  - Dermoid cysts are often associated with bony remodeling.

  - Dermoid cysts may have fluid and fat levels internally with variable internal density in the lumen.
- MRI:
  - T1 images typically are hypointense internally.
  - T2 images typically are hyperintense internally.
- Ultrasound and color Doppler imaging (CDI):
  - Dermoid cysts generally have a smooth border with either an echogenic or hypoechogenic lumen.
  - CDI is useful to differentiate between vascular and cystic lesions.

CT scans are best suited for imaging bony abnormalities; while MRIs provide better images of soft tissues. Because MRIS do not use radiations, they are generally preferable in children.

SURGICAL PROCEDURE: EXCISIONAL BIOPSY OF DERMOID CYST

Simple cysts outside the skull are excised through an incision in the skin. If a cyst is more complex and extends deeply with attachments inside the orbit or extension to the brain, it may be necessary to consult otolaryngology, neurosurgery, or oculoplastics to assist with the cyst removal.

- Consider a preoperative dose of IV antibiotics for orbital surgeries.
- Prep the surgical site with a Betadine scrub.
- Infiltrate local anesthesia around the lesion (1%-2% lidocaine or 0.25%-0.5% Marcaine with 1:200,000 epinephrine).
- Perform the skin incision.
  - Superficial lateral periorbital dermoids can be approached by lid crease, sub-brow (Wright), or orbital rim incisions. Lid crease incisions offer the best cosmetic outcome (Figs. 33.1 and 33.2).
  - Superficial medial periorbital dermoids can be approached through a sub-brow, lid crease, or frontoethmoid incision (modified Lynch) (Fig. 33.2).
  - The superficial skin incision is generally made with a scalpel (Bard Parker no. 15 blade).
  - Endoscopic removal of superficial periorbital dermoid cysts can be performed using brow-lift endoscopes and incisions superior to the hairline. Care must be taken not to damage the temporal branch of the facial nerve during lateral dissection and the supratrochlear or supraorbital nerves during medial dissection.[2]
- Dissect carefully through the deep dermal and subcutaneous tissue with blunt tip scissors until the smooth yellowish cyst wall is identified. Bluntly dissect the cyst free from soft tissue attachments (blunt tip scissors, a hemostat, and cotton tip applicators can all be helpful). Leaving a bit of tissue on the surface of the cyst to grasp can help later with elevating the cyst.

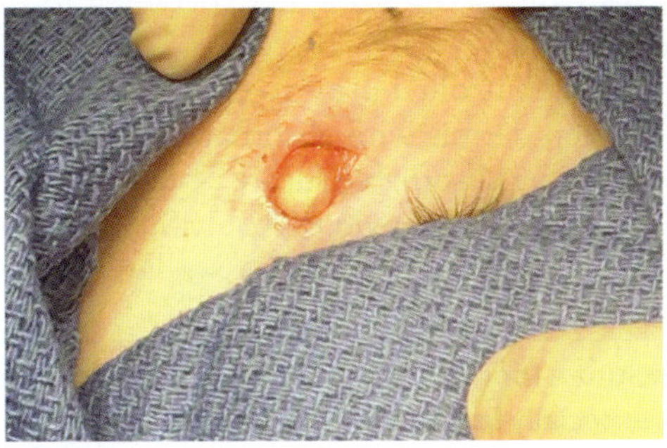

FIGURE 33.1. Sub-brow incision for a periorbital frontozygomatic dermoid cyst excision. (Courtesy of Tammy Yanovitch, MD.)

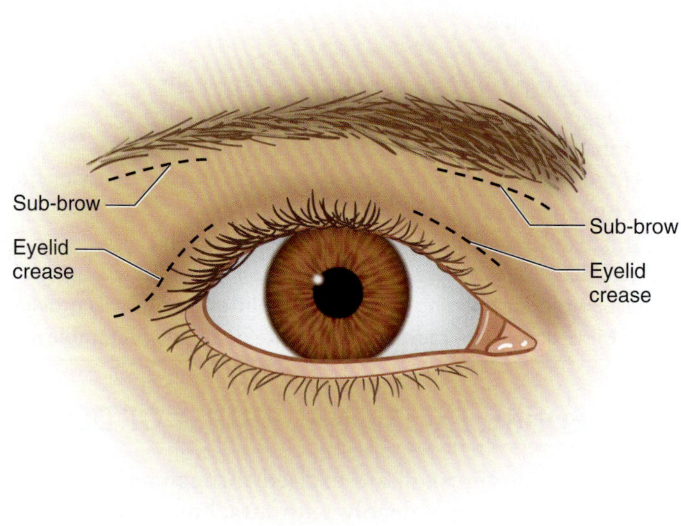

FIGURE 33.2. Incision sites for dermoid cyst removal.

Dermoid cysts are usually tethered to the periosteum near the bony suture lines and may be nestled down into a bony hollow. They are often bigger than they initially appear. Ensure that the dermoid cyst is free from all other soft tissue attachments prior to freeing the dermoid cyst from the periosteum as the cyst wall is often thin, friable, and may rupture at the base.

- Once the cyst is free from all other soft tissue attachments, use a freer elevator to lift the cyst. Cryoextraction with a retinal CryoProbe may be used to grasp the cyst during the final stage of excision. Apply the CryoProbe to the cyst wall and ensure that an ice ball forms on the cyst. A CryoProbe can also be used to seal a ruptured section of the cyst.
- If the dermoid cyst ruptures during excision, excise the cyst wall completely and copiously irrigate the cyst contents from the wound. Consider using suction to decompress the cyst contents if rupture occurs.

Most ruptured cysts do not result in postoperative inflammation if the cyst contents are adequately irrigated.[3]

- Dermoid cysts have a very typical appearance, and the diagnosis is usually easily confirmed during surgery (Fig. 33.3). Consider sending the specimen to pathology in formalin for confirmation of diagnosis.
- Use cautery to make sure all bleeding is controlled prior to closing the wound.
- Close all deep tissue spaces and the deep dermis with absorbable suture (4-0 to 6-0 Vicryl). Close the superficial skin with either absorbable suture (4-0 to 6-0 Gut or fast-absorbing gut) or nonabsorbable suture (4-0 to 6-0 nylon). Apply Steri-Strips to cover the wound, consider a pressure bandage if there is concern for swelling or bleeding.

An obvious advantage to using an absorbable suture for closure is that it does not require removal, which may be difficult to do without sedation, especially in younger children or children with special needs.

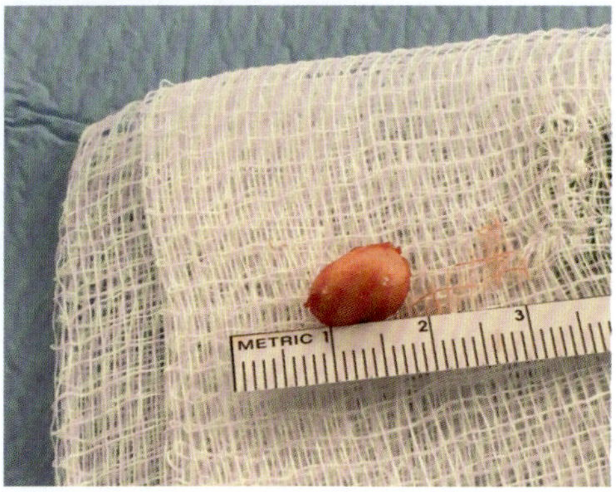

FIGURE 33.3. Typical appearance of a periocular dermoid cyst.

POSTOPERATIVE CONSIDERATIONS

Use an antibiotic ointment to the wound until healed. Remove nonabsorbable skin sutures in 5-10 days. Good sun protection in the first year after surgery can help with scarring. Expect a dent in the bone in the location of the dermoid. This can remodel over time.

ACKNOWLEDGMENTS

The views expressed in this chapter are those of the author and do not necessarily reflect the official policy or position of Fort Belvoir Community Hospital, the Defense Health Agency, Department of Defense, or U.S. Government.

References

1. Shields JA, Shields CL. Orbital cysts of childhood—classification, clinical features, and management. *Surv Ophthalmol*. 2004;49:281-299.
2. Chater-Cure G, Hoffman C, Knopman J, et al. Endoscopy-assisted removal of periorbital inclusion cysts in children. *J Neurosurg Pediatr*. 2011;7:161-164.
3. Siah WF, Al-Muhaylib AA, Rajak S, et al. Clinical outcomes of ruptured periorbital and orbital dermoid cysts. *Ophthal Plast Reconstr Surg*. 2017;33:264-267.

CHAPTER 34

Lid Lesions

Alice A. Lin, MD

PEDIATRIC LID LESIONS

Preoperative Considerations

One of the main preoperative considerations with pediatric lid lesions is whether there is need for surgical treatment at all. Many lid lesions will get better with time and nonsurgical treatments. Given most caregivers' aversion to surgery and general anesthesia for their child, try to maximize all nonsurgical options first.

Many lesions may also be treated under local anesthesia. The ability to safely remove a lid lesion without sedation depends on the individual patient. Children and even some teenagers often will not be able to tolerate the procedure without sedation due to anxiety and stress.

If performing the procedure with local anesthesia in the clinic setting, place 1 drop of topical anesthetic in the eye on the affected side so the patient will not experience stinging from the Betadine prep. Then, slowly inject 2% lidocaine with epinephrine around the affected area. Use a 27G to 30G needle on a 3- or 5-cc syringe. The local injection requires time (~5-8 minutes) for the lidocaine to induce anesthesia and for the epinephrine to induce vasoconstriction.

When the patient is under general anesthesia, a local anesthetic with epinephrine should still be used. If used early, the local anesthetic can control bleeding but can sometimes make it more difficult to localize a small lesion. Consider using a marking pen to delineate lesions prior to injection of local anesthetic. Be careful not to remove marks during the sterile prep. Alternatively, the anesthetic can be injected at the end of the case to provide postoperative hemostasis and anesthesia.

CHALAZION

Preoperative Considerations

There are many options for treating acute chalazia that span from over-the-counter (OTC) or home-based treatments to surgical interventions. Chronic and recurrent chalazia are increasingly felt to be related to a Demodex infestation/overgrowth[1] so long-term treatment is aimed at decreasing the mite burden around the eyelids and eyelashes.

Home-based treatments include frequent warm compresses and eyelid scrubs. Blepharitis and chalazia may respond to daily eyelid scrubs with baby shampoo. Other non-prescription options include tea tree oil scrubs and OTC hypochlorous acid sprays. A daily dose of 500-1500 mg of a good-quality omega-3 supplement can be added to address meibomian gland dysfunction.

Prescribed medical treatments may include topical antibiotic/steroid drops or ointment, topical azithromycin (Azasite), and oral antibiotics such as oral azithromycin, erythromycin, or doxycycline (over 8 years of age only). LipiFlow or MiBiFlow treatments can also be administered in the office in some cooperative children.

Surgical interventions include Kenalog injections as well as incision and drainage of chalazia. Depending on the patient, these procedures can be performed in the office under local anesthesia or in the operating room under general anesthesia.

Surgical Planning

- Manage patient and caregiver expectations. Warn caregivers that the incision and drainage of chalazia only treats the current lesion(s) and does not prevent future chalazia from forming.
- Consider consent for treatment of both eyes or all four eyelids if the patient is under general anesthesia. Perform a thorough examination under anesthesia and drain any chalazia present. The 67808 CPT code includes the incision and drainage under anesthesia of multiple chalazia on multiple eyelids.
- If a chalazion is external, excise the chalazion externally and remove all affected skin. Warn caregivers that they will see an open wound or defect in the eyelid but that this typically heals well with minimal scarring.
- Surgical instruments:
  - a Bard Parker no. 11 blade or a no. 15-degree stab blade, chalazion lid clamp, chalazion curettes, sterile cotton tipped applicators, 4 × 4 gauze pads, 2% lidocaine with epinephrine on a 27G needle, a 1- or 3-cc syringe, triamcinolone acetonide (Kenalog) (10, 20, or 40 mg/mL), fine toothed forceps, Westcott scissors.

Surgical Procedure

- Inject local anesthesia with epinephrine (see Chapter 1) around each chalazion if desired. Consider marking small chalazia with a permanent marker prior to injection.
- Clean and prep each affected eyelid with Betadine prep.
- Center and apply chalazion clamp to affected area. In most cases, it is preferable to evert the eyelid and incise the tarsal conjunctiva. However, external chalazia should be addressed externally, with all affected skin removed.
- For intralesional steroid injections, draw up 0.1-0.2 cc of the steroid and inject the affected area using a 27G needle, either transcutaneously or transconjunctivally.
  - May repeat in 2 weeks if not resolved.
  - Consider using triamcinolone acetonide 10 or 20 mg/mL or injecting transconjunctivally in patients with pigmented skin because of the risk of skin depigmentation.

Be aware that any intralesional injection carries the risk of vision loss due to a steroid embolus causing a central retinal artery occlusion (CRAO).

- Surgical incision and drainage:
  - Internal chalazion—make a vertical incision over the center of the chalazion with a sharp blade. Take care not to extend the incision to the lid margin to avoid creating a notch. Express the contents using sterile cotton tipped applicators and a curette. Use a curette to ensure that there are no further pockets that need to be cleared. If there is fibrotic scar tissue, consider using triamcinolone acetonide

to augment the treatment. 0.1-0.2 cc of triamcinolone acetonide can be dripped over the area or injected around the cavity. Any steroid injection carries the risk of CRAO, skin depigmentation, and fat atrophy.

- External chalazion—often, the pressure from the chalazion lid clamp itself will rupture the scab, opening the cavity. If it does not, use toothed forceps and Westcott scissors to remove the scab, then clear the cavity using cotton tipped applicators and a curette. All affected skin should be removed to heal effectively. Use low temp cautery as needed for hemostasis. Leave the wound open to heal by secondary intention.

Postoperative Considerations

- Apply antibiotic-steroid ointment to the affected area.
- If desired, apply a pressure eye patch; to promote hemostasis, reduce edema and prevent children from rubbing the area as they awaken from anesthesia. The patch can be removed after a few hours.

If removing chalazia on both eyes, consider incising the smaller chalazion first and pressure patching that eye while operating the second eye. Remove the first pressure patch as the child is being extubated and leave the pressure bandage over the second eye (larger chalazion) for several hours.

CAPILLARY HEMANGIOMA

Preoperative Considerations

The location and size of a capillary hemangioma will dictate whether observation only or interventional treatment is required. Any capillary hemangioma that interferes with the visual axis, causes significant astigmatism, or causes exposure keratopathy, requires treatment. For example, a large capillary hemangioma in the center of the upper eyelid can push on the eye and induce significant astigmatism. This needs to be treated, whereas a small capillary hemangioma on the lower eyelid near the lateral canthus can often be closely monitored without intervention. Determine if the patient needs to be screened for PHACES syndrome (>5 visible hemangiomas, large segmental facial hemangioma).

PHACES syndrome is the association of a segmental facial hemangioma, usually large, in combination with one or more other birth defects. Patients with PHACES syndrome may have posterior fossa brain malformations, hemangioma, arterial lesions, cardiac abnormalities, eye abnormalities (relatively rare and varied), and sternal/midline abnormalities.

Treatment Options

- Oral propranolol (2 mg/kg/day in divided doses) can be given to most patients[2]; it is usually initiated and monitored by the pediatrician or pediatric dermatologist. The pediatric ophthalmologist will continue to monitor for induced astigmatism and amblyopia. Even though the capillary hemangioma may shrink within a few months, the current recommendations are to continue oral propranolol until 1 year of age as the hemangioma may continue to grow throughout the first year of life.
- Topical timolol maleate 0.5% gel-forming solution administered directly to the hemangioma twice daily can be effective for small, superficial hemangiomas.[3]
- Steroids can be injected locally or given systemically. Injection consists of a combination of triamcinolone acetonide 40 mg + betamethasone 6 mg or methylprednisolone 25-40 mg + triamcinolone acetonide 40 mg. These are most effective

for an early subcutaneous lesion. The total amount of steroid injected should be limited to 1.5 mL. Evaluate at 6 weeks, and repeat if necessary. Systemic steroids (1.5-5.0 mg/kg/day, generally 3 mg/kg/day) are given over several weeks and are most effective for hemangiomas with a large orbital component.

Intralesional steroids have been associated with systemic side effects, local skin depigmentation, local fat atrophy, and CRAO. Slow injections at low pressures, followed by fundus examination are recommended. Systemic steroids are associated with many systemic side effects.

- Lasers can also be used to shrink and treat superficial hemangiomas. Pulsed dye laser treatment is most often used, although Nd:Yag lasers have also been used. The hemangiomas are treated over several sessions by pediatric dermatologists.
- Sclerosing agents like interferon-alpha 2 have been used to rapidly shrink hemangiomas. This injection is usually performed by interventional radiologists and pediatric dermatologists.
- Well-circumscribed hemangiomas are rarely surgically removed.

EPIDERMAL INCLUSION CYSTS

Preoperative Considerations

These often occur after a scratch or minor trauma. A scroll of epithelial cells involutes and then continues to grow under the epidermis, forming a small cyst filled with keratin. They may be easily removed in the clinic using minimal local anesthesia in older children.

Surgical Planning

- Manage patient and caregiver expectations.
- Consider sending specimen for pathological analysis.
- Surgical instruments:
  - Bard Parker no. 11 blade and handle, curved mosquito clamp, smooth or toothed forceps, dermal punch, 4 × 4 gauze pads, 27G or 30G needle, 1- or 3-cc syringe, 2% lidocaine with epinephrine, 6-0 gut or Vicryl suture, pathology specimen jar.

Surgical Procedure

- Inject anesthesia subcutaneously around the lesion.
- Make an incision over the center of the lesion. This can be accomplished using a Bard Parker no. 11 blade to create a 2- to 3-mm incision or using a dermal punch.
- Use forceps or a mosquito clamp to stretch the incision and decrease pressure in the area.
- Gently squeeze the cyst back and forth to loosen it and try to express the cyst intact.
- If the cyst ruptures, simply clear the cavity of the cyst contents and then remove the cyst wall. This is important as the cyst will have a high rate of recurrence if not completely removed.
- Use forceps or the mosquito clamp to grasp the cyst wall at the bottom center of the cyst and remove.
- Leave the wound open to heal by secondary intention or place a single absorbable suture.

Postoperative Considerations

- Antibiotic ointment may be useful for small children who may pick at the area.
- No further follow-up needed.

MOLLUSCUM CONTAGIOSUM

Preoperative Considerations

Molluscum lesions are elevated with a pink and pearly appearance (Fig. 34.1). They have a characteristic central dimple and can be associated with ipsilateral follicular conjunctivitis. Children often induce spreading of the vesicles by scratching. The immune system will eventually contain the virus and the lesions will self-resolve, but it can take several months to years. Any treatments involve irritation of the lesion to stimulate the immune system to work against the virus. This is usually signaled by the lesion and surrounding skin becoming red and inflamed. It is rare for molluscum to become secondarily infected; the redness is a sign that the immune system is working, and the lesion should resolve shortly. Treatment and resolution can take several months, especially if the child is self-spreading by itching or has more sensitive, eczematous skin.

There are several home remedies that caregivers can try. Most are topical, although some are systemic. Due to the risk of damaging the eye, it is important to warn caregivers to be cautious with potentially caustic topical agents, such as vinegar.

OTC treatments: Topical options should be applied regularly. Options such as vinegar, tea tree oil, or clear nail polish can be applied daily, while OTC adapalene (Differin) gel should be applied 2-3 nights per week. Duct tape may also be applied to lesions and changed nightly until resolved. There are also several nonpharmaceutical grade "treatments" available for purchase online.

Prescription treatments: May be applied in the office by a physician or at home a few nights a week as tolerated. These include tretinoin cream 0.025%, cantharidin ("beetle/bug juice"), salicylic acid, and potassium hydroxide. Imiquimod (Aldara) cream is no longer recommended.

Surgical treatment options: Several different methods have been used to remove molluscum lesions. These include cryotherapy, cautery, laser, curettage, and shave excision. Cryotherapy is typically not performed around the eyelids.

Surgical Planning

- Manage patient and caregiver expectations.
- Can be done in the office but depending on age and number of lesions, may need to be performed under general anesthesia.
- Surgical instruments:
  - Bard Parker no. 11 blade or no. 15 stab blade, 15G needle, toothed forceps, chalazion curette, 4 × 4 gauze pads.

Surgical Procedure

- Grasp the lesion with toothed forceps and then use the blade to remove the lesion at the base.
- Alternatively, unroof the lesion with toothed forceps and a blade or needle tip. Express contents of the cyst by squeezing or using a curette. Be sure to remove the central crystal-like or soft white core.

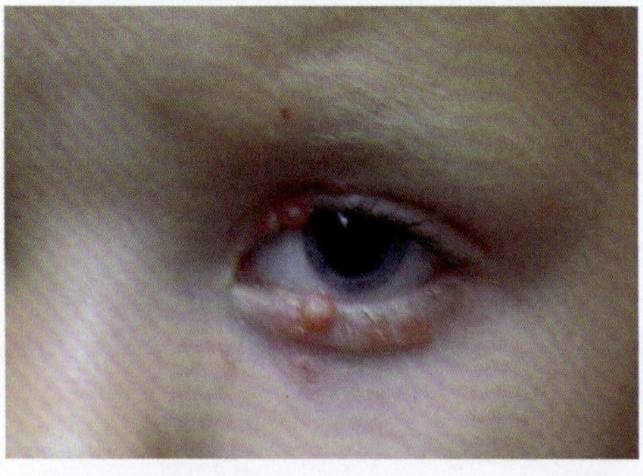

FIGURE 34.1. *Molluscum contagiosum* lesions of upper and lower eyelid in a 4-year-old healthy child. (Courtesy of Laura B. Enyedi, MD.)

Postoperative Considerations

- Apply antibiotic ointment to site.
- No further follow-up needed.

PAPILLOMA

Preoperative Considerations

Papillomas are benign masses that are commonly found in the periorbital skin and the eyelid margins. These can easily be removed under local anesthesia in many cases and should always be sent for pathological analysis.

Surgical Planning

- Manage patient and caregiver expectations.
- Determine whether patient is able to tolerate removal in the office under local anesthesia vs. need for general anesthesia.
- Surgical instruments:
    - Toothed forceps, Westcott scissors, low-temperature cautery, 3- or 5-cc syringe, 27G or 30G ½ inch needle, 2% lidocaine with epinephrine, pathology specimen container.

Procedure

- Inject 2% lidocaine with epinephrine around the affected area.
- Clean and prep the affected area.
- Use toothed forceps to pick up the papillomatous lesion and locate the point of attachment to the eyelid.
- Use Westcott scissors to excise the lesion at its base and the point of attachment.
- Send specimen for pathological analysis.
- There is typically minimal bleeding from the area, and the skin will heal well, but use low-temperature cautery and pressure for hemostasis if needed.

Postoperative Considerations

- Apply antibiotic ointment to operative site.
- Follow-up with pathology results.

PYOGENIC GRANULOMA (LOBULAR CAPILLARY HEMANGIOMA)

Preoperative Considerations

A sterile inflammatory response can be seen after a ruptured chalazion, trauma, or surgery. It will look like a fleshy mass and is sometimes pedunculated. They are often found along the tarsal conjunctiva. If surgical excision is planned, there is always the risk of inducing another pyogenic granuloma. For this reason, a trial of topical timolol should be tried initially to involute the vasculature. Timolol maleate 0.5% drops or gel-forming solution is instilled in the affected eye twice a day.[4] The lesion usually starts to involute within a few weeks, but it can take several weeks to fully involute. Recheck the patient after 1 month to see if the lesion is getting smaller.

Surgical Planning

- Manage patient and caregiver expectations.
- Determine whether the patient is able to tolerate removal in the office under local anesthesia or requires general anesthesia.
- Surgical instruments:
    - Toothed forceps, scissors, low-temperature cautery, 2% lidocaine with epinephrine, 3- or 5-cc syringe, 27G or 30G ½ inch needle, pathology specimen jar.
- Try to avoid excess manipulation in the area so another granuloma is not induced.

Procedure

- Inject 2% lidocaine with epinephrine around the affected area.
- Clean and prep the affected area.
- Use toothed forceps to gently pick up the lesion.
- Use Westcott scissors to excise the lesion at the point of attachment.
- Send specimen for pathological analysis.
- There is typically minimal bleeding from the area and will heal well, but use low-temperature cautery and pressure for hemostasis if needed.

Postoperative Considerations

- Apply antibiotic ointment to operative site.
- Follow-up with pathology results.

References

1. Liang L, Ding X, Tseng SC. High prevalence of demodex brevis infestation in chalazia. *Am J Ophthalmol.* 2014;157(2):342-348.
2. Missoi T, Lueder GT, Gilbertson K, et al. Oral propranolol for the treatment of periocular infantile hemangioma. *Arch Ophthalmol.* 2011;129:899-903.
3. Ni N, Langer P, Wagner R, et al. Topical timolol for periocular hemangioma: report of further study. *Arch Ophthalmol.* 2011;129(3):373-379.
4. Oke I, Maan A, Petersen R, et al. Treatment of ocular pyogenic granuloma with topical timolol. *JAMA Ophthalmol.* 2017;135(4):383-385.

CHAPTER 35

Tarsorrhaphy

Michelle S. Go, MD

PREOPERATIVE CONSIDERATIONS

When deciding whether or not the patient needs a tarsorrhaphy, it is helpful to think of the reasons for corneal decompensation. If the problem lies with the ocular surface, can it be managed with aggressive lubrication, medications, or scleral contact lenses? If the patient has paralytic lagophthalmos, would a gold weight or Botox to the upper eyelid be preferable? Is corneal protection required temporarily or long-term? What part of the eyelid requires closure? It is important to rule out infection prior to performing a tarsorrhaphy. Make sure that the tarsorrhaphy does not completely cover the eye if serial examinations are needed or eye drops are necessary. Also take into consideration that there may be a significant risk of amblyopia depending upon the patient's age and the size of the tarsorrhaphy.

Surgical Planning

- Temporary vs permanent:
  - Consider a temporary tarsorrhaphy when the condition is expected to improve or will last only a few weeks. The following materials can be used:
    - Adhesive tape (several hours).
    - Suture (weeks).
    - Glue (weeks).
    - Botox (several weeks to months).
  - A permanent tarsorrhaphy can be considered for patients requiring corneal protection for 3 months or greater.
- Suture choice:
  - Double-armed sutures are preferable.
  - Absorbable (Vicryl) suture may be used for permanent tarsorrhaphies, and nonabsorbable sutures (silk, Prolene, and nylon) may be used for temporary tarsorrhaphies.
- Location:
  - Determine where the cornea is exposed as well as what part of the eyelid and how much should be closed.
  - Temporal location usually results in good closure, allows the patient to see, and lets the surgeon examine the eye.
  - Central or medial tarshorrhaphies can also be used.

Tape tarsorrhaphy: Using a piece of medical paper tape ~½" by 1 ½ to 2" long, tape the lateral lower lid up toward the edge of the brow to decrease the palpebral fissure until the upper lid is able to close fully. Tape can also be applied directly over the upper and lower lids, but the patient will be unable to open the eyes unless the tape is removed. These techniques may be appropriate for nocturnal lagophthalmos.

Botox tarsorrhaphy: Inject 10 units of Botox into the center of the upper eyelid near the lid crease.

Glue tarsorrhaphy: Squeeze cyanoacrylate in between the eyelid margins and hold the eyelids closed for about 1 minute until the glue sets.

SURGICAL PROCEDURE

Temporary Tarsorrhaphy

- Optional: use a pen to mark points on the upper and lower lids where the tarsorrhaphy will begin and end.
- Clean the skin surface with an alcohol swab.
- Inject lidocaine, preferably with epinephrine, into the eyelids at the intended location of the tarsorrhaphy. Also inject into the tarsal plate.
- If using a bolster to prevent cheese-wiring through the skin, cut two pieces of butterfly tubing a few millimeters longer than the intended length of the tarsorrhaphy.
- Pass one arm of a double-armed 4-0, 5-0, or 6-0 nonabsorbable suture in this order: 1st bolster → upper eyelid skin → upper eyelid grey line → lower eyelid grey line → lower eyelid skin → 2nd bolster (Fig. 35.1).
  Note: The initial pass through the skin can be made on either the upper or lower eyelid and on either the nasal or temporal edge of the intended tarsorrhaphy based on preference.
- Repeat the pass with the second arm of the suture several millimeters away from the initial pass (Fig. 35.1).
- Tie the suture down on the bolster.

The use of a bolster is optional. The suture can also be passed through the lumen of the butterfly tubing instead of through the plastic. A sliding/locking bolster can also be placed on a drawstring to allow for easy separation and closure of the eyelids.[1]

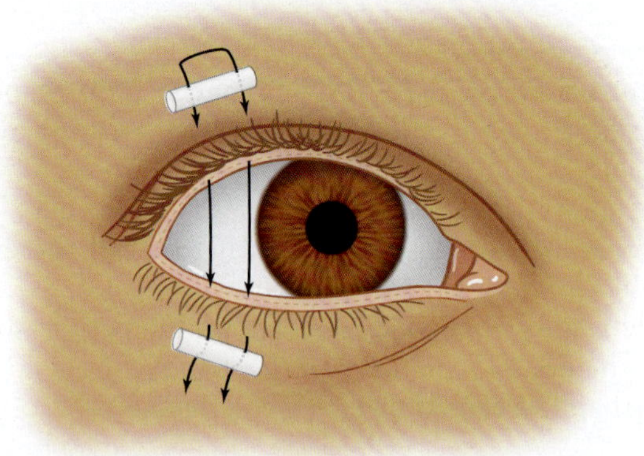

FIGURE 35.1. One arm of the double-armed suture is passed through the first bolster, upper eyelid skin surface, upper eyelid grey line, lower eyelid grey line, lower eyelid skin surface, and second bolster. The process is repeated several millimeters from the first pass with the second arm of the suture. *Dashed lines* represent the grey line.

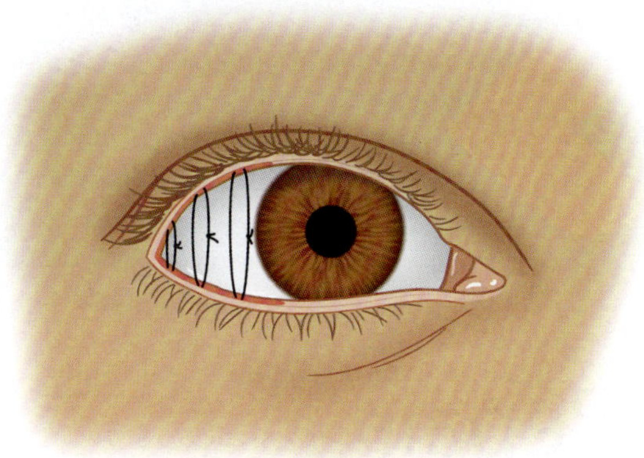

FIGURE 35.2. Interrupted horizontal mattress sutures are placed through the de-epithelialized posterior lamellae of the upper and lower lids.

Permanent Tarsorrhaphy[1,2]

- Optional: mark where the tarsorrhaphy is to begin and end on the upper and lower lids.
- Clean the skin surface with an alcohol swab.
- Inject lidocaine with epinephrine into the eyelids and tarsal plate at the intended location of the tarsorrhaphy.
- Prep and drape the eyelids.
- Use a no. 15 or no. 11 blade to score the upper and lower eyelid margins at the grey line for the length of the intended tarsorrhaphy.
- Using Westcott scissors, remove the posterior lamellae of the upper and lower lids where the margin was scored.
- Suture the posterior lamella of the upper eyelid with that of the lower eyelid with 5-0 or 6-0 Vicryl sutures in a simple interrupted or horizontal mattress fashion along the length of the de-epithelialized lid margin (Fig. 35.2). Avoid passing the sutures full thickness through the tarsal conjunctiva.
- Suture the anterior lamellae of the upper and lower eyelids with interrupted 6-0 or 7-0 Vicryl sutures.
- Clear the lashes from the sutures.

An effective simplified approach is to use one layer of closure rather than two. The initial steps are the same. After scoring the eyelid margins at the grey line and removing epithelium over the posterior lamellae of the upper and lower eyelids, a 5-0 or 6-0 Vicryl suture is passed from skin to tarsus on one eyelid then tarsus to skin on the opposing eyelid in a simple interrupted or a sinusoidal mattress fashion. The suture is tied to itself, bringing the de-epithelialized tarsal edges together.

POSTOPERATIVE CONSIDERATIONS

Reversal of Tarshorrhaphy

- Temporary tarsorrhaphies can be easily removed by cutting the suture.
- Permanent tarsorrhaphies can be reversed by cutting along the adhesion with scissors.

References

1. Rajak S, Rajak J, Selva D. Performing a tarsorrhaphy. *Community Eye Health*. 2015;28(89):10-11.
2. Periocular malpositions and involutional changes. In: Foster JA, ed. *Basic and Clinical Science Course (BCSC) Section 7: Orbit, Eyelids, and Lacrimal System*. San Francisco, CA: American Academy of Ophthalmology (AAO); 2015:225.

CHAPTER 36

Epiblepharon Repair

Michelle T. Cabrera, MD

PREOPERATIVE CONSIDERATIONS

In an eye with lower lid epiblepharon, identify whether the patient has been symptomatic from trichiasis. If possible, perform a careful slit lamp examination to identify trichiasis and other signs of corneal issues. Look for punctate epithelial erosions, frank corneal epithelial defects, and/or scarring. Occasionally children will adopt abnormal head postures to keep lashes off the cornea or out of the visual axis (Fig. 36.1). Age-appropriate visual acuity assessment and refraction are also critical to understanding the clinical impact, while ensuring that appropriate refractive and amblyopic treatments are pursued.

Indications for Surgery

Epiblepharon (overriding orbicularis but not entropion) with significant trichiasis identified on slit lamp examination or careful penlight examination plus any of the following:

- Symptoms of:
  - Eye redness.
  - Tearing.
  - Eye rubbing.
  - Pain and/or foreign body sensation.
- Recurrent corneal erosion.
- Corneal scarring.
- Associated significant refractive error: induced astigmatism and/or anisometropia.
- Associated induced amblyopia.
- Associated abnormal head postures (occasional):
  - Head turn away affected side in unilateral cases (keeps medial lashes off the cornea).
  - Chin down in bilateral cases (Fig. 36.1).

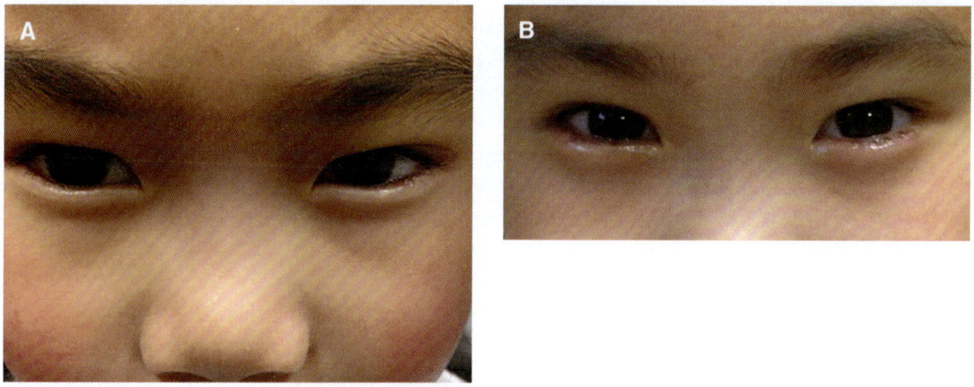

FIGURE 36.1. A 6-year-old child bilateral epiblepharon. Both corneas had significant keratopathy. **A.** Preoperative chin down head position. **B.** One week postoperative appearance. Head is straighter with lashes no longer touching the cornea. (Courtesy of Laura B. Enyedi, MD.)

Conservative Therapy for Patients Who Do Not Require Surgery

Most children tolerate epiblepharon with trichiasis quite well and do not require surgery.[1] These patients may benefit from conservative measures:

- Prescribe topical artificial tears if visible punctate epithelial erosions.
- Provide clinical follow-up including age-appropriate visual acuity and refraction assessment.
- Advise families/patient regarding warning signs to seek treatment (symptoms and signs of corneal erosion).
- Advise families that many young children, particularly infants, may grow out of this condition.
- Advise families/patient that surgery may be necessary in the future.

> **Older symptomatic children and adults may tolerate mechanical epilation with forceps; however, lashes grow back in 3-6 weeks and can be more irritating than mature lashes.**

Surgical Planning

- Manage patient/family expectations by discussing the risk of failure/recurrence/scarring following surgery (all possible but uncommon).
- If only a few lashes (2-3 per lid) are touching the eye, consider radiofrequency ablation; however, this approach will likely require more than one session.
    - Radiofrequency ablation can be performed for both the upper and lower eyelids, while surgical approach is only for lower eyelids.
    - Radiofrequency ablation can be performed without a sterile operating room environment; it requires a radiosurgical cautery instrument such as an Ellman Surgitron. The procedure requires general anesthesia for children or uncooperative adults. Local anesthetic works for cooperative adults. See details of the procedure below.
- For more numerous lashes, or to avoid multiple anesthetics, plan for incisional surgery.
- Consider bilateral incisional surgery, even if only unilateral trichiasis, in order to achieve a cosmetically symmetric result.
- Document keratopathy and symptoms and consider external photographs for insurance coverage.

SURGICAL PROCEDURE: LOWER LID INCISIONAL EPIBLEPHARON REPAIR WITH OR WITHOUT ROTATING SUTURE TECHNIQUE (VIDEO 36.1)

- Following induction of anesthesia and prior to injection with local anesthetic, pull down the lower lids to remove redundancy of eyelid skin and mark the medial one-third of the lower lids, ~1 mm from the lower lid margin. Ensure symmetry between eyes.
- Inject lidocaine with epinephrine.
- Perform routine Betadine prep, and drape of both eyes.
- Place sterile corneal protector.
- Perform incision along previously placed markings using no. 15 Bard Parker blade.
- Continue to dissect posteriorly using the monopolar cautery with Colorado needle in cut mode or Westcott scissors, avoiding full-thickness incision through the posterior lamellae.

There is no need to repair a full-thickness hole through the posterior lamellae. If a full-thickness hole is identified during dissection, create a new dissection plane anteriorly to access the anterior tarsal surface.

- Perform dissection inferiorly along the anterior surface of the tarsus in the suborbicularis plane.
- For more severe cases, place rotating sutures using 5-0 or 6-0 Mersilene or Vicryl suture (or similar).[2] Take a bite through the inferior tarsus. Evert the eyelid to ensure that the suture is not full thickness. Take a vertical bite through the subcutaneous tissues at the superior lip of the wound, posterior to anterior, ensuring that the needle exits just under the skin, then tie the suture down tightly to pull the lid margin toward the inferior tarsus (Fig. 36.2). After tying the suture, ensure that the eyelid is still opposed to the globe.

Rotating sutures allow for less aggressive skin removal and may be helpful in more severe cases. Aggressive skin removal can lead to ectropion or eyelid retraction.

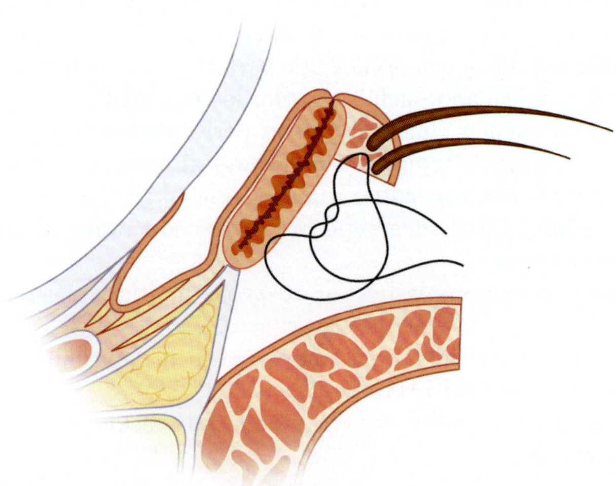

FIGURE 36.2. Rotational sutures from inferior tarsus to subcutaneous tissues.

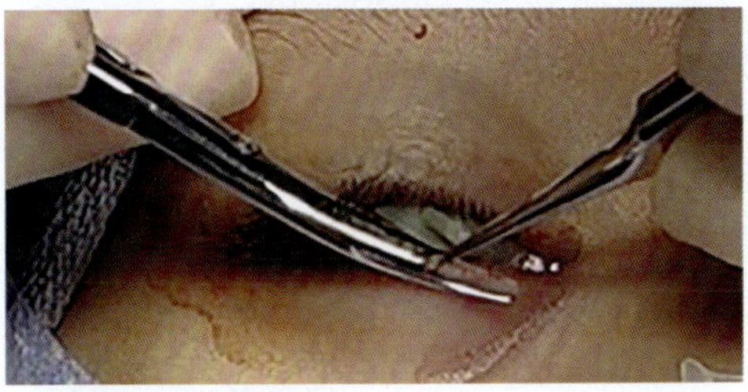

FIGURE 36.3. Removal of a small overriding crescent of skin.

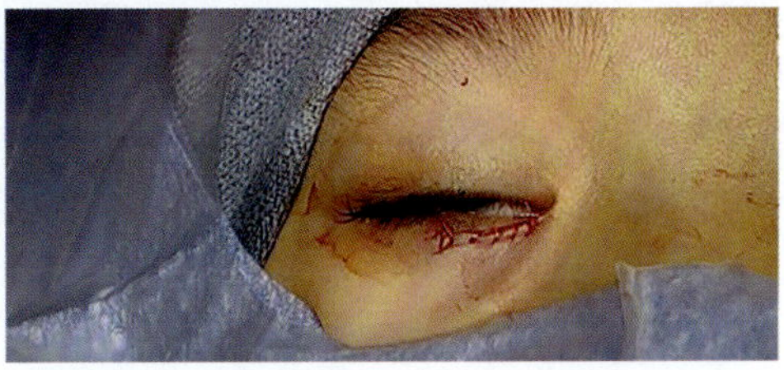

FIGURE 36.4. Appearance of closed wound.

- Place 1-2 more rotating deep sutures along the length of the wound.
- Use Westcott scissors to excise a crescent-shaped portion of orbicularis overlying the wound, 1-2 mm in width.
- Use Westcott scissors to excise a crescent-shaped portion of skin, 1-2 mm in width (Fig. 36.3).
- Close the skin with running or interrupted 6-0 fast absorbing or plain gut (Fig. 36.4).
- Remove corneal protector.
- Repeat the procedure for the contralateral eye.

SURGICAL PROCEDURE: RADIOFREQUENCY ABLATION OF LASHES

- The settings tend to vary from machine to machine, and it is best to check with the manufacturer for specific information on settings.
- Place a corneal protector.
- Put the radiofrequency ablation needle into the follicle.
- Energize the tip while in place, usually for about 1 second.
- When appropriately treated, the hair will easily pull out with Jeweler forceps without force.
- Treat all offending lashes.
- Remove the corneal protector.

POSTOPERATIVE CONSIDERATIONS

- Most patients are comfortable returning to work/school the day after surgery.
- Ophthalmic antibiotic ointment should be applied to the wound for 7 days postoperatively following incisional eyelid surgery but is not required for ablation.
- Recurrence of eyelash growth usually occurs following lash ablation for 50% of lashes, requiring 1-2 repeat treatments.
- Radiofrequency ablation can result in eyelid edema, erythema, and thickening of the lid margin.
- Incisional reoperations are likely to result in increased bruising, hematoma, and prolonged recovery compared to first-time procedures.

References

1. Simon JW, Williams KH, Zobal-Ratner JL, Barry GP. Conservative management of lower eyelid epiblepharon in children. *J Pediatr Ophthalmol Strabismus*. 2017;54(1):15-16.
2. Woo KI, Yi K, Kim YD. Surgical correction for lower lid epiblepharon in Asians. *Br J Ophthalmol*. 2000;84:1407-1410.

CHAPTER 37

Enucleation

Arthika Chandramohan, MD, MPH • Dilraj S. Grewal, MD • Prithvi Mruthyunjaya, MD, MHS

PREOPERATIVE CONSIDERATIONS

Indications for enucleation in children are rare, but most commonly include the following[1]:

- Blind, painful eye
- Following severe trauma (ie, irreparable open globe injury; concern for risk of sympathetic ophthalmia)
- Intraocular tumor (specifically as primary or secondary treatment for retinoblastoma)
- Rarely congenital or progressive phthisis bulbi (ie, chronic poorly controlled uveitis from juvenile idiopathic arthritis). Unexplained phthisis bulbi should be investigated for retinoblastoma.

Surgical Planning

- Have a detailed discussion with patient's parents or guardian regarding the goals of the enucleation (ie, tumor staging, prevention of sympathetic ophthalmia, pain control), and plans for postoperative steps for reconstruction with an ocularist.
- Select device for severing the nerve (ie, snare, curved enucleation scissors +/– Wells enucleation spoon).
- Select type of implant (ie, porous implants are more commonly used in developed countries[2] vs. nonporous implants; Table 37.1 describes more commonly used implants).

SURGICAL PROCEDURE: ENUCLEATION (VIDEO 37.1)

- Ensure that the correct eye is marked and draped using a redundant check system among multiple team members to eliminate the possibility of removing the wrong eye. Once the patient is under general anesthesia, the nonsurgical eye is taped closed by the surgeon.
- In cases where the select eye is not readily identifiable externally (ie, intraocular tumors, posterior globe rupture) prior to surgical incision, indirect ophthalmoscopy or repeat B-scan ultrasound is performed to ensure that the appropriate eye is being removed.

TABLE 37.1. Various Available Orbital Implants

Implant Type	Implant Material	Benefits	Drawbacks
Nonporous	Glass Acrylic Silicone	• Improved prosthesis movement with myoconjunctival technique (each muscle sutured to respective fornix) compared to porous implants[3]	• Muscle reattachment to a scleral shell rather than the implant itself can result in implant displacement and migration • Higher rates of extrusion and infection[4]
Porous	Hydroxyapatite Synthetic hydroxyapatite Bioceramic Medpor	• Provide improved implant movement because of direct attachment of extraocular muscles to the implant • Associated with less migration, extrusion, and lower risks of infection[5]	• More expensive • More prone to implant exposure[6] and postoperative inflammation
Other	Dermis fat graft	• Maintains orbital bone growth with soft tissue volume expansion over time • Can be used with implant in older children (>5 years old)[7]	• Can result in contracted fornices and cosmetically significant enophthalmos[4] (though less common in children) when used independently
	No implant	• Allows for follow-up of tumor extension prior to implant placement (can also stage implant placement at a later date)	• No prevention of socket contraction or stunted orbital bone development resulting in poor orbital cosmesis and development

- Though the child is under general anesthesia, a peribulbar or retrobulbar block may be given to both positionally elevate the globe within the orbit and for postoperative pain management.
- Once the patient is prepped and draped, consider the placement of a double-armed 4-0 silk suture passed from the conjunctival surface within the fornix, full thickness through the lid and tied externally to preserve the superior and inferior fornices.[8]

Consider using a surgical marking pen to ink the limbus 360 degrees, which will aid in identification of the conjunctival edges to ensure independent layered closure of Tenon capsule and conjunctiva at the end of the case.

- Complete a 360-degree conjunctival peritomy using blunt Westcott scissors. Once complete, use the same instrument to dissect away Tenon capsule in all four quadrants between the muscle insertions (avoid direct spreading over muscle insertions to prevent excessive bleeding).
- Each rectus muscle is identified using a muscle hook, cleaned, and secured with a 6-0 double-armed Vicryl suture in a manner similar to strabismus surgery (see Chapter 42). Once tagged, the rectus muscles are disinserted at the insertion with high temperature cautery.
- A muscle hook is used to bluntly dissect any posterior connective tissue attachments to the globe.
- The inferior and superior oblique muscles are then identified, isolated, and transected with cautery. The inferior oblique may also be clamped for 10 seconds prior to transecting to avoid additional bleeding. Some surgeons prefer to secure the oblique muscles and reattach to the prosthesis.

- Enucleation snare technique:
  - Once all muscles are disinserted, 4-0 silk sutures are passed in a lamellar fashion near the muscle insertions medially and laterally.
  - An enucleation snare is then placed around the globe and guided by a hemostat (held by the assistant), while upward counter traction is applied on the globe by silk sutures.
  - Once the snare is appropriately and as posteriorly positioned as possible, release the hemostat and tighten the snare until the optic nerve is transected. This technique tends to minimize bleeding after globe removal.
- Enucleation scissor technique:
  - The globe is turned laterally and a curved heavy hemostat is inserted along the medial globe wall and clamped around a distal portion of the optic nerve. The hemostat is used to "strum" the nerve to ensure proper identification.
  - Enucleation scissors are then passed posterior to the clamp, which is then released.
  - Scissors are deployed, and the nerve is transected.
- The globe is examined externally, optic nerve length recorded, and then placed in formalin and sent for histopathologic examination. Communication with the pathologist is critical in cases of suspected intraocular tumor to ensure proper tissue processing.
- The orbit is packed with epinephrine-soaked neurosurgical sponges or iced gauze pads, and external pressure is placed to ensure hemostasis, usually requiring 2-4 minutes.
  - If the bleeding persists after removing the gauze, identifiable bleeding sites can be cauterized with bipolar cautery, or gel foam placed in thrombin can also be placed over the severed optic nerve to aid in hemostasis.
- Once bleeding has stopped, sizing balls are placed in the orbit to determine the size of implant needed. Try to use the largest size implant that will allow for adequate closure (usually at least a 20-mm implant is favored in children over 2 years of age) to prevent enophthalmos and superior sulcus deformity.[9]

Donor sclera can be used to wrap the implant and is necessary for muscle reattachment with nonporous implants (Fig. 37.1). Windows are cut into the scleral wrap to approximate the insertion of the rectus muscles. A drill may be used to reshape the posterior surface of the implant and to make small holes to promote vascular ingrowth.

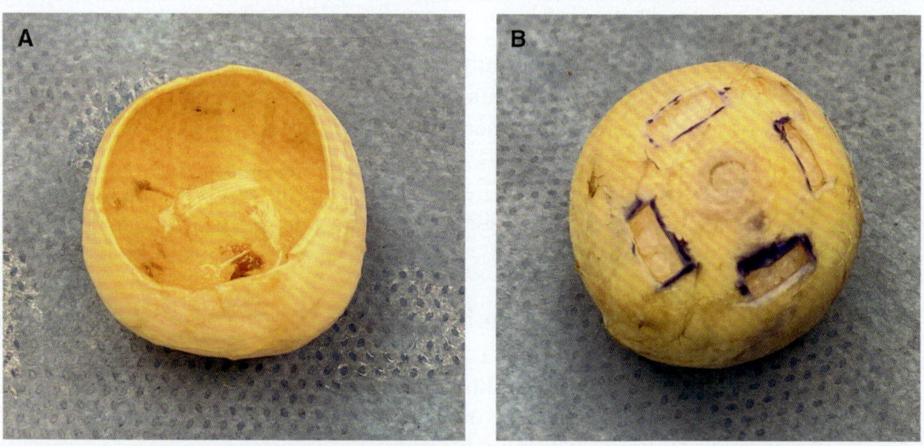

FIGURE 37.1. A. Donor sclera. **B.** Scleral-wrapped implant with windows cut for muscle reattachment to the implant itself. (Images courtesy of Dr. Benjamin Erickson, MD)

- The implant is selected and soaked in dilute antibiotic (ie, 2 mg/mL gentamicin solution). Porous implants, like hydroxyapatite, benefit from suction exchange of the antibiotic via the porous channels within the implant. This is accomplished by placing the implant into a 60-cc syringe and aspirating the antibiotic bath. Air is drawn into the syringe allowing the solution to permeate the pores of the implant.[10]
- The implant is then placed in the orbit using a sphere introducer, and rectus muscles are reattached to the implant or to the scleral covering by passing the two arms of the 6-0 Vicryl through the implant or shell anterior to the implant equator.
- Perform a layer-by-layer closure of Tenon capsule and conjunctiva separately using 5-0 and 6-0 Vicryl suture, respectively, in an interrupted or running fashion.
- An appropriately sized conformer is then placed in the socket with antibiotic ointment (ie, erythromycin or tobramycin/dexamethasone), and wound tension is double checked with the lids closed to reduce the risks of wound dehiscence and/or implant extrusion. If forniceal sutures were placed at the beginning of the case, release these prior to placement of the conformer.
- A pressure dressing is then applied.

POSTOPERATIVE CONSIDERATIONS

- The pressure patch is left in place for 1-5 days, and once removed, antibiotic ointment is applied to socket 2-3 times a day.
- Remind the patient and caretaker of the importance of maintaining the conformer in the orbit to prevent forniceal contracture; if the patient and/or parents are unable to replace the conformer if it dislodges from the orbital surface, they must present for replacement within 72 hours.
- The socket can be fit for a prosthesis on average 6 weeks following enucleation so long as no further immediate therapies (ie, orbital antibiotics, adjuvant radiation) are necessary.

References

1. Moshfeghi DM, Moshfeghi AA, Finger PT. Enucleation. *Surv Ophthalmol.* 2000;44(4):277-301.
2. Mourits DL, Hartong DT, Bosscha MI, et al. Worldwide enucleation techniques and materials for treatment of retinoblastoma: an international survey. *PLoS One.* 2015;10(3):e0121292.
3. Shome D, Honavar SG, Raizada K, et al. Implant and prosthesis movement after enucleation: a randomized controlled trial. *Ophthalmology.* 2010;117(8):1638-1644.
4. Yousef YA. Enucleation surgery—orbital implants and surgical techniques. *Enucleation.* 2016;9(1):46-48.
5. Hornblass A, Biesman BS, Eviatar JA. Current techniques of enucleation: a survey of 5,439 intraorbital implants and a review of the literature. *Ophthal Plast Reconstr Surg.* 1995;11(2):77-86; discussion 87-88.
6. Shields CL, Shields JA, De Potter P, et al. Problems with the hydroxyapatite orbital implant: experience with 250 consecutive cases. *Br J Ophthalmol.* 1994;78(9):702-706.
7. Mitchell KT, Hollsten DA, White WL, et al. The autogenous dermis-fat orbital implant in children. *J AAPOS.* 2001;5(6):367-369.
8. Katowitz JA, Katowitz WR. *Pediatric Oculoplastic Surgery.* Switzerland: Springer; 2017.
9. Ababneh OH, AboTaleb EA, Ameerh MAA, et al. Enucleation and evisceration at a tertiary care hospital in a developing country. *BMC Ophthalmol.* 2015;15(1):120.
10. Badilla J, Dolman PJ. Methods of antibiotic instillation in porous orbital implants. *Ophthalmic Plast Reconstr Surg.* 2008;24(4):287-289.

CHAPTER 38

Pediatric Ptosis Repair: Frontalis Suspension

Roshni Ranjit-Reeves, MD

Frontalis suspension is the procedure of choice for patients with significant ptosis with poor levator function (Fig. 38.1). Often, it is performed to prevent and/or treat amblyopia due to obstruction of the visual axis (deprivation amblyopia) and/or significant induced astigmatism (refractive amblyopia) secondary to the eyelid position. Surgery may also be performed to alleviate a chin up head position, which can interfere with gross motor development (sitting in an infant and walking in a toddler or older child). While the primary goal of the procedure is to improve visual function, aesthetics and facial symmetry should also be addressed.

Indication for procedure: Significant ptosis with poor levator palpebrae superioris function (<4 mm).

PATHOPHYSIOLOGY OF POOR LEVATOR FUNCTION

- Congenital:
  - Idiopathic (most common).
  - Blepharophimosis-Ptosis-Epicanthus Inversus syndrome (BPES) (see chapter 41).
  - Double elevator palsy (monocular elevation deficiency).
  - Duane retraction syndrome (see Chapter 52)
  - Marcus-Gunn jaw winking (trigemino-oculomotor/maxillopalpebral synkinesis).

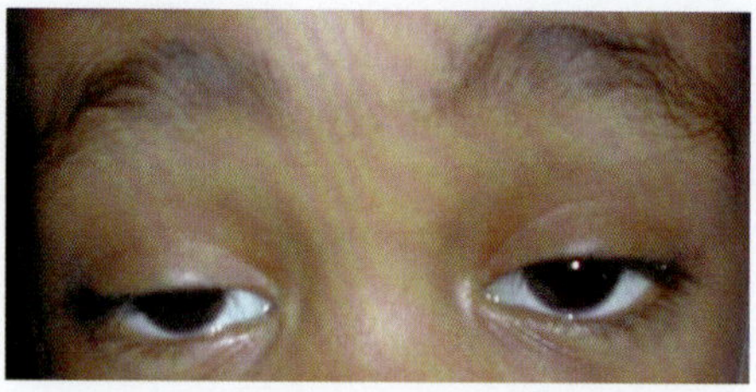

FIGURE 38.1. Bilateral congenital ptosis in a 5-year-old boy. Notice use of brow and lack of lid crease (courtesy of Laura B. Enyedi, MD).

- Rare congenital disorders.
  - Abetalipoproteinemia.
  - Congenital fibrosis of the extraocular muscles (CFEOM).
  - Moebius syndrome (Congenital oculofacial paralysis).
  - Refsum disease.
- Myogenic:
  - Kearns-Sayre syndrome.
  - Myotonic dystrophy.
  - Oculopharyngeal muscular dystrophy.
- Neurogenic:
  - Cranial nerve III palsy.
  - Endocrine exophthalmos.
  - Eyelid apraxia.
  - Muscular dystrophy.
  - Myasthenia gravis, occasionally, after maximal medical therapy.
  - Progressive supranuclear palsy.
- Traumatic:
  - Contact lens intolerance.
  - Eyelid foreign body.
  - Eyelid laceration.
  - Orbital fracture.
- Mechanical:
  - Tumors.
  - Primary tumors (ie, capillary hemangioma).
  - Metastasis.
- Infection:
  - Preseptal cellulitis.
  - Orbital cellulitis.
  - Chalazion/hordeolum.

Wait at least 6 months in traumatic ptosis for recovery of levator palpebrae superioris function to allow for appropriate surgical planning.

HISTORY

- Age of onset.
- Progressive vs stable.
- Static vs variable.
- Family history.
- History of strabismus or amblyopia.
- Recent trauma or ophthalmologic surgical procedure.
- Associated findings—lagophthalmos when sleeping, use of brow or head position.
- Gross motor development (ie, determine if head position interfering with sitting or walking).
- Old photo evaluation for comparison.

PREOPERATIVE ASSESSMENT

Complete eye examination.

- Visual acuity—assess specifically for amblyopia, which can be bilateral or unilateral.
- External exam—assess for chin up head position and/or use of brow to elevate the lids. Assess blink and lagophthalmos.

Use of the brow and/or a compensatory head position can indicate that the child is trying to gain binocularity and use the ptotic eye in unilateral cases.

Blowing a quick puff of air in a baby's face is a good way to assess the blink.

- Confrontation visual fields—assess for ptosis affecting the superior field.
- Ocular motility and alignment—assess all positions of gaze, especially upgaze. Assess for strabismus, which may accompany ptosis or may occur as a result of amblyopia.

The superior rectus may be abnormal in cases of congenital ptosis. Superior rectus function is critical for a normal Bell response. Abnormal function of the superior rectus may predispose to exposure keratopathy. Positioning an infant prone is a good way to assess eye elevation and superior rectus function. Eye elevation can be difficult to elicit even in normal infants.

- Pupils—assess for anisocoria. In Horner syndrome, there is usually mild ptosis and good levator function, in addition to miosis, on the affected side.
- Anterior segment—assess for preoperative exposure keratopathy. Perform Schirmer testing if possible.
- Cycloplegic refraction—assess for with-the-rule astigmatism, which can cause refractive amblyopia and may require spectacle treatment. Astigmatism secondary to ptosis may or may not improve postoperatively.
- Fundus examination—look for abnormalities of the optic nerve and retina as those findings may be helpful in determining if the ptosis is associated with an underlying condition.
- Obtain preoperative photos for documentation of ptosis, insurance approval of surgery, and intraoperative guidance on height and contour of lids.
- Eyelid measurements.
    - Frontalis strength—intact frontalis function is essential to the success of the procedure. Look for use of the brow to elevate lid preoperatively.*
    - Lagophthalmos—observing the patient while sleeping or asking parents about eyelid closure during sleep is helpful.
    - Levator excursion/function—measurement of levator function is critical in determining the most appropriate surgical procedure for ptosis (see chapter 39).*
    - Margin crease distance—typically, the eyelid crease is poorly formed in congenital ptosis.
    - Margin fold distance.
    - Margin reflex distance 1 (MRD1).*
    - Palpebral fissure.
    - Palpebral fissure on downgaze—patients with idiopathic congenital ptosis will often exhibit lid lag where the upper eyelid is higher than normal with the globe in downgaze because of fibrosis of the levator. This lid lag may worsen after ptosis surgery.
    - Presence of Bells phenomenon—tested by opening the eyelids widely while the baby is forcibly trying to close them.*
    - Synkinesis (eg, Marcus Gunn jaw-wink)—best observed when the baby is feeding.*

*Indicates the most critical elements for surgical planning.

TABLE 38.1. Frontalis sling materials

Surgical Material	Advantage	Disadvantage
Autogenous fascia lata	Harvested from fascia Good tensile strength Rejection risk is rare	Creation of second donor site Difficult to harvest tissue in a child under the age of 3 years
Allogenic fascia lata	Can be used in children under 3	Potential risk of rejection from donor to recipient
Gore-Tex (polytetrafluoroethylene)	Can be used in any age group Micropores allow for tissue integration	Biofilm can form over material
Supramid suture (4-0 polyfilament)	Does not require a donor Can be used in any age group	Increased risk of ptosis recurrence due to hydrolysis of the suture
Silicone rod	Sling can be more easily adjusted if needed over time Can be used in any age group	Risk of biofilm formation over silicone

PREOPERATIVE COUNSELING

- Counsel patient and family specifically on postoperative lagophthalmos and increased palpebral fissure on downgaze, which is especially common in congenital ptosis from fatty infiltration of the levator palpebrae superioris. Discuss the fact that the lid function will never be "normal" because the levator muscle is abnormal. Explain that the lid position will vary with effort and that there is potential for the lid to change over time. Discuss risk of additional surgery to address height or contour of lid, and small risk of sling exposure, infection, and/or need for removal of sling. Discuss increased risk of corneal exposure, especially with a poor Bell phenomenon and need for long-term lubrication.

SURGICAL PLANNING

- Select preferred sling material (see Table 38.1).

SURGICAL PROCEDURE: FRONTALIS SLING WITH SILICONE ROD (SEE ALSO CHAPTER 41) (VIDEO 38.1)

VIDEO

- Remove the sleeve from the silicone rod (FCI Ophthalmic, SKU S3.1000u, Sling length 300 mm, Needles: 58 mm long) and soak the silicone rod and sleeve in antibacterial solution (cefazolin) to help prevent postoperative infection. Consider preoperative IV antibiotics to further reduce infection risk.

The cefazolin will leave harmless white residue on the silicone.

- Wound marking:
  - Triangular pattern (Fig. 38.2). Mark two points 1-5 mm above the lash line. The marks should be in line with the medial and lateral limbus, using the pupil for centration.

Variations to the triangular pattern are noted in Figure 38.2.

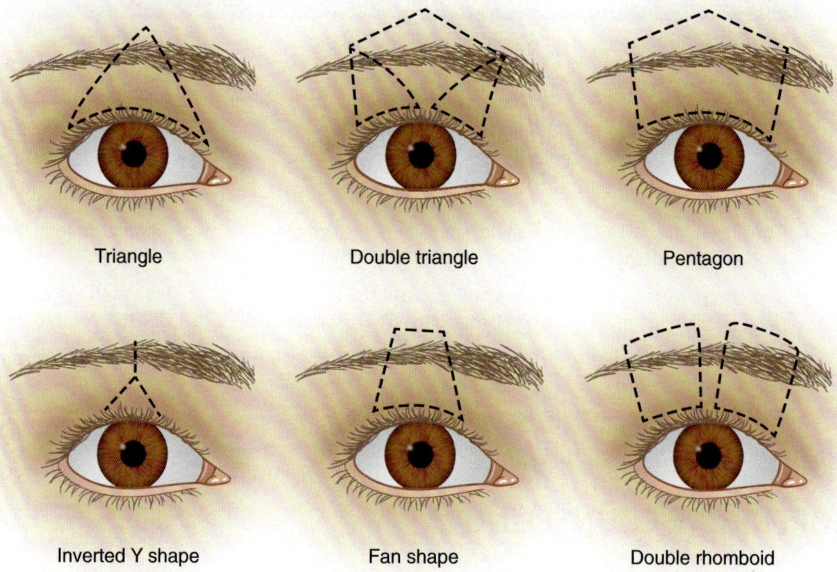

FIGURE 38.2. Various configurations for frontalis suspension procedure.

The lower the stab incisions, the more lift you will get but if the incisions are too close to the lid margin, the eyelid may pull away from the globe. Higher stab incisions (closer to the natural location of a lid crease) may look more natural but may not achieve as much lift. Usually the two stab incisions are ~10 mm apart (in a normal sized child). The further apart the incisions are, the more squared off the lid contour will be. The closer together the incisions, the more "peaked" the contour will be. Many factors will influence the exact location of the stab incisions including contour of the lids, severity of ptosis, whether the ptosis is unilateral or bilateral, need for lid crease (eg, Asian children may not need as much of a lid crease to look natural), and superior rectus function (eg, be very conservative lifting the lid with a poor Bell response). Place a third mark just superior to the brow hair follicles between the two lid marks. The supraorbital notch should be palpated and marked to avoid this area during the surgery. The upper portion of the wound may vary between 0.5 and 4 mm above the brow hair follicles depending on frontalis function. It is important to take into account facial asymmetry and wound placement for improved functional and cosmetic outcomes.

- Inject local anesthetic with epinephrine and wait ~5 minutes for improved hemostasis (see Chapters 1 and 42).
- Prep and drape the patient, taking care to not remove the previously placed marks. Use a no. 15 or no. 64 Bard-Parker blade to create incisions through skin and orbicularis muscle of the eyelid and brow as the globe is protected with a Jaeger plate.
- Optional step: Preplace a simple absorbable suture at each of the lid wounds to later close the skin and anchor the sling in place during healing. Some surgeons feel this reduces the tendency of the sling to migrate upwards in the lid, reducing the lid lift.
- Pass the silicone sling material attached to a spear needle into the medial eyelid wound to include a partial-thickness tarsal bite, as the globe is protected with a Jaeger plate. The needle should exit the lateral eyelid wound. Check to be sure you did not go full-thickness and that the lid contour is nicely curved.
- Using the Jaeger plate and/or a conformer to protect the globe, pass the medial needle superiorly and slightly medially toward the brow incision just under the septum, leaving the needle in place in the brow incision so that the second needle does not spear the sling ("crossed-swords"). Pass the lateral needle, similarly.

- Bring both needles out of the brow wound and pass them carefully through the silicone tube connector (Watzke sleeve) in a "crossed-swords" manner so that the sling is not cut by the needle. A cross-action forceps can be used in the sleeve to facilitate this maneuver. Tighten the rod to position the upper eyelid height at the corneal limbus if there is a good Bell reflex preoperatively. Expect the lid to fall a bit when the sleeve is tucked in and with the effects of gravity.

An alternative to using the Watzke sleeve is to simply tie the ends of the sling together. A potential advantage to knotting the sling is that it may be less likely to slip, but it may be bulkier and might make potential future adjustments more difficult.

- Optional: tie a Prolene suture tightly around the sleeve with the knot on the underside to make identifying the sleeve easier in the event of a re-operation.
- Once the position is confirmed, pass the needles, which are now crossed and held together by the connector, through the brow wound and exit through the skin just medial and lateral to the brow wound.
- Cut the ends flush with the skin, leaving a few mm beyond the sleeve so that the sling can be tightened or loosened. Tuck the sleeve completely into the wound, ensuring it is well covered by the overlying frontalis muscle.
- Close the wound with 5-0 or 6-0 plain gut suture using a vertical mattress stitch centrally and two interrupted sutures medially and laterally or with a nonabsorbable 5-0 Prolene suture tied in the same fashion to close the brow wound (note: only use nonabsorbable sutures in a child that will cooperate with removal of sutures in clinic). The eyelid stab incisions will heal by secondary intention or tie the sutures if you preplaced the optional lid sutures.

POSTOPERATIVE INSTRUCTIONS

- Ice the wounds to help decrease swelling for 24-48 hours.
- Use antibiotic ointment on all skin wounds.
- Lubricate the eye with ointment for lagophthalmos long term.
- Recheck cycloplegic refraction ~6 weeks post-op.

POSTOPERATIVE COMPLICATIONS

- Dry eye/exposure keratopathy—prevent and treat with aggressive lubrication.
- Granuloma.
- Infection—often requires removal of sling material.
- Overcorrection—if the lid is significantly too high after 6 weeks, downward massage of the lid may help the sling loosen or migrate in the lid to reduce the effect.
- Undercorrection—suspension material may dissolve or break, reducing the lid lift.
- Sling exposure—requires repositioning of sling or removal and replacement.

Suggested Readings

Elsamkary MA, Roshdy MM. Clinical trial comparing autogenous fascia lata sling and Gore-Tex suspension in bilateral congenital ptosis. *Clin Ophthalmol.* 2016;10:405-409.

https://www.aao.org/oculoplastics-center/frontalis-suspension

Lin LK, Uzcategui N, Chang EL. Effect of surgical correction of congenital ptosis on amblyopia. *Ophthal Plast Reconstr Surg.* 2008;24(6):434-436. [Medline].

Morris CL, Buckley EG, Enyedi LB, et al. Safety and efficacy of Silicone Rod Frontalis Suspension Surgery for Childhood Ptosis Repair. *J AAPOS.* 2008;45:280-290.

Raza Rizvi SA, Gupta Y, Yousuf S. Evaluation of safety and efficacy of silicone rod in tarso-frontalis sling surgery for severe congenital ptosis. *Ophthal Plast Reconstr Surg*. 2014;30:11-14.

Shimizu Y, Nagasao T, Shido H, et al. Intra-eyebrow frontalis suspension using inverted Y-shaped short autogenous fascia lata for blepharoptosis with poor levator function. *J Plast Reconstr Aesthet Surg*. 2015;68(1):49-55.

Tannenbaum RE, Shi W, Johnson TE, et al. Frontalis suspension with supramid suture: longevity results in very young patients with congenital ptosis. *Ophthal Plast Reconstr Surg*. 2014;30:110-115.

CHAPTER 39

Pediatric Ptosis Repair: Levator Resection

Meghan S. Flemmons, MD

PREOPERATIVE CONSIDERATIONS

Levator resection may be performed if there is fair to good levator function. This is determined by measuring upper eyelid margin excursion when looking from downward to upward with manual fixation of the upper brow. Classic teaching requires >4 mm of levator function for levator resection; however, typically, levator function of at least 6-7 mm correlates to better results with less under correction. Levator function of 4 mm or less usually requires a frontalis suspension procedure. Minimal ptosis (2 mm or less) with normal levator function and good response to phenylephrine may be corrected with a mullerectomy.

Deciding the amount of levator muscle to resect is the most important preoperative consideration in repairing congenital ptosis. The amount of ptosis, levator function, and intraoperative lid position will help determine the final amount of levator resection. Beard[1] described resection amount based on levator function and severity of ptosis (Table 39.1), whereas Berke[2] emphasized intraoperative lid position after resection based on preoperative levator function (Table 39.2). Carraway[3] promoted a standard 4-mm resection for every 1 mm of ptosis. Using a combination of these guidelines and considering individual patient needs and characteristics is usually the most helpful approach. In general, the better the levator function, the more postoperative rise is expected. However, the appearance of the muscle including dystrophy, thickness, fibrosis, or fatty infiltration should also be considered when determining the amount of resection. It is important to communicate with caregivers that the procedure may result in over or undercorrection, asymmetry of height and/or contour, and possible need for revision in the future.

TABLE 39.1. Beard[1] approach to levator resection

Amount of Ptosis	Levator Function	Levator Resection
Mild (2 mm)	Usually good	10-13 mm (mild)
Moderate (~3 mm)	Good (8-16 mm)	14-17 mm (moderate)
	Fair (5-7 mm)	18-22 mm (large)
	Poor (≤4 mm)	30 mm (maximum)
Severe (4 mm)	Usually poor	Maximum or frontalis suspension (preferred)

TABLE 39.2. Amount of levator resection based on levator function and intraoperative eyelid height under general anesthesia[2,4]

Levator Function	Intraoperative Eyelid Position[a]
Good (>10 mm)	Target: 3-4 mm below the limbus; 2-3 mm under correction (2-3 mm postoperative rise expected)
Fair (8-9 mm)	Target: 2 mm below the limbus; 1-2 mm under correction (1-2 mm postoperative rise expected)
Fair (6-7 mm)	Target: 2 mm below the limbus; full correction (no postoperative rise expected)
Fair (5-6 mm)	Target: 1 mm below the limbus; 1-2 mm over correction (postoperative drop expected)
Poor (0-4 mm)	Frontalis suspension preferred

[a]The greater the levator function, the more postoperative rise you can expect when the patient awakens from anesthesia. Lagophthalmos will be present at the end of the procedure despite general anesthesia (as with a frontalis sling), which is used to determine the intraoperative lid height.[2,4]

SURGICAL PROCEDURE (VIDEO 39.1)

- Mark the central peak (in preoperative area if possible). Mark desired lid crease (equal to normal contralateral side or ~8-10 mm above to lid margin) (Fig. 39.1).
- Inject lidocaine 1% with epinephrine 1:100 000 into upper eyelid using a 27 G needle on a 3-cc syringe (see Chapter 42).

Marking and injection may occur prior to or after the sterile prep. Allow ~10 minutes for epinephrine to constrict vessels and for edema to subside.

- Place a conformer in the eye (for protection and lubrication of the eye).
- Use a Bard Parker no. 15 blade to make skin incision at lid crease marking.

The blade makes a clean, smooth skin incision; however, hemostasis should be achieved quickly as bleeding into the surgical field may make identifying important structures more difficult. For further dissection, the Colorado tip monopolar cautery provides cutting and coagulation for a clean surgical field.

- Use Colorado tip monopolar cautery on "blend" setting to dissect carefully through orbicularis muscle to the orbital septum. Start with both the cut and coagulation settings at 3. Increase setting if not cutting efficiently (rarely exceeding a setting of 5).

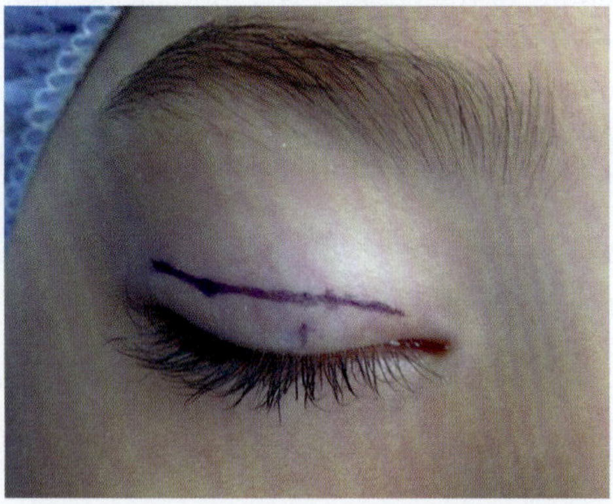

FIGURE 39.1. Vertical marking at desired central peak. Lid crease marking matches height of left upper eyelid crease.

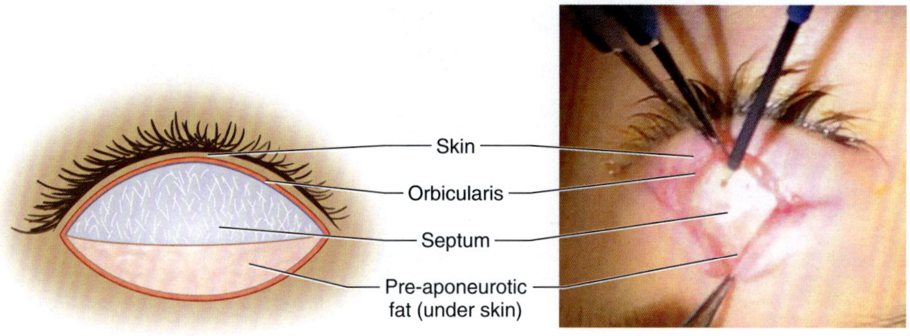

FIGURE 39.2. Orbital septum anatomy.

> **The orbital septum in children is very thick. Look for the landmark of preaponeurotic fat. Gentle pressure on the globe will push fat and septum forward (Fig. 39.2).**

- Once the orbital septum is entered centrally and the preaponeurotic fat is identified, extend the orbital septum opening laterally and medially. Then gently dissect the fat from the levator aponeurosis that is immediately posterior. The Colorado tip and/or a cotton tip applicator may be used.
- Turn your attention to inferior aspect of the incision and dissect with either scissors or the Colorado tip to expose the central and lateral aspects of the tarsus.
- Mark the desired resection amount using calipers and a surgical marker from the superior edge of the tarsus upward onto the levator.
- Identify the levator attachment onto the tarsus, then use high temperature cautery to detach the levator from the underlying Mueller muscle upward to the marking. Your assistant can help by pulling inferiorly on Mueller muscle during the dissection.
- With a 5-0 double-armed nylon suture, make a 2-3 mm partial-thickness pass centrally through the tarsus with one of the needles at the location of the desired central eyelid peak. After the pass, evert the eyelid to ensure the suture is not full thickness through the tarsus. Pass each arm of the suture through the levator at the previously marked site and tie a temporary knot. Remove the conformer and check the lid height.

> **If the procedure is bilateral, detach the levator on each side first, then pass the suture on each side sequentially, using a temporary tie, to compare lid height. Keep in mind that if the ptosis is asymmetric, the amount of resection and intraoperative lid height target may also be asymmetric.**

- Adjust the lid higher or lower as desired. This should be done carefully, as the levator may be dystrophic and thin and may tear easily. Once at the desired height, cut the loop of the temporary knot and tie permanently.
- Children often have a temporal eyelid droop, and a second suture may needed temporal to the original suture to advance/resect the lateral aspect of the levator. This will make the eyelid contour more natural and avoid temporal hooding.
- Excise excess levator with the high temperature cautery.
- Close the skin using 6-0 fast-absorbing or plain gut suture using interrupted or a running suture. If desired, prior to skin closure, 2-3 sutures may be placed subcutaneously through orbicularis muscle including a small bite of the levator edge to accentuate the lid crease (Fig. 39.3).

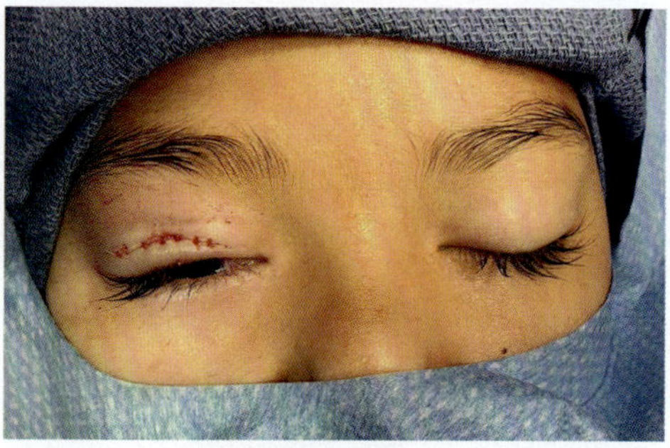

FIGURE 39.3. Postoperative eyelid position (patient with moderate ptosis and good levator function).

POSTOPERATIVE CONSIDERATIONS

Antibiotic ophthalmic ointment is applied to the skin incision and the eye 2-3 times daily. Liquid gel artificial tear drops should be used frequently if there is lagophthalmos. Ice packs applied to the operated lid 10-15 minutes at time, 2-3 times a day, for 2-3 days will help decrease postoperative swelling. Acetaminophen is usually sufficient for postoperative pain management. If the patient had good levator function prior to surgery, postoperative fall is not expected. However, if the patient had poor levator function, postoperative fall may occur (see Table 39.2). Final lid position is most often achieved by 3 months postoperatively.

In the immediate postoperative period, the patient has a high risk of complications from corneal exposure; therefore, aggressive lubrication (artificial tears every 2 hours, ointment prior to naps/bedtime) should be emphasized. Often, lagophthalmos will improve over 1-3 months. Hematoma, excessive edema, and infection are less common, but may occur. The most common long-term postoperative complication is under correction or asymmetry. Given that many cases of congenital ptosis have abnormal levator structure and function, the limitations of the repair, regardless of type of ptosis procedure, must be accepted by the surgeon and communicated well to the caregivers.

References

1. Beard C. The surgical treatment of blepharoptosis: a quantitative approach. *Trans Am Ophthalmol Soc*. 1966;64:401-487.
2. Berke RN. Results of resection of the levator muscle through a skin incision in congenital ptosis. *AMA Arch Ophthalmol*. 1959;61:177-201.
3. Carraway JH, Vincent MP. Levator advancement technique for eyelid ptosis. *Plast Reconstr Surg*. 1986;77:394-403.
4. Heher KL, Katowitz JA. In: Katowitz JA, ed. *Pediatric Oculoplastic Surgery*. New York, NY: Springer; 2002:253-288.

Suggested Reading

Kim CY, Lee SY. Determination of the Amount of Ptosis Correction in Levator Resection Surgery for Pediatric Congenital Ptosis. *Aesth Plast Surg*. 2018;42:201. https://doi.org/10.1007/s00266-017-0982-0.

CHAPTER 40

Pediatric Ptosis Repair: Muller Muscle Conjunctival Resection

Paramjit K. Bhullar, MD • Jason A. Liss, MD

PREOPERATIVE CONSIDERATIONS

Select Appropriate Patients

- Muller muscle conjunctival resection is uncommonly performed in children.
- Procedure advantages:
  - Can be done under local or general anesthesia, a distinct advantage in the pediatric population.
  - There is no visible skin scar.
- Candidates should meet the following criteria:
  - Have between 1 and 2.5 mm ptosis.
  - Have a 1.5-mm improvement in ptosis with phenylephrine testing (ie, 5 minutes after placing 1 drop of phenylephrine 2.5% onto the ptotic eye).

> **A less than 1.5-mm improvement in ptosis with phenylephrine testing may be acceptable in some cases; that is, if it places the eyelid in a position that the patient would consider an improvement.**

  - Have greater than 10 mm levator function.
  - Have a defined lid crease.

> **Patients with congenital ptosis may not have a defined lid crease and would be suboptimal candidates for Muller muscle conjunctival resection, as they would require a separate procedure to create an eyelid crease.**

Preoperative Documentation

- Record the distance between the upper eyelid margin and the corneal light reflex (MRD1) and consider photos before and after phenylephrine testing.
- Record levator function.
- Determine the amount of tissue to be resected.

Numerous nomograms and strategies exist for the amount of tissue to be resected, based the on degree of ptosis; a commonly used strategy is to resect 4 mm of conjunctiva per 1 mm of desired ptosis correction.

Preoperative Counseling

In addition to usual surgical risks, patients should be counseled on the following:

- Foreign body sensation until suture dissolution.
- Undercorrection or overcorrection of ptosis, with need for revision ~15% of the time.

SURGICAL PROCEDURE

- Ensure that the OR has a Putterman clamp.
- If the patient allows, mark the skin of the upper eyelid margin corresponding to the pupillary position while the patient is in primary gaze.
- Evert the eyelid and inject lidocaine 2% with 1:100,000 epinephrine and 200 USP units hyaluronidase per 20 cc anesthetic, into the conjunctiva, superior to the tarsal plate. Alternatively, local anesthetic may be injected inferior to the brow, with the eyelid in normal position.
- Prep and drape the patient in a sterile fashion.
- Place a 4-0 silk suture through the upper eyelid margin, at the level of the tarsus (Fig. 40.1).
- Evert the upper eyelid over a Desmarres retractor (Fig. 40.2).
- Use calipers to measure half the desired resection of conjunctiva superior to the superior border of the tarsus, and mark this distance centrally, medially, and laterally. Note: Allow for at least 5 mm of space between the central mark and the medial mark, as well as between the central mark and lateral mark (Fig. 40.3).
- Use forceps to lift conjunctiva and Muller muscle (it will naturally separate from the underlying levator muscle), place a 6-0 nylon traction suture through each of the three marked areas, and pull up on these traction sutures to elevate the tissue to be clamped and resected (Fig. 40.4).
- Place a Putterman clamp such that it engages the tented conjunctiva at the level of the superior border of the tarsus (Fig. 40.5).

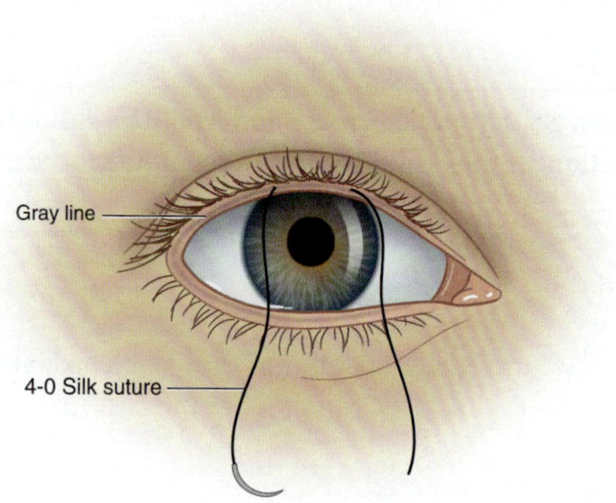

FIGURE 40.1. A 4-0 silk suture is placed through the upper eyelid margin, at the level of the tarsus.

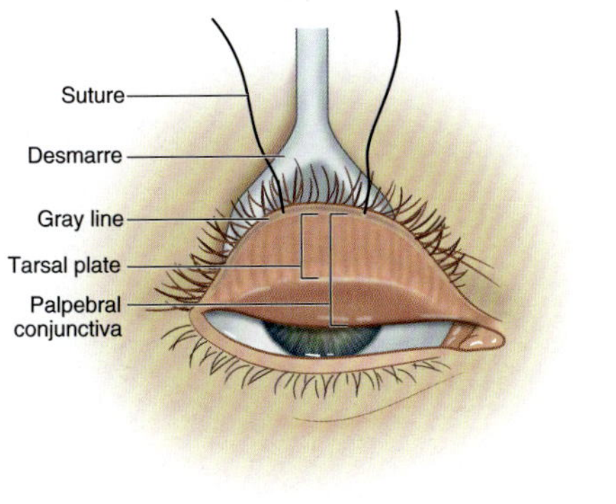

FIGURE 40.2. The upper eyelid is everted over a Desmarres retractor.

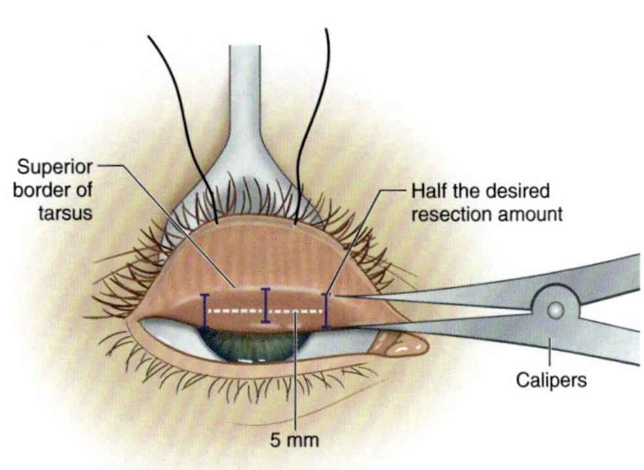

FIGURE 40.3. Calipers measure half the desired resection of conjunctiva superior to the superior border of the tarsus, and this distance is marked centrally, medially, and laterally.

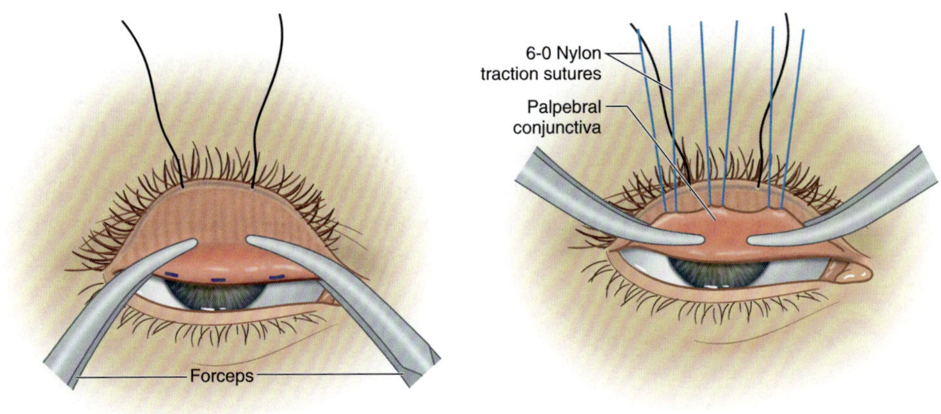

FIGURE 40.4. Forceps lift conjunctiva and Muller muscle and a 6-0 nylon traction sutures are placed through each of the three marked areas, and tissue to be clamped and resected is elevated via tension on the traction sutures.

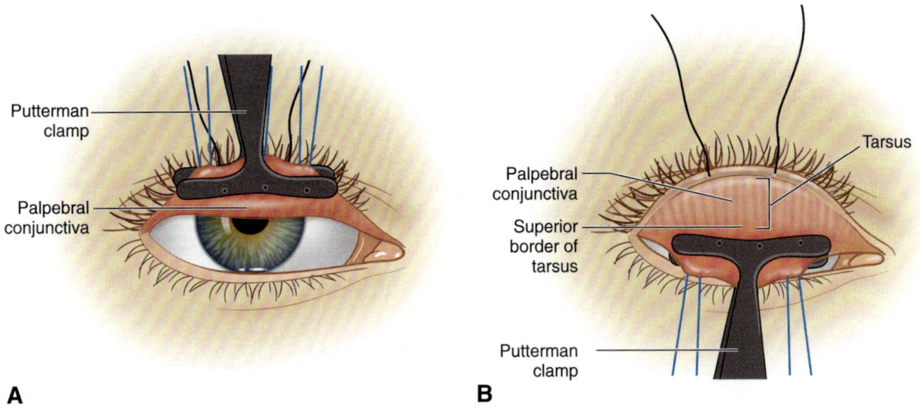

FIGURE 40.5. The Putterman clamp is placed such that it engages the tented conjunctiva at the level of the superior border of the tarsus. (**A:** Putterman held superiorly. **B:** Putterman held inferiorly)

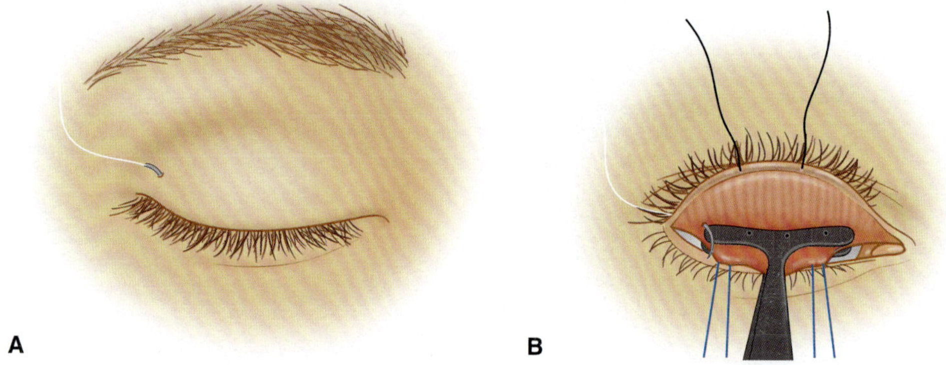

FIGURE 40.6. A 6-0 plain gut suture is passed full-thickness from the skin of the upper eyelid **(A)** to the palpebral conjunctiva, with the exit site of the suture resting lateral but just adjacent to the Putterman clamp **(B)**.

- Place a full-thickness pass of 6-0 plain gut suture from the skin of the upper eyelid to the palpebral conjunctiva, with the exit site of the suture resting lateral, but just adjacent, to the Putterman clamp (Fig. 40.6).
- Run the 6-0 plain gut suture in a horizontal fashion along the length of the eyelid to the other end of the Putterman clamp. Then, turn the suture around and repeat this process until returning to the starting point. Note: the suture should rest just inferior to the Putterman clamp. Tip: It can be helpful to use a sticker to hold the tail of the suture so that it does not get pulled into the eyelid during suturing (Fig. 40.7).
- Pass the needle out beneath (superior to) the tarsus through the skin, near the entry point (Fig. 40.8).

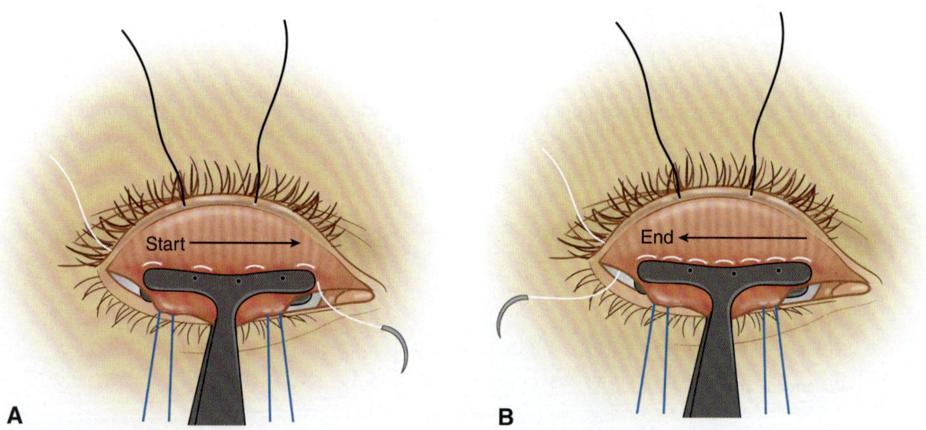

FIGURE 40.7. A 6-0 plain gut suture is placed in a horizontal fashion along the length of the eyelid to the other end of the Putterman clamp **(A)** and back to the starting point **(B)**.

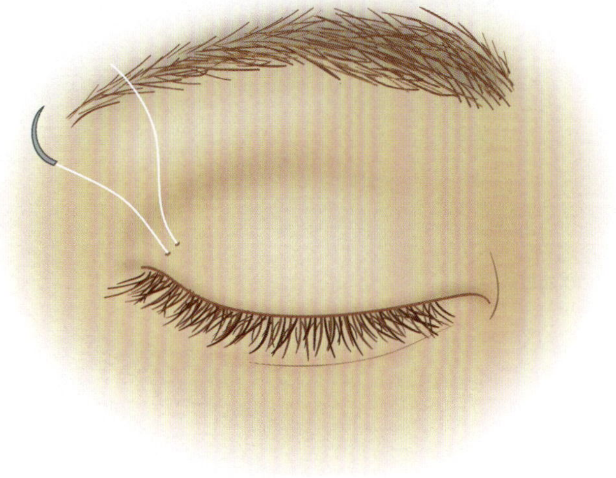

FIGURE 40.8. The needle tip exits superior to the tarsus, through the skin, near the entry point.

- Use a Bard Parker no. 15 blade to make metal-on-metal contact along the Putterman clamp, and cut through the tissue, being careful not to cut the plain gut suture. Pull on the ends of the suture to ensure it was not cut (Fig. 40.9).
- Tie the 6-0 plain gut suture down at the level of the skin (Fig. 40.10).
- Remove the 4-0 silk sutures.
- Place antibiotic ointment onto the globe.

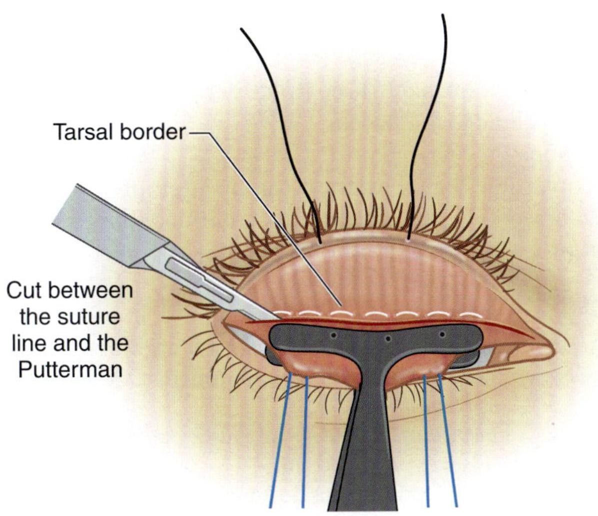

FIGURE 40.9. A 15-blade is used to make metal-on-metal contact along the length of the Putterman clamp, resecting tissue, with care not to cut the suture.

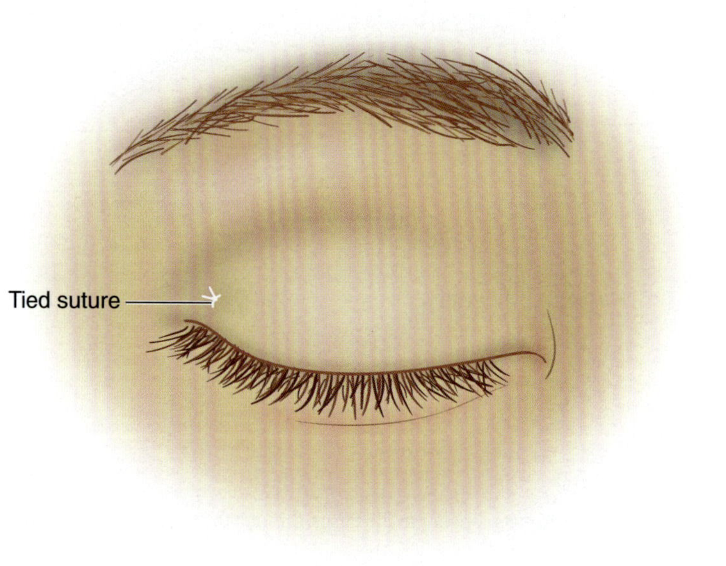

FIGURE 40.10. The 6-0 plain gut suture is tied down at the level of the skin.

Some surgeons like to bury the suture knot under the conjunctiva rather than externalize it. Instead of passing the 6-0 plain suture through the skin, make a small cut in the conjunctiva lateral, but just adjacent to, the Putterman clamp. From this incision, start running the 6-0 plain gut suture horizontally along the Putterman clamp and back as described above, and exit near the entry point of the suture, within the conjunctival incision. Tie the ends to bury the knot within the incision.

POSTOPERATIVE CONSIDERATIONS

- The patient should:
  - Use antibiotic ointment three times per day.
  - Return to clinic in 1-2 weeks.
- Complications:
  - Overcorrection: digital massage can be attempted to lower the eyelid.
  - Undercorrection: usually requires additional surgery, for example, a Fasanella-Servat procedure or a levator advancement or resection (see Chapter 39).

Suggested Readings

American Academy of Ophthalmology. *Muller Muscle Resection in Basic Techniques of Ophthalmic Surgery*. 2nd ed. United States of America: Academy of Ophthalmology; 2015: 433-436.

Korn B, Kikkawa D. *Video Atlas of Oculofacial Plastic and Reconstructive Surgery*. 2nd ed. Amsterdam, Netherlands: Elsevier; 2016:33-36.

Putterman AM, Urist MJ. Müller muscle-conjunctiva resection: technique for treatment of blepharoptosis. *Arch Ophthalmol*. 1975;93(8):619-623.

CHAPTER 41

Pediatric Ptosis Repair: Blepharophimosis Syndrome

Michael J. Richard, MD

Blepharophimosis syndrome is a rare disorder either inherited as an autosomal dominant trait or occurring sporadically. The major findings of the syndrome include severe congenital ptosis, horizontal narrowing of the palpebral fissures, and epicanthal folds extending superiorly from the lower eyelid (epicanthus inversus). Other findings may include telecanthus, absence of a lid crease, low nasal bridge, and euryblepharon (Fig. 41.1). Female blepharophimosis patients can have primary ovarian insufficiency, which may affect menstruation and fertility.

EXAMINATION AND SURGICAL PLANNING

- Assess for degree of ptosis including levator function by measuring MRD1 and levator function. Ptosis is typically severe (MRD1 < 1 mm), and levator function is extremely poor (<4 mm), and correction necessitates a frontalis sling procedure.
- Note presence and degree of anomalous head position (chin up) and any effect this position is having on development (sitting in an infant, walking in toddler or older child).
- Measure visual acuity with attention toward amblyopia.

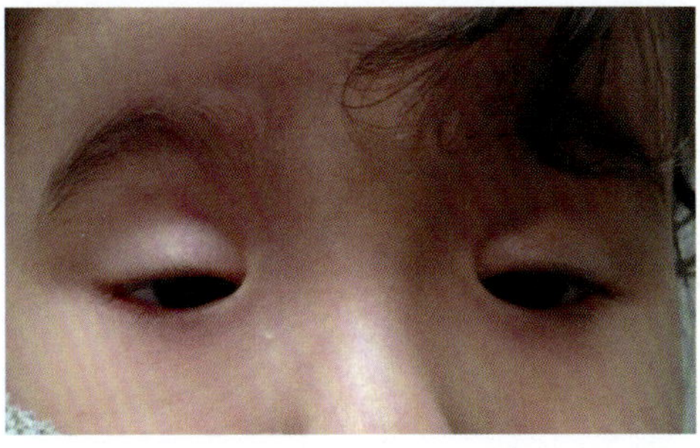

FIGURE 41.1. Patient with blepharophimosis syndrome findings of congenital ptosis, epicanthus inversus, and telecanthus.

- Perform cycloplegic refraction as ptosis can cause significant astigmatism (usually with-the-rule).
- Assess degree of telecanthus and epicanthus inversus. Severe telecanthus may require transnasal wiring, but more moderate degrees can be addressed by epicanthoplasty and medial canthal tendon plication.

Some authors advocate staging the procedures. Alternatively, treatment of the ptosis, epicanthal deformities, and telecanthus can be performed concurrently during a single surgery, usually around the age of 1 year. Earlier surgery may be necessary if ptosis is causing deprivational amblyopia or an anomalous head position that is affecting the child's development.

In an infant, the maximum safe doses of local anesthetic are relatively small, and if performing the ptosis and epicanthus surgery simultaneously and bilaterally, the injection volumes desired for hemostasis in multiple wounds can easily exceed the maximum doses. It is important to calculate the total maximum volume of anesthetic based on weight and not exceed that amount (see Chapters 1 and 42). For example, the maximum dose of lidocaine with epinephrine is 7 mg/kg. In a 6-kg baby, the maximum volume of 2% epinephrine with lidocaine would be 2.1 cc. One way to reduce the amount of anesthetic and still achieve hemostasis is to reduce the percentage of lidocaine from the typical 2% to 1% (which will double the volume that can be safely administered). Another approach would be to inject the needed anesthetic for the first part of the procedure (eg, bilateral epicanthus repair), perform that procedure, and later (after time for drug metabolism) inject for the second procedure (eg, frontalis slings). The anesthesia team can be very helpful in calculating weight-based maximum doses and volumes.

PTOSIS

Materials-BD Visitec Frontalis Suspension set (Seiff) consisting of a 0.9 mm by 6.3-cm silicone rod with swaged needles (20G × 2½ inches) on each end and a 10-mm long silicone sleeve with which the silicone rods can be secured.

The most common frontalis sling suspensory materials include autogenous fascia lata, preserved fascia lata, and 1-mm silicone rods (see chapter 38). Silicone rods produce less lagophthalmos because of the elastic nature of the material and are also adjustable.

Frontalis Sling Surgical Procedure

Many configurations have been described based on the location and number of stab incisions—including triangular, rhomboid, pentagonal, double triangular, and double rhomboid (see chapter 38). The pentagonal configuration (described here) utilizes five stab incisions with a single strand of silicone tubing as the suspensory material.

- Mark the planned incisions prior to injecting local anesthetic with epinephrine (Fig. 41.2).
- Place a corneal protector in the operative eye.

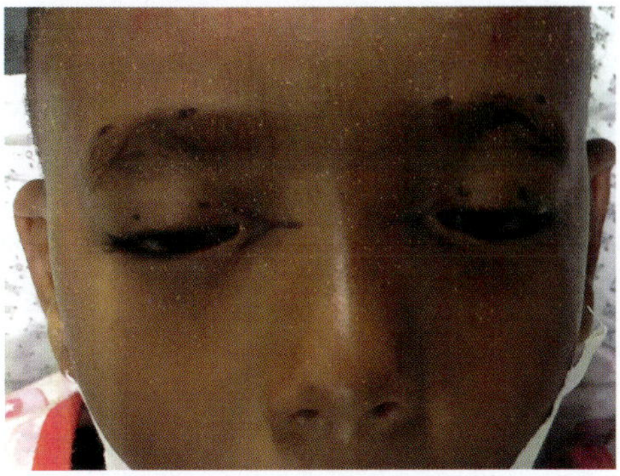

FIGURE 41.2. Preoperative markings for repair of blepharophimosis by frontalis sling procedure and Y-to-V advancement.

- Make a central brow incision using a Bard-Parker no. 15 or no. 64 blade at the superior border of the brow cilia in line with the pupil. Enlarge the incision slightly so that it is just larger than the width of the blade. The stab should be made down to the level of the frontalis muscle, which is adherent to the periosteum at this level. Once the incision is made, use a Stevens scissor to bluntly dissect a pocket in this tissue plane to allow room for the silicone sling.
- Make two paramedian brow incisions at the superior border of the brow and just outside the corresponding limbus. Each of these is only the width of the blade. Again, use a Stevens scissor to bluntly dissect a small pocket beneath the skin and subcutaneous tissues.
- Make two horizontal eyelid incisions ~2-6 mm above the lash line (corresponding to the upper half of the tarsal plate) and just inside the corresponding limbus. Sharply dissect down to the epitarsus using Westcott scissors. Alternatively, use a no. 64 blade to make a stab incision down to epitarsus.

Placing these incisions closer together will result in a more peaked lid contour, while placing the incisions further apart will result in a flatter lid contour. Placing these incisions closer to the lid margin may give more lift but may also be more likely to result in entropion.

Use a Webster needle driver and bend the needle to approximate a 3/8 curve suture needle, which gives some mechanical advantage in passing through the tissue.

- Introduce one of the needles from the suspension set through the medial eyelid incision and gain purchase of the epitarsus.
- Pass the needle along the length of the tarsus until the lateral incision and pull the sling until equal segments are visible from each eyelid incision.
- Pass the lateral needle back into the lateral eyelid incision aiming vertically for the lateral paramedian brow incision. Attempt to pass the needle in a postseptal plane and then gain purchase of the arcus marginalis at the superior orbital rim before passing the needle out of the lateral brow incision. This directs the vectors of lift in the most natural and advantageous directions and also minimizes the possibility of seeing the sling through the skin. It is helpful to introduce a partially opened Adson forceps into the brow incision with downward pressure against the frontal bone to receive the needle as you pass it out the incision. This stabilizes the tissues and

prevents you from grasping more superficial tissues, which may lead to dimpling of the skin and soft tissues overlying the sling.

- Pass the medial needle from the medial eyelid incision to the medial brow incision in the same manner.

Each pass of the needle significantly dulls the tip of the needle. In this case, the needle extending from the lateral eyelid incision will have already passed through tissue and will be noticeably duller than the medial needle.

- Pass the lateral needle in through the lateral brow incision and out through the lateral aspect of the central brow incision. Make the pass deep to the subcutaneous tissues in the plane just anterior to the frontalis muscle. Introduce an Adson forceps into the central brow incision to help receive the needle just as in the previous step. You can leave the needle in place for the next step so that the needles pass in a "crossed swords" technique to avoid spearing the sling as the second needle is passed.
- Pass the medial needle in through the medial brow incision and out through the medial aspect of the central brow incision in the same manner.
- Use a heavy hemostat or Webster to straighten the previously bent needles.
- Pass each needle through the silicone sleeve provided in the set. A Watzke sleeve spreading forceps is helpful to gain access to the inner diameter of the sleeve and to facilitate the passage of the needle. The lateral needle should be passed from lateral to medial through the sleeve, and the medial needle should be passed opposite the lateral needle. A "crossed swords" technique can prevent spearing the sling with the needle. Once the needles are passed through the sleeve, remove the needles.
- Pull the silicone ends to tighten the sling while checking for appropriate height and contour. Aim for the lid height to be at the superior limbus intraoperatively.

The lid height typically drops between 1 and 2 mm postoperatively.

- Adjust the lid contour by pulling more or less on one of the silicone ends. Pulling on the more medial silicone end after it has passed through the sleeve will raise the lateral aspect of the eyelid and vice versa. It is common to have to pull more on the sling that controls the lateral eyelid, but this should be adjusted as dictated by the intraoperative lid position. Trim the ends of the sling, leaving a few millimeters on each side in case the sling needs to be tightened or loosened.
- Tuck the sleeve into the wound, making sure both the sleeve and the ends are well covered and not going to extrude out of the wound. Check to make sure the lid did not drop excessively after the sleeve was tucked into the wound.
- Close each of the stab incisions with interrupted 6-0 plain gut suture. The central brow incision usually requires two sutures, while the remainder of the incisions require only one.

Postoperative Care

Apply ophthalmic ointment to all incisions and into each eye three times per day. Use ice 15 minutes per hour for 48 hours while awake only as tolerated by the child. See the patient in 7-10 days for follow-up.

EPICANTHAL FOLDS

Treating the epicanthal folds prior to the frontalis sling can be helpful to give a bit more horizontal length and improve the contour of the lid with a sling. Several techniques have been described for the treatment of epicanthal folds. The Y-to-V advancement flap described by Dutton for mild to moderate folds and a four flap or "running man" technique for moderate to severe folds (a Y-to-V advancement flap with the addition of a Z-plasty on either side) are described below.

Y-TO-V ADVANCEMENT FLAP WITH MEDIAL CANTHAL TENDON PLICATION

Surgical Procedure

- Mark a horizontal V-shaped incision with the apex of the V 5-7 mm medial to the medial canthal angle. The arms of the V should be parallel to the upper and lower lid margins and should extend for 8-10 mm approximately 2-3 mm from the lid margin. Mark a horizontal line from the point of the V for a length of 5-7 mm to create a Y-shaped incision. The longer the limbs of the incision, the more correction you will achieve (Figs. 41.2 and 41.3).
- Cut along the marked skin sites with a no. 15 blade. Use Westcott scissors to dissect a skin-muscle flap and undermine slightly in all directions. This will expose the medial canthal tendon.
- Pass each arm of a double-armed 4-0 Mersilene suture lateral to medial through the medial canthal tendon near the canthal angle. Then pass each arm of the suture through the periosteum at the anterior lacrimal crest.

Remember that the lacrimal sac lies just deep to the medial canthal tendon and just posterior to the anterior lacrimal crest. You want to pass as deep as possible so as to not pull the lower lid away from the globe but not so deep as to damage the lacrimal sac. Passing a Bowman probe can be helpful if there is any doubt about the location of the lacrimal sac.

- Advance the skin-muscle flap medially into the defect. If needed, excise some of the excess subcutaneous tissue from beneath the V portion of the flap for cosmesis.
- Close the apex with a 6-0 chromic suture and the remainder of the incisions with 7-0 chromic suture (Fig. 41.4).

Postoperative Care

Apply ophthalmic ointment to all incisions three times per day. Use ice 15 minutes per hour for 48 hours while awake only as tolerated by the child. See the patient for follow-up in 7-10 days.

FIGURE 41.3. A Y-shaped incision is marked as described in the surgical procedure section. After incising the marked site, the tissue is undermined widely and point A is advanced to appose point B.

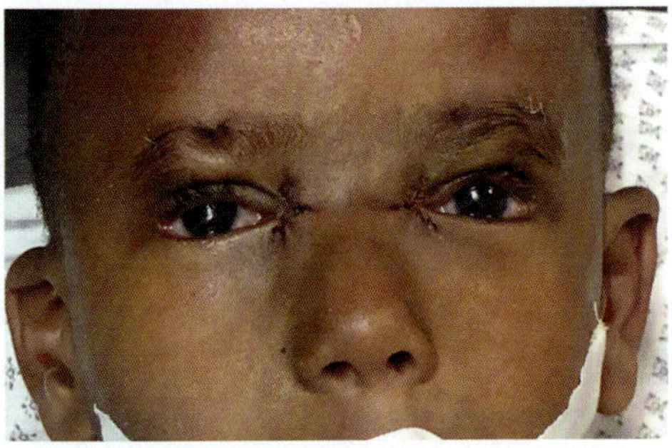

FIGURE 41.4. Photo showing the immediate postoperative position of lids and medial canthus following frontalis sling and Y-to-V advancement.

FOUR FLAP OR "RUNNING MAN" TECHNIQUE

This technique is the exact same as the aforementioned Y-to-V advancement flap but with an added Z-plasty incision on either side of the Y to V. When drawn, it looks like a stick figure flexing both arms (Fig. 41.5).

Surgical Procedure

- Mark the Y-to-V as described previously.
- Mark the midpoint of the horizontal line and draw a V with its point oriented laterally on either side. These Vs are the "flexing arms" of the stick figure. Each of these Vs will form a Z-plasty with the lateral half of the horizontal segment (the lower half of the trunk of the stick figure). Each limb of the V should be ~1-2 mm longer than the lateral half of the horizontal segment. The angle of the V segment should be ~60 degrees with the horizontal segment and 45 degrees with itself (Fig. 41.5).
- Once the incision sites are drawn, incise along the marked sites with a no. 15 blade.
- Dissect a skin-muscle flap and undermine gently using Westcott scissors.
- Plicate the medial canthal tendon using double-armed 4-0 Mersilene suture as described in the Y-to-V section.
- Transpose each of the four skin-muscle flaps and close them with interrupted 7-0 chromic sutures (Fig. 41.6).
- Advance the point of the V medially into the base of the Y and close with a single 6-0 chromic suture (Fig. 41.6).

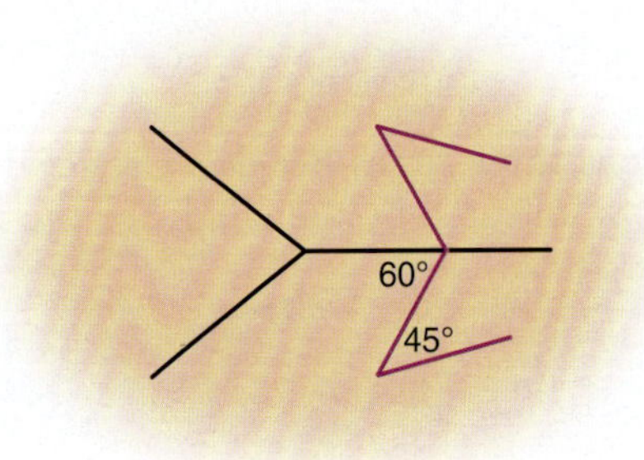

FIGURE 41.5. The "running man" flap orientation involves the standard Y-to-V composition with the addition of Z-plasties (shown in purple). Each limb of the Z-plasty is 1-2 mm longer than half of the horizontal segment of the Y.

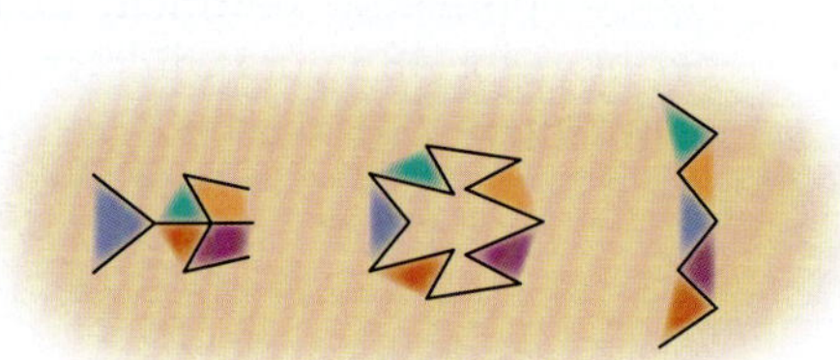

FIGURE 41.6. Color-coded diagram demonstrating the transposition of each flap segment in the "running man" technique.

Postoperative Care

Apply ophthalmic ointment to all incisions three times per day. Use ice 15 minutes per hour for 48 hours while awake only as tolerated by the child. See the patient in 7-10 days for follow-up.

TELECANTHUS

Transnasal Wiring Surgical Procedure

- Materials
  - 16G spinal needle with trocar.
  - 28G, 30G, or 32G stainless steel wire.
  - Supramid sheet 0.3 mm thickness.
  - Drill with 2-mm rotary burr.
- Pack the nose with neurosurgical patties soaked in oxymetazoline hydrochloride (Afrin) 0.05%.
- Mark a V-shaped skin incision with the point of the V ~7 mm medial to the medial canthal angle. Extend each arm ~8-10 mm parallel to the lid margin.
- Incise the marked skin sites with a Bard-Parker no. 15 blade.
- Dissect a skin-muscle flap to expose the medial canthal tendon.
- Undermine anteriorly from the anterior lacrimal crest in a preperiosteal plane to provide exposure for the transnasal wire from the opposite side later in the procedure.
- Cut the medial canthal tendon close to its periosteal insertion at the anterior lacrimal crest.
- Incise the periosteum just posterior to the anterior lacrimal crest with a scalpel and elevate the periorbita within the lacrimal sac fossa using a Freer elevator.
- Reflect the periorbita and the lacrimal sac laterally.
- Punch through the lacrimal bone with a small hemostat taking care not to disturb the nasal mucosa. Enlarge the ostium using 2-mm Kerrison rongeurs until the opening is ~5 mm in diameter. The ostium should remain posterior to the anterior lacrimal crest.
- Perform the same dissection on the opposite side.
- Drill a 2-mm hole through the nasal bone just anterior to the anterior lacrimal crest.
- Pass a 16G spinal needle with trocar into the drill hole and then through the nasal septum and out through the ostium on the opposite side. Take care to protect the globe on the contralateral side with a corneal protector and a small malleable while the needle is being passed. Remove the trocar and pass the two free ends of a piece of 28G, 30G, or 32G stainless steel wire into the bore of the spinal needle and pull the needle and wires out the opposite nasal bone. Hold the wires and remove the spinal needle. Repeat these steps on the opposite side. On each side, you will have a wire loop that passes into the nasal bone, passes through the nasal septum and into the ostium on the contralateral side where it loops back on itself through the same path and emerges again from the nasal bone (Fig. 41.7).
- Pass a double-armed 4-0 Mersilene suture through the medial canthal tendon close to its tarsal attachment and then tie the suture through the looped end of the wire.
- Cut a small sheet of Supramid to a size of ~4-5 mm diameter and pass the free ends of the wire through the sheet. The sheets may need to be pierced with a 25G needle to aid in passing the wire.
- Pull the wires until the opposite canthal tendon is pulled into the bony ostium and into the desired position. Twist the wire ends together to secure the tension on them. Cut the ends and bend them toward the Supramid sheet so as to not cause irritation in the surrounding soft tissue.

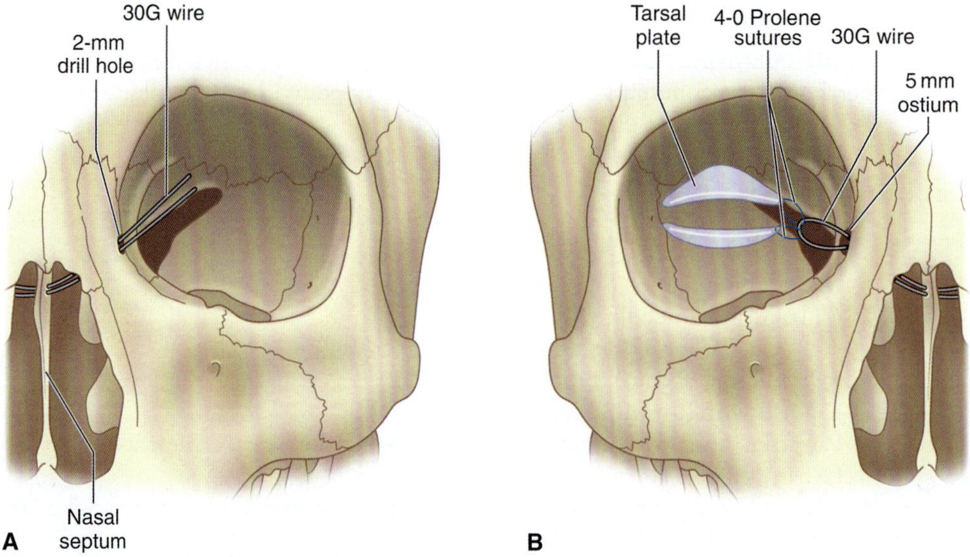

FIGURE 41.7. Schematic for transnasal wiring to repair severe telecanthus of the right eye in blepharophimosis syndrome. **A.** A 2-mm hole is drilled on the left side just anterior to the anterior lacrimal crest. A stainless steel wire is passed through the drill site, through the nasal septum, and out the 5 mm ostium that has been created in the lacrimal bone on the right side. This wire is then passed back through the same course where it is again retrieved through the 2-mm drill hole on the left side. **B.** A 4-0 Prolene suture is passed from the medial edge of the upper and lower tarsal plates to the loop of stainless steel wire as it exits the 5 mm ostium on the right side. This provides purchase of both the upper and lower eyelids and will allow for their repositioning medially and posteriorly when the stainless steel wire is tightened and secured on the left side.

- Pass a 6-0 chromic suture through the center of the skin-muscle flap and then pass through the medial canthal tendon and back out the skin more medially. Tie this suture in a mattress fashion to help reform the normal concavity of the medial canthus. The remainder of the skin is closed with interrupted 7-0 chromic sutures.

Postoperative Care

Apply ophthalmic ointment to all incisions three times per day. Use 15 minutes per hour for 48 hours while awake only as tolerated by the child. See the patient in 7-10 days for follow-up.

Suggested Readings

Dutton JJ. Medial and lateral canthal reconstruction. In: Dutton JJ, ed. *Atlas of Ophthalmic Surgery, Volume II: Oculoplastic, Lacrimal, and Orbital Surgery*. St. Louis, MO: Mosby-Year Book; 1992:199-203, 214-215.

Foster JA, Katowitz JA. Developmental eyelid abnormalities. In: Katowitz JA, ed. *Pediatric Oculoplastic Surgery*. New York, NY: Springer-Verlag; 2002:212-213.

McCord CD Jr, Codner MA. Pediatric eyelid anomalies. In: McCord CD Jr, Codner MA, eds. *Eyelid and Periorbital Surgery*. St. Louis, MO: Quality Medical Publishing, Inc; 2008:776-779.

Section IX

Strabismus Surgery

CHAPTER 42

The Basics

Lucas Bonafede, MD

ANATOMY[1,2] (FIG. 42.1)

- All the extraocular muscles except the inferior oblique muscle originate from the orbital apex. The inferior oblique muscle originates from the anterior orbital floor lateral to the lacrimal sac.
- The rectus muscles form the muscle cone in the orbit with the apex at their origin and base at their penetration of Tenon capsule.
- The muscles are surrounded by fibrous capsules that are attached by a thin continuous membrane called the intermuscular septum.
- The superior rectus and inferior rectus muscles have attachments to the upper and lower eyelids, respectively.

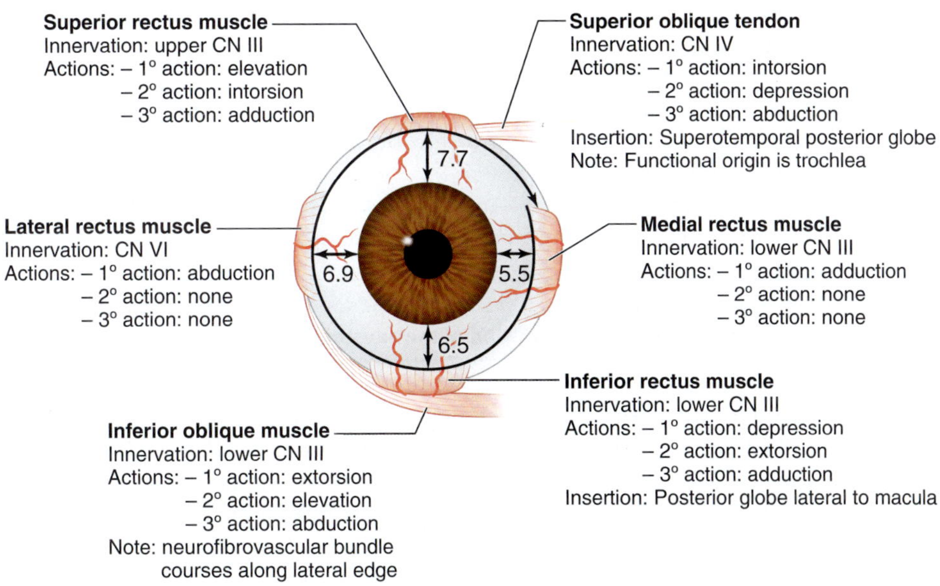

FIGURE 42.1. Anatomic representation of extraocular muscle insertions, innervations, and function.

Because of attachments to the upper and lower eyelids, vertical rectus muscle strengthening or weakening procedures can change the eyelid position.

- The arterial blood supply to the rectus muscles is from the medial and lateral muscular branches of the ophthalmic artery, which give rise to the anterior ciliary arteries. Variable number of anterior ciliary arteries emerge from the rectus muscle tendons and enter the episclera by the limbus to perfuse the anterior segment.

Anterior segment ischemia is a risk of strabismus surgery, especially when operating on multiple muscles and in patients with risk factors (see Chapter 54).

ANESTHESIA (SEE CHAPTER 1)

The choice of anesthesia depends on patient factors (age, level of anxiety, ability to cooperate with surgery, comorbidities), surgical plan (ie, adjustable sutures, reoperation, bilateral), and surgeon preference.

- General anesthesia:
  - Best option for children and uncooperative adults.
  - Risks of general anesthesia should be reviewed with the patient.
  - May limit ability to accurately test ocular alignment until full recovery.
  - Most suitable for pediatric patients, complex cases, reoperations, and bilateral surgery.
- Topical anesthesia:
  - Good option for cooperative patients, patients in whom general anesthesia is contraindicated, and adjustable suture cases.
  - Usually administered in conjunction with light sedation.
  - Typically performed with tetracaine and lidocaine gel; reapplications may be necessary.
  - May require conversion to general or retrobulbar anesthesia if unable to complete surgery safely with topical anesthesia.
  - Most suitable for routine cases; use cautiously for reoperations or complicated strabismus.
- Retrobulbar anesthesia:
  - May limit ability to accurately test ocular alignment until anesthetic has reversed.
  - Risks scleral perforation and/or retrobulbar hemorrhage (especially if the patient is on blood thinners).
  - Relative contraindications—increased axial length, bleeding diathesis, thyroid eye disease, space-occupying lesion within the orbit, and previous scleral buckling.

Because CN IV travels outside the muscle cone, the superior oblique may not be affected by a retrobulbar block until there is adequate diffusion of the anesthetic.

Take care to limit the volume injected of retrobulbar anesthesia to avoid excess sub-Tenon and subconjunctival fluid, which can make surgery more difficult. A modified Van Lint block can be used in conjunction with a retrobulbar block in order to provide akinesia to the orbicularis oculi.

- Local anesthetic dosing:[3]
  - It is important to consider maximum doses for safe administration of anesthetics. This is particularly relevant in infant surgery, especially oculoplastics procedures such as frontalis sling and blepharophimosis repair.
  - Maximum dose recommendations are based on systemic toxicity, not local toxicity.

- Toxicity: CNS dysfunction and depression, including respiratory and cardiovascular dysfunction.
- Maximum single dose should be determined by the clinical judgment of the physician administering the medication. General guidelines based on the cited reference are as follows:
  - **Lidocaine with epinephrine:** 6-7 mg/kg (max 500 mg/dose).
  - **Bupivacaine with epinephrine:** 2.5-3 mg/kg (max 225 mg/dose).

POSITIONING—SURGEON AND PATIENT

- Position the patient in the supine position with his or her neck extended (slight "sniffing position") so that the operative area is flat.
- Maintain close communication with the anesthesia team to ensure any head positioning is performed in a safe manner.
- Tilt the bed and/or head to improve exposure if necessary.

Turning the head toward the surgeon can be especially helpful for scleral passes when recessing the horizontal rectus muscles.

- Consider using a bed with a headrest in order to aid in patient positioning and comfort. Additionally, wrist rests or chairs with armrests may help provide support for the surgeon's arms.
- For most rectus muscles, sit across from the operative muscle to provide optimal exposure. Sit superiorly or on the opposite side if operating on the inferior oblique muscle. For the superior rectus or superior oblique muscles, determine the position that optimizes exposure and facilitates use of the dominant hand (eg, a right-handed surgeon can access superior muscles most easily when seated on the patient's right).

PREPPING AND DRAPING

- Some surgeons prefer exposing only the operative eye, others prefer having both eye exposed. This may be dependent on the choice of anesthesia.
- Prep the operative eye, both eyes, or the upper face with 5% povidone-iodine, per surgeon preference.
- Place a towel or gauze over the laryngeal mask airway (LMA) or endotracheal tube to prevent inadvertent extubation of the patient during drape removal.
- Some surgeons use a bladed speculum, others prefer a wire speculum. If a wire speculum is planned, use Tegaderm or a plastic drape to isolate the lashes from the operative field.

Installation of povidone-iodine in fornices pre- and postsurgery decreases bacterial colonization and may reduce risk for infection.[4,5]

Surgeries performed under topical anesthesia may benefit from prepping and draping both eyes in order to test alignment intraoperatively without needing to re-prep for adjustments.

Covering the eyebrows with Tegaderm can reduce risk of accidental removal of brow hairs when taking off an adhesive drape.

FORCED DUCTION AND EXAGGERATED TRACTION TESTING

The forced duction and exaggerated traction tests can be helpful to detect restrictions or laxity (especially superior oblique laxity). These tests are performed either with topical anesthesia (tetracaine drops or lidocaine gel) or after the induction of general anesthesia.

The benefit of using topical anesthesia is the ability to also test for force generation, which is helpful to identify paralytic strabismus.

- Description of procedure:
  - Use toothed forceps to grasp close to limbus where the conjunctiva and Tenon capsule fuse 90 degrees away from the muscle being tested.
  - Put the muscle being tested on stretch to isolate its field of action when testing for restriction (ie, tightness appreciated in lateral gaze indicates possible medial rectus muscle restriction).
    - For horizontal and vertical recti, proptose the globe.
    - For oblique muscles, retropulse the globe.
  - Observe how the muscle behaves and what position it returns to after its release for information regarding restriction and the elastic properties of the muscle.
- Complications include subconjunctival hemorrhage, tearing or stretching of conjunctiva, and corneal abrasions/lacerations from a slipped instrument.

When testing the superior oblique muscle, a "popping" sensation may be felt when rotating the eye in an elevated and adducted position as the globe slips over the superior oblique tendon.[6] The degree of tightness during this test correlates with clinical overaction.

SUTURES/NEEDLES/INSTRUMENTS

- Suture/needles:
  - Traction suture: 4-0 to 6-0 silk.
  - Muscle: 6-0 absorbable suture (ie, Vicryl or Polysorb, single or double armed depending on surgical technique). A spatulated needle (S14, S24) is commonly used.
    - Load the needle with a second instrument as opposed to using hands or fingers to decrease the risk of postoperative infection and needle sticks.
    - Avoid holding the needle with the needle holder during tying or manipulating the suture, as it may dull the needle tip and/or lead to accidental needle sticks.
    - Single or double lock the knots at each pole to ensure the muscle is secured.
    - Secure sutures with 2-1-1 knot (Figure 42.2).
  - Conjunctival closure: 8-0 Vicryl/Chromic gut/Plain gut.

In cases where the conjunctiva is thin and friable (ie, older patients), use a BV-1 taper needle, which is very small and delicate and less likely to damage fragile tissues.

When tying the 2-1-1 knot, leaving one side of the suture longer than the other facilitates tying a square knot; always start a throw by grabbing the longer side of suture (Fig. 42.2).

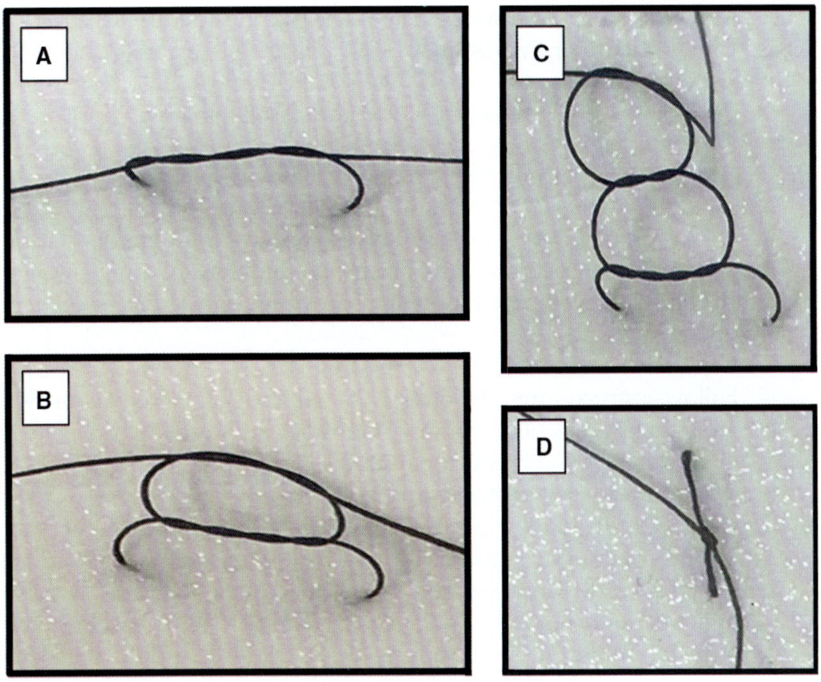

FIGURE 42.2. **A-D.** Square knot 2-1-1 technique.

- Instruments (Fig. 42.3):
  - Locking or nonlocking forceps—eg, Bishop Harmon, Castroviejo 0.5 mm (locking and nonlocking), Curved Moody.
  - Needle holder—locking or nonlocking, curved or straight.
  - Scissors—eg, blunt-tip Westcott scissors.
  - Muscle hooks—eg, Stevens "small," Jameson, Green, Wright, Von Graefe, Culler.

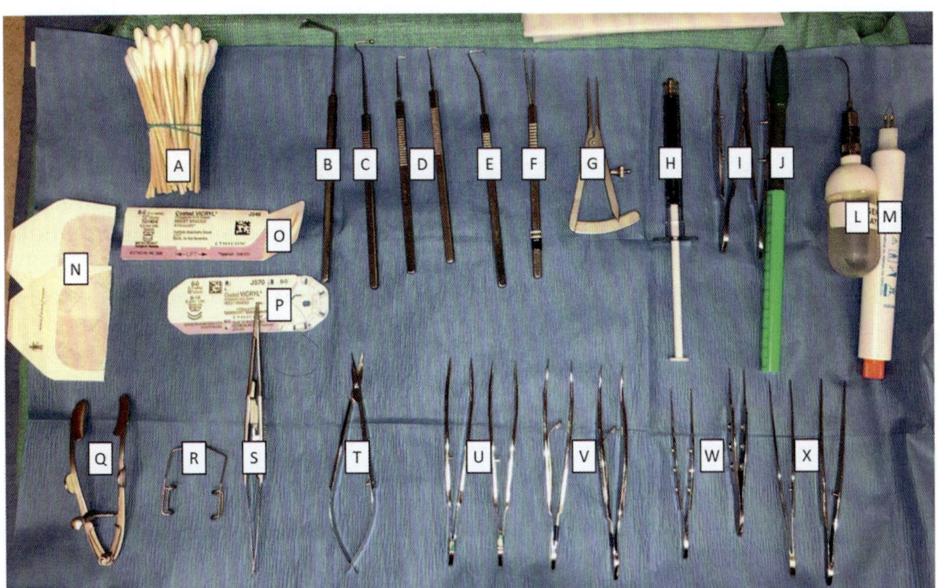

A: Cotton-tip applicators. B. Fisson retractor. C. Jameson hook. D. Stevens "small" hook. E. Green "square" hook. F. Velez hook. G: Calipers. H. Dilute povidone-iodine. I: 0.5mm Castroviejo Forceps. J. Marking pen. L: Irrigation bulb. M: Cautery. N: Tegaderm. O: 8-0 Vicryl suture on TG-140-6 needle. P: 6-0 Vicryl suture on S-14 needle. Q. Bladed speculum. R: Wire speculum. S. Locking needle-holder. T. Wescott scissor. U: Tying forceps. V: Moody fixation forceps. W: Tissue forceps. X: Smooth forceps.

FIGURE 42.3. Strabismus surgery set.

- Measuring device—calipers, ruler, scleral ruler (Scott curved).
- Muscle clamp or hemostat.
- Eyelid speculum.
- Retractors—eg, Desmarres, Helveston, Fison, etc.

SPECIAL CONSIDERATIONS

- Consider preoperative, intraoperative, and/or postoperative antibiotics in special populations, such as those with a history of previous filtering/shunt surgery, immune compromise, developmental delay, previous or concurrent infection (skin, ear, rhinitis).[7]
- Postoperative care:
  - Follow-up recommendations vary significantly between providers, ranging from 1 day to 6 weeks postoperative. Consider initial follow-up visits for:
    - Children: 1-3 days postoperative.
    - Adults: 1 week postoperative.
  - Activity restrictions typically include no swimming or water near/in the eyes for 2 weeks and no strenuous activities, including trampolines and heavy weight lifting for 1 week. Most children can return to school in 2-3 days after surgery. Adult patients can resume driving once they are able to perform quick eye movements without hesitation and vision is appropriate. The decision to return to driving may vary depending on local regulation and should be made on a case-to-case level by the physician and patient.
  - Instruct patients and patient families to call immediately for increased redness and swelling of the eyes, pain, discharge, decreased vision, eyelid pain or swelling, fever, or lethargy as these suggest infection. They should also be told to call immediately for abrupt change in eye position with reduced ductions, which may indicate a slipped muscle (see Chapter 54).
  - Medications:
    - Topical antibiotic and steroid, if desired.
    - Acetaminophen and/or ibuprofen per package insert. Narcotics are rarely indicated.
    - Consider an antiemetic (eg, ondansetron) in patients at high risk for postoperative nausea and vomiting.

SURGICAL GUIDELINES FOR STRABISMUS SURGERY

The following tables are abstracted from the Atlas of Ophthalmic Surgery: Volume III[1] and are frequently used by the Pediatric Ophthalmology and Strabismus faculty at Duke Eye Center for surgical planning. There are many different guidelines available with different approaches to surgical planning (Tables 42.1-42.9). These tables present suggested numbers for routine surgery and are based on the technique used by the authors. Individual surgeons should determine the best guideline for their surgical style.

TABLE 42.1. Bilateral Surgery

Esotropia[a,b] Prism diopter	Medial rectus recession Both eyes (mm)	OR	Lateral rectus resection Both eyes (mm)
15	4.0		4.0
20	4.5		5.0
25	5.0		5.5
30	5.5		6.0
40	6.0		7.0
50	6.5		8.0
>50	Three muscle surgery (Table 42.3)		
Exotropia[a] Prism diopter	**Lateral rectus recession Both eyes (mm)**	**OR**	**Medial rectus resection Both eyes (mm)**
15	5.0		3.0
20	6.0		4.0
25	6.5		5.0
30	7.0		5.5
35	7.5		6.0
40	8.0		6.0
45	9.0		6.0
50	10.0		6.0
>50	Three muscle surgery (Table 42.3)		

[a]*Subtract 1 mm from each muscle for <12 months of age.*
[b]*For high AC/A ratio, add 1 mm to medial rectus recession.*

TABLE 42.2. Unilateral Surgery

Esotropia[a] Prism diopter	Medial rectus recession (mm)	AND	Lateral rectus resection (mm)
15	4.0		4.0
20	4.0		5.0
25	5.0		5.0
30	5.0		6.0
35	5.0		7.0
40	6.0		7.0
50	6.0		8.0
Exotropia[a] Prism diopter	**Lateral rectus recession (mm)**	**AND**	**Medial rectus resection (mm)**
15	4.0		3.0
20	5.0		4.0
25	6.0		4.0
30	7.0		5.0
35	8.0		5.0
40	9.0		6.0
50	10.0		6.0

[a]*Subtract 1 mm from each muscle for <12 months of age.*

TABLE 42.3. Three Muscle Surgery

Esotropia Prism diopter	Medial rectus recession (mm) Both eyes	AND	Lateral rectus resection (mm) One eye
60	6.0		5.0
70	6.0		7.0
80	6.0		9.0
90	6.5		10.0
>90	Four muscle surgery		
Exotropia Prism diopter	**Lateral rectus recession (mm) Both eyes**	**AND**	**Medial rectus resection (mm) One eye**
60	9.0		4.0
70	10.0		5.0
80	10.0		6.0
>80	Four muscle surgery		

TABLE 42.4. Hang-back Recession

Prism diopter	Esotropia Medial rectus recession Both eyes (mm)	Exotropia Lateral rectus recession Both eyes (mm)
15	N/A	3.5
20	4.0	4.0
25	4.5	5.0
30	5.0	6.0
35	5.5	7.0
40	6.0	8.0
50	6.5	9.0
60	7.0	10.0

TABLE 42.5. Vertical Deviations[a]

Hypertropia (prism diopter)	Superior rectus recession (mm)		Inferior rectus resection (mm)		Superior rectus resection (mm)		Inferior rectus recession (mm)
5	3		N/A		N/A		3
10	4-5		N/A		N/A		4-5
15	4	AND	3	OR	3	AND	4
20	5		4		4		5
25	6		5		5		6
30	7		5		6		6

[a]*For thyroid myopathy with tight inferior rectus, use only recession of inferior rectus and decrease amounts by 1 mm or use adjustable sutures.*

TABLE 42.6. Dissociated Vertical Deviation (DVD) Surgery

Prism diopters	Superior rectus hang-back recession (mm)
<10	5.0
10	6.0
15	7.0
20	8.0
25	9.0

TABLE 42.7. Adjustable Suture Guidelines[a,b,c,d]

Diagnosis	Operation	Post-adjustment deviation
Esotropia	Bilateral medial rectus recession	Ortho—5 ET
	Unilateral recess/resect	Ortho—10 XT
Exotropia	Bilateral lateral rectus recession	Ortho—5 ET
	Unilateral recess/resect	Ortho—8 ET
Hypertropia	Recess or recess/resect	Ortho—1-2 over
Restrictive	Recess or recess/resect	2-7 under

[a]*Avoid incomitancy (>10 PD) in gaze positions.*
[b]*Undercorrect sensory esotropia/exotropia by 2-5 PD.*
[c]*Watch for duction weakness in recessed muscle.*
[d]*May need to adjust targets in patients with thyroid eye disease or other special considerations.*

TABLE 42.8. A-/V-Patterns (no oblique dysfunction)[a]

Difference (upgaze-downgaze) in prism diopters	Tendon width displacement
10	¼
15	½
20	¾
25	1

[a]*A-pattern—medial rectus displaced upward; lateral rectus displaced downward. V-pattern—medial rectus displaced downward; lateral rectus displaced upward (see Chapter 51).*

TABLE 42.9. Kestenbaum Procedure for Nystagmus[a]

	Esotropic eye (Right head turn/left gaze = right eye) (Left head turn/right gaze = left eye)		Exotropic eye (Right head turn/left gaze = left eye) (Left head turn/right gaze = right eye)	
	Lateral rectus resection (mm)	Medial rectus recession (mm)	Medial rectus resection (mm)	Lateral rectus recession (mm)
Classic	8	5	6	7
+40%	11	7	8.5	10
+60%	13	8	9.5	11

[a]*In a patient with a right head turn/left gaze, the right eye is esotropic and the left eye is exotropic. In a patient with a left head turn/right gaze, the left eye is esotropic and the right eye is exotropic (see Chapter 53).*

References

1. Buckley EG, Freedman SF, Shields MB. In: Waldrop TG, ed. *Atlas of Ophthalmic Surgery: Volume III: Strabismus and Glaucoma*. 1st ed. St. Louis, MO: Mosby; 1995.
2. Lueder GT, et al. "Section 6: Pediatric ophthalmology and strabismus." In: Cantor LB, et al., eds. *Basic and Clinical Science Course*. San Francisco, CA: American Academy of Ophthalmology; 2016.
3. Hoffman H, Dondelinger K, Worthington G, et al. *Iowa head and neck protocols: maximum recommended doses and duration of local anesthetics.* https://medicine.uiowa.edu/iowaprotocols/maximum-recommended-doses-and-duration-local-anesthetics
4. Koederitz NM, Neely DE, Plager DA, et al. Postoperative povidone-iodine prophylaxis in strabismus surgery. *J AAPOS*. 2008;12(4):396-400.
5. Benson CE, Rogers KL, Suh DW. Dual application versus single application of povidone-iodine in reducing surgical site contamination during strabismus surgery. *J AAPOS*. 2014;18(4):347-350.
6. Guyton DL. Exaggerated traction test for the oblique muscles. *Ophthalmology*. 1981;88(10):1035-1040.
7. House RJ, Rotruck JC, Enyedi LB, et al. Postoperative infection following strabismus surgery: case series and increased incidence in a single referral center. *J AAPOS*. 2019;23(1):26.e1-26.e7.

CHAPTER 43

Conjunctival Incisions and Muscle Isolation

Tanya Glaser, MD

PREOPERATIVE CONSIDERATIONS

All strabismus surgery requires an incision through the conjunctiva and Tenon capsule to allow access to the extraocular muscles in the episcleral space. The two most common incisional approaches are the limbal approach and the fornix (cul-de-sac) approach. Key questions to consider when selecting an incision type include patient age and conjunctival integrity, history of prior surgery (strabismus, glaucoma, or retinal detachment), number of muscles needing to be accessed, and potential for discomfort or scarring. For instance, an inferotemporal fornix incision might be optimal for a young patient undergoing a lateral rectus muscle recession and inferior oblique myectomy because it provides easy access to both muscles. On the other hand, a limbal incision might be used in an older patient with conjunctival scarring who needs a medial rectus muscle advancement for overcorrection after a prior recession. Regardless of which type of incision is used, a drop of topical 2.5% phenylephrine prior to starting strabismus surgery helps to provide vasoconstriction and prevents bleeding. A 6-0 silk traction suture (in older patients with thinner, fragile conjunctiva) or Moody locking forceps (in younger patients with thicker conjunctiva and Tenon capsule) may be used prior to creating an incision to help stabilize the globe and improve exposure.[1,2,3]

A well-placed conjunctival incision is critical to successful strabismus surgery as it will determine exposure, ease of muscle manipulation, and closure. While there are pros and cons to each incision type (Table 43.1), two surgeons may use different incisions for the same surgical procedure.

SURGICAL PROCEDURE: LIMBAL INCISION AND MUSCLE ISOLATION (VIDEO 43.1)

- In the limbal approach, the initial incision is made at the limbus with the base of the incision at the fornix. The incision is made where conjunctiva and Tenon capsule are fused, thus maintaining alignment of these structures and limiting adhesions between conjunctiva, Tenon capsule, and sclera.

- Using a toothed forceps, elevate the conjunctiva and Tenon capsule about 2 mm from the limbus and to one side of the muscle insertion. Use Westcott scissors perpendicular to the limbus to make a single cut (large enough to insert the Westcott tips) through these tissues down to bare sclera.
- Turn the Westcott scissors so they are flush with the globe, enter the incision and bluntly dissect to create a space between the sclera and overlying tissues, parallel to the limbus for ~2-3 mm.
- Release the tissue from the limbal edge by placing one blade into the dissected space, one blade above and against the limbus, and cutting in a single smooth motion along the limbus for ~2 clock hours (to access a single rectus muscle, larger if accessing adjacent rectus muscles).
- Reapproximate the edge of the conjunctival incision/flap. Extend the initial radial incision (currently 2-3 mm in length) to about 8 mm using the Westcott scissors. If accessing the medial rectus, stop the radial incision proximal to the plica semilunaris (semilunar fold).
- Make a similar radial incision on the other side of the limbal opening. The two radial incisions should be at an obtuse angle to the limbus, creating a rhomboid shape (Fig. 43.1).
- At each side of the base, lift the edge (placing Tenon capsule on stretch) and push the closed Westcott scissors into the oblique quadrant between adjacent rectus muscles. Bluntly dissect until an opening is made through Tenon capsule and bare sclera is seen. Be sure to point the scissors *between* muscles, not over the muscle.
- Use muscle hooks and the two openings in Tenon capsule to isolate the rectus muscle insertion. This can often be done with direct visualization of the muscle edge.

One technique uses a small Stevens tenotomy hook to initially engage the muscle. Next, a Jameson muscle hook is inserted and passed just posterior to the Stevens tenotomy hook, isolating the entire rectus muscle insertion. If done correctly, the Jameson muscle hook should pass through the first opening in Tenon capsule, then under the muscle, and then out the second opening in Tenon capsule.

- Elevate the conjunctival flap to allow further dissection of the Tenon capsule and intermuscular septum from the muscle body anteriorly. Avoid opening posterior Tenon capsule as this will result in orbital fat coming forward.
- To close the limbal incision, identify the conjunctival edge of the flap and reapproximate its location at the limbus. At each corner, place an 8-0 Vicryl (or other absorbable suture) 1 mm posterior to the conjunctival edge of the flap and suture this to the limbal conjunctiva. It is important to avoid including Tenon capsule with this suture pass. In some cases, it may be difficult to distinguish Tenon capsule from the conjunctiva, and, in these instances, it can be helpful to hydrate the tissue to provide more contrast between the tissues. In addition, the conjunctival edge will occasionally fold under the flap and grasping the Tenon on the underside of the flap will help delineate the conjunctival corner. There is often redundant conjunctiva and Tenon capsule after a resection, advancement, or plication. Care should be taken to not mistake the plica for the edge of conjunctiva, and a very small amount of conjunctiva may need to be trimmed to prevent overhang of redundant tissue at the limbus.[1,2,4,5]

Potential complications include dellen formation, conjunctival cyst formation, prolapse of Tenon capsule, and advancement or distortion of the plica semilunaris (see Chapter 54).

SURGICAL PROCEDURE: FORNIX (CUL-DE-SAC) INCISION AND MUSCLE ISOLATION (VIDEOS 44.1 AND 45.1)

- In the fornix approach, the globe is rotated to expose the incision site, which is made in any of the oblique quadrants.
- Using a toothed forceps, the conjunctiva is placed under anterior traction about 8 mm posterior to the limbus laterally.

While an incision 8 mm from the limbus is made when accessing the lateral rectus, an incision 5 mm from the limbus should be used when accessing the medial rectus to avoid the plica semilunaris.

The fold created from this traction should be perpendicular to the limbus. Use Westcott scissors to create an opening in the conjunctival tissue parallel to the limbus and eyelid margin. On the medial side, care should be taken to avoid the plica by orienting the incision more horizontally and/or locating the incision a few mm closer to the limbus.

- Rotate the forceps 90 degrees, elevate the underlying intermuscular septum and Tenon capsule and cut down (now perpendicular to limbus) all the way to bare sclera. In younger patients with a significant amount of Tenon capsule, two toothed forceps can be used to grasp the intermuscular septum and Tenon capsule to make this cut down to sclera and the triangles of tissue held by each forceps can then be excised at the base with Westcott scissors.
- A small (Stevens tenotomy) hook is then passed into the episcleral space just under the edge of the muscle. A second larger hook (Jameson or Square or Double Bend) is then passed behind the small hook to the far side of the rectus muscle. The tip of the hook should be able to rotate freely up to the limbus. If the hook is unable to rotate easily, the entire insertion has not been isolated. Pass additional hooks as needed or lift the edge of the muscle over the hook with a heavy toothed forceps.
- Use a second hook to stretch the conjunctival tissue over the first hook, exposing the leading edge of the hook and overlying intermuscular septum.
- Rotate the first hook slightly upward placing the Tenon capsule and intermuscular septum on tension. Elevate these tissues with forceps and using Westcott scissors make a small opening exposing the toe of the first hook and bare sclera. Pass the first hook through this opening.
- Place a tenotomy hook in the opening and pass it along the bare sclera around the edge of the muscle. If the hook catches, there is likely more muscle that needs to be isolated. Be wary of blood at this stage, as it is often a sign that the muscle has been split.
- Using forceps and Westcott scissors, excise the remaining anterior Tenon capsule from the muscle with sharp dissection while being careful not to damage the muscle capsule and anterior ciliary blood vessels. Many surgeons do minimal muscle "cleaning" in fornix cases. A little more dissection is necessary in resections/plications than in recessions.
- To close the fornix incision, identify and reapproximate the cut conjunctival edges, while carefully avoiding Tenon capsule. Moody locking forceps can be placed at the edges of the wound in order to oppose the conjunctiva while allowing Tenon capsule to fall back. Close with an absorbable suture. The number of sutures needed depends on the size of the incision. In cases where the incision is small and well-hidden in the fornix, suture may not be required.[1,2]

Potential complications include conjunctival cyst formation, prolapse of Tenon capsule, fat adherence syndrome (due to unintentional violation of posterior Tenon capsule with fat prolapse), and lid fissure abnormalities (due to symblepharon formation or scarring) (see Chapter 54).

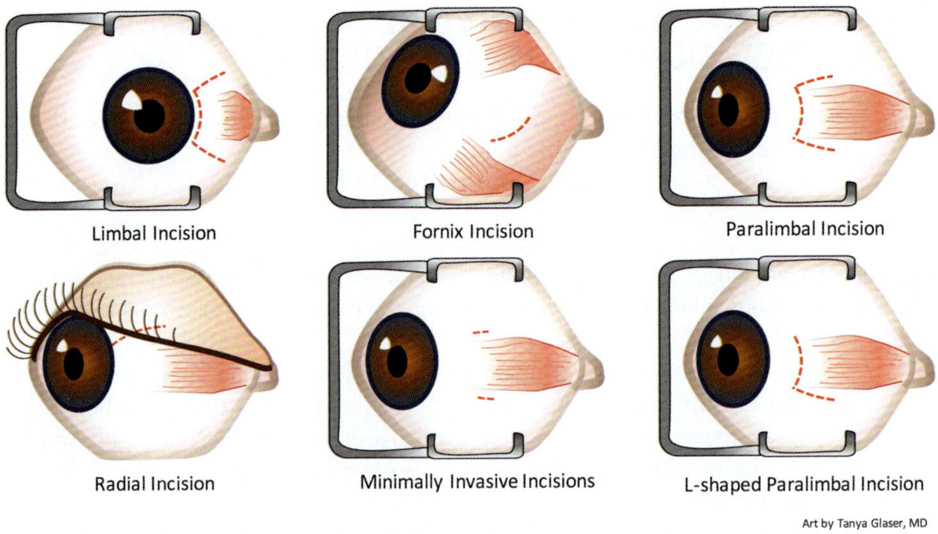

FIGURE 43.1. Diagram of different types of strabismus incisions.

OTHER TYPES OF INCISIONS (FIG. 43.1; TABLE 43.1)

- Paralimbal incision: The conjunctival incision is placed just anterior to the muscle insertion and parallel to the limbus, while the Tenon capsule incision is made posterior to the muscle insertion and perpendicular to the limbus, sometimes along only one side of the muscle, creating an L-shaped wound. The L-shaped modification of the paralimbal incision is particularly useful for adjustable sutures. The benefit of this approach is that it offers excellent exposure and visibility of the muscle insertion, but it risks injury to the muscle and vasculature.
- Radial incision: The conjunctival incision starts at the limbus and extends radially along the lateral border of the muscle. This incision is smaller than a limbal incision and provides better visualization than a fornix incision. It can also be used with an adjustable suture.[6]
- Minimally invasive strabismus surgery (MISS): An incisional approach where muscles are accessed through several small keyhole incisions instead of a single larger incision. The benefits of this technique include less tissue manipulation, preservation of perilimbal episcleral vessels, decreased scarring, and reduced redness. The downsides to this technique include a steep learning curve, requirement of a surgical microscope, and decreased visualization of the anatomy.[7]

TABLE 43.1. Pros and cons of different strabismus incisions

	Limbal approach	Fornix (cul-de-sac) approach
Pros	• Ideal for reoperations • Good for older patients with thinner conjunctiva • In some instances, preferable for adjustable suture technique • Better exposure, especially when operating without an experienced assistant	• Tends to be more comfortable since away from limbus • Avoids damage to episcleral perilimbal vessels • Often faster to close
Cons	• More discomfort from closing conjunctival sutures • Possibility of more visible conjunctival scarring • More likely to have corneal dellen formation	• Avoid in older patients with thin conjunctiva that is more likely to tear • Requires greater anatomic expertise • More challenging in reoperations

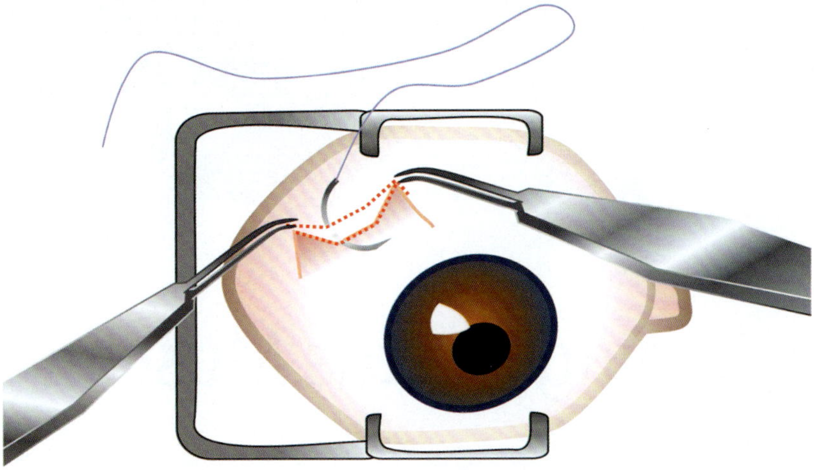

FIGURE 43.2. Method of conjunctival closure using Moody locking forceps.

CHALLENGES IN CONJUNCTIVAL CLOSURE AND OTHER PEARLS

The conjunctiva can be closed with simple interrupted or buried 8-0 Vicryl sutures. The robust Tenon capsule in children can at times make conjunctival closure challenging. It is important to avoid incorporating Tenon capsule into conjunctival closure. It is also crucial to ensure you have approximated the very edges of the conjunctival tissue, as buried epithelium can result in a conjunctival cyst (see Chapter 54), which usually requires excision. One methods of conjunctival closure that works well for fornix incisions is using two Moody locking forceps to grasp each corner of the incision and lift up. This makes the conjunctival edge easy to visualize and allows Tenon capsule to fall away from the wound edge (Fig. 43.2).

Conjunctival closure in elderly patients or those with prior surgery can be particularly challenging as the conjunctiva can be thin, friable, and easily tear. In such cases, it can be helpful to use an 8-0 Vicryl on a BV needle (vascular needle). It is also helpful to pass the needle completely through the conjunctiva on each side of incision (ie, two separate passes) rather than carry the tissue on the needle to the distal conjunctiva. Sometimes the conjunctiva may need to be recessed if there is not adequate tissue for closure, such as in cases of a large recession with fragile conjunctiva. In this situation, it is most important to cover the muscle and muscle stitch. Lastly, taking a bite of episclera as you close the conjunctiva can take tension off fragile conjunctiva, minimizing the risk of tearing as you tie down the suture.

With large medial rectus resections or advances, consider tacking the conjunctiva down to the surface of the muscle or to the sclera anterior to the insertion using a double armed 8-0 Vicryl to keep the plica from advancing forward and the redundant conjunctiva from bulging forward.

References

1. Buckley EG, Freedman S, Shields MB, et al. *Atlas of Ophthalmic Surgery. Volume III, Strabismus and Glaucoma*. 1st ed. St. Louis, MO: Mosby; 1995.
2. Lambert SR, Lyons CJ. *Taylor & Hoyt's Pediatric Ophthalmology and Strabismus*. 5th ed. Edinburgh; New York: Elsevier; 2017.
3. Sami DA. Conjunctival incisions for strabismus surgery: a comparison of techniques. *Tech Ophthalmol*. 2007;5:125-129.
4. Von Noorden GK. The limbal approach to surgery of the rectus muscles. *Arch Ophthalmol*. 1968;80(1):94-97.
5. Von Noorden GK. Modification of the limbal approach to surgery of the rectus muscles. *Arch Ophthalmol*. 1969;82(3):349-350.
6. Velez G. Radial incision for surgery of the horizontal rectus muscles. *J Pediatr Ophthalmol Strabismus*. 1980;17(2):106-107.
7. Mojon DS. Review: minimally invasive strabismus surgery. *Eye (Lond)*. 2015;29(2):225-233.

CHAPTER 44

Weakening Rectus Muscles

Megan X. Law, MD

PREOPERATIVE CONSIDERATIONS

Recessions move the muscle insertion to a new location closer to its origin to weaken the effect of the muscle. There is an exponential increase in effect with large recessions as reflected in standard strabismus surgical charts (see Chapter 42).[1,2] Recessing a single rectus muscle will induce incomitance, with a greater effect in the muscle's field of action. Asymmetric bilateral recessions will also induce incomitance, with greater effect in the field of action of the more recessed muscle. Great caution should be taken in recessing a rectus muscle posterior to the equator as this can significantly impair the muscle's function.[3] A guideline for the maximal recession of the four rectus muscles without inducing duction limitation is listed in Table 44.1.[1,2,3,4]

TABLE 44.1. Maximal recession (approximate) from the limbus

	Maximal recession (mm)
Medial rectus	7
Lateral rectus	10
Superior rectus	10
Inferior rectus	6

SURGICAL PLANNING

In most cases, a traditional recession is performed. Alternative weakening procedures include the hang-back recession and marginal myotomy[1-6] (Table 44.2).

- **Traditional recession:** muscle tendon is disinserted from the sclera and fixated at a new location posterior to the original insertion.
- **Hang-back recession:** muscle tendon is disinserted from the sclera and suspended by sutures through the original insertion.
- **Marginal myotomy (Z-plasty):** muscle tendon is partially cut at two parallel locations in opposite directions leading to elongation and lengthening.

TABLE 44.2. Pros and cons of three rectus muscle weakening techniques

	Traditional recession	Hang-back recession	Marginal myotomy
Pros	Most predictable effect (standard surgical tables)	Safety: small deep-set eye, high myopia, staphyloma, scleral buckle, or glaucoma drainage device	Safety: small deep-set eye, high myopia, staphyloma, scleral buckle or glaucoma drainage device, previous recession
		Easy access to knots for adjustable sutures	Can combine with recession for a "double" weakening effect
		Standard surgical tables are available	Can further weaken a "maximally recessed" rectus muscle
		Useful in large superior rectus recessions, "bypassing" the superior oblique insertion	Avoids scleral passes
Cons	Posterior scleral passes can be challenging	Risk of muscle slip posteriorly with small recessions (greater than intended effect)	Less predictable effect (no standard surgical tables)
		Risk of muscle slip anteriorly with large recessions (smaller than intended effect)	Risk of severing the muscle
		Risk of muscle slip perpendicular to the recession (eg, induced vertical deviation with a horizontal recession)	Cannot be easily reversed

SURGICAL PROCEDURE: RECESSION[1] (VIDEO 44.1)

1. Once the muscle has been isolated (see Chapter 43), apply light cautery (optional) to the large vessels on the muscle and sclera to prevent bleeding.
2. Use a double-armed 6-0 Vicryl suture (or alternative absorbable suture, such as Polysorb) on a S-14 or S-29 spatulated needle to make a partial-thickness pass crossing 2/3 of the muscle width (Fig. 44.1). The suture should be no more than 1 mm from the muscle insertion.

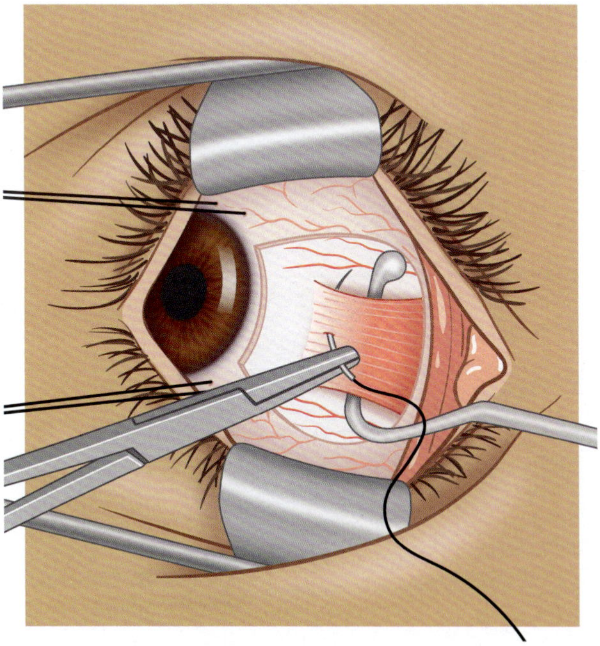

FIGURE 44.1. Partial-thickness transverse suture pass.

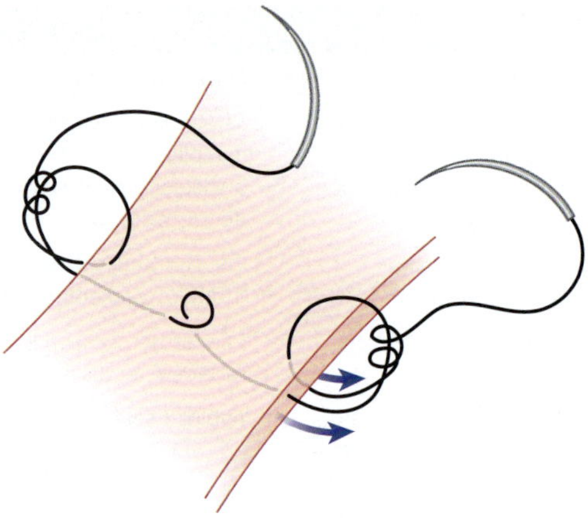

FIGURE 44.2. Central overlap of transverse sutures with locking bites at the muscle borders.

3. Make a full-thickness suture pass at the border of the muscle (~1/3 the width of the insertion) near the insertion in an anterior-to-posterior direction. This pass should be slightly posterior to the initial transverse suture pass. Use the needle holder to grasp the suture end and pull it through the loop once or twice in the same direction to create a locking bite.

It is important not to pull the suture anteriorly or posteriorly at this point as it can change the position of the suture in the muscle, altering the effect of the recession.

4. Using the other end of the same suture, repeat the above procedure in the opposite direction. There should be an overlap of the transverse sutures by 1-2 mm centrally (Fig. 44.2).
5. Disinsert the muscle from the globe with blunt-tipped Westcott scissors while placing traction on the muscle hook and sutures (Fig. 44.3).

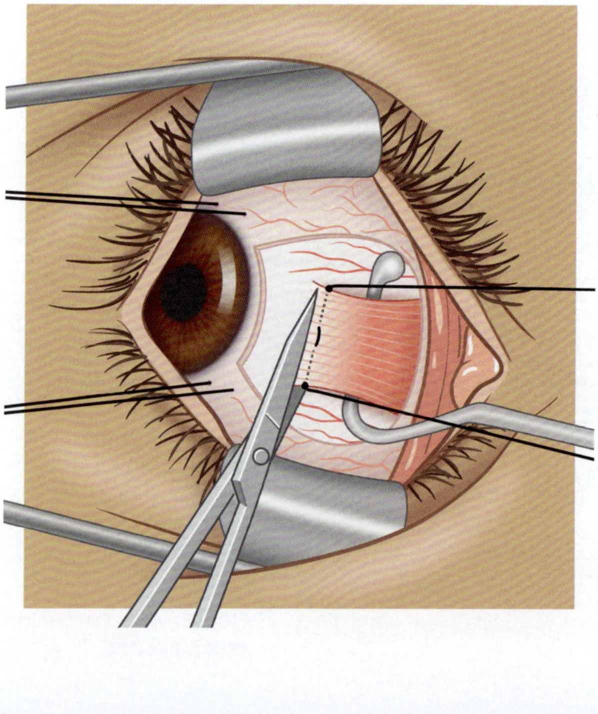

FIGURE 44.3. Disinsertion of the muscle from the globe.

During this maneuver, hold the ends of the suture between your thumb and the muscle hook, keeping the suture taut between your thumb and index finger to avoid inadvertently cutting it.

If the insertion is very tight, using the scissors with the tips down can make disinsertion easier and safer.

6. Cauterize bleeding of the scleral stump with a low temperature cautery if necessary.

If the muscle starts to bleed after it has been cut from the globe, pressure from a small Desmarres retractor or cotton tip applicators soaked in 2.5% phenylephrine may be used to stop bleeding prior to performing the scleral pass. Cauterizing the muscle at this point risks burning through the suture.

7. Using calipers, mark the planned amount of recession posterior to the insertion. Dry the sclera with a cotton tip applicator to prepare for the scleral pass.

For large recessions, consider rotating the patient's head toward the surgeon to optimize exposure. Make sure the anesthesia team is aware of any manipulations involving the patient's head.

Position the caliper so that it is perpendicular to the limbus to ensure an accurate measurement. A deep mark can be used to help get the proper depth of scleral pass.

For larger recessions, a Scott ruler is more accurate due to curvature of the globe.

8. Using the same needles, make partial thickness passes through the sclera at the designated location, usually heading toward the insertion. The point where the needle enters is more important than the direction of the needle pass (Fig. 44.4).

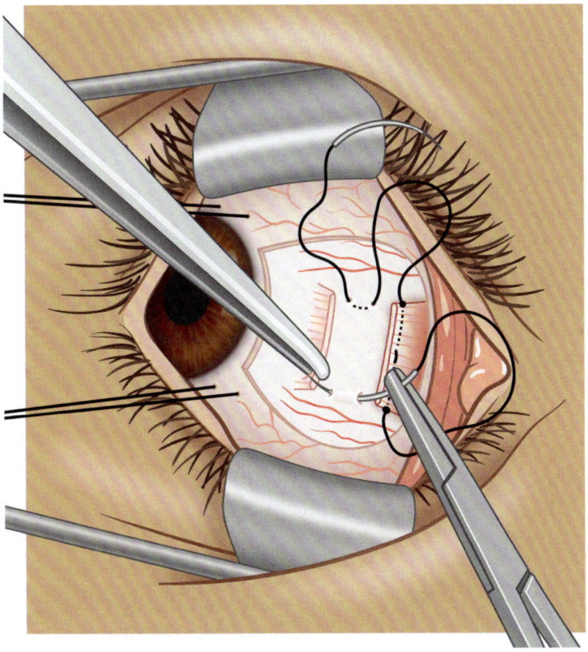

FIGURE 44.4. Partial-thickness scleral pass for traditional recession.

The point of scleral entry determines the recession amount. The direction of the scleral pass has no effect. In some instances, where exposure is difficult, it may be easier and safer to pass the needle angled superior or inferior to the insertion. Angling the pass enables the avoidance of passing the needle through the thinnest part of the sclera which is just posterior to the muscle insertion.

9. Using needle holders or tying forceps, pull the sutures to bring the muscle to the new position on the sclera and tie the sutures using a 2-1-1 square knot.

Avoid incorporating Tenon capsule into the scleral pass as this can result in an inclusion cyst (see Chapter 54). One way to do that is to have the assistant place a retractor or hook over the conjunctiva and Tenon's and hold it back while you tighten the suture.

If the central muscle belly is sagging at this point, an additional bite can be taken through the center of the muscle to pull it forward.

When tying a square knot, it is often helpful to leave one end of the double-armed suture slightly longer than the other. Start each throw by grasping the longer end.

10. If necessary, close the conjunctiva (see Chapter 43).

SURGICAL PROCEDURE: HANG-BACK RECESSION[1]

- Following step 6 from above (Surgical procedure: Recession), pass the same needles through sclera at the scleral ridge of the original muscle insertion (Fig. 44.5).
- Pull the sutures so that the muscle is at the sclera and hold the sutures taut to measure the desired amount of recession along the length of the suture. Be sure that both sutures are of equal length.
- Use a locking straight needle driver to clamp the sutures at this location.

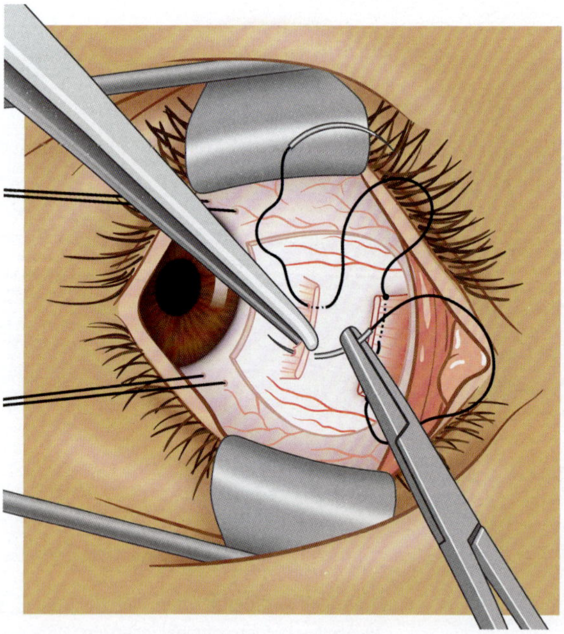

FIGURE 44.5. Partial thickness scleral pass for hang-back recession.

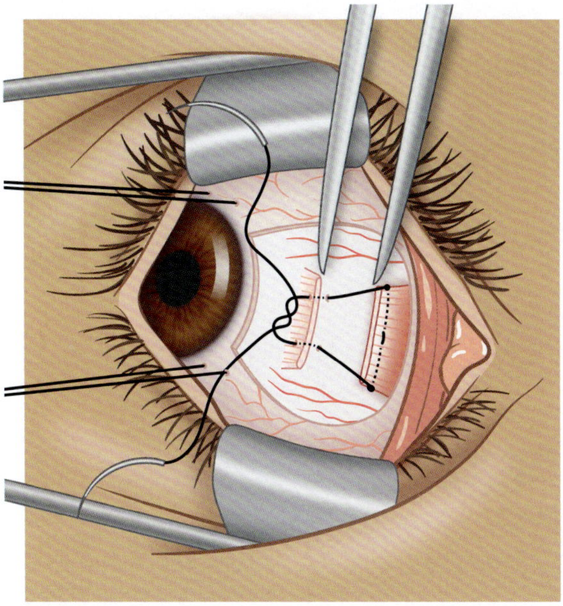

FIGURE 44.6. Verification of recession amount using hang-back technique.

- Tie the sutures with a 2-1-1 square knot over the needle driver and then release the needle driver to allow the muscle to hang back posteriorly. Alternatively, position the muscle at the desired location. Perform the first throw and check the distance from the insertion. Once the position of the muscle is verified, proceed with the remaining throws, taking care to not move the position of the muscle (Fig. 44.6).
- Close the conjunctiva (see Chapter 43).

Marginal Myotomy/Z-Plasty[1,6]

- Once the muscle has been isolated (see Chapter 43), use a hemostat to clamp 50%-80% of the tendon width ~4 mm from the muscle insertion.
- Use a second hemostat to clamp 50%-80% of the tendon width ~4 mm from the first hemostat in the opposite direction (Fig. 44.7).

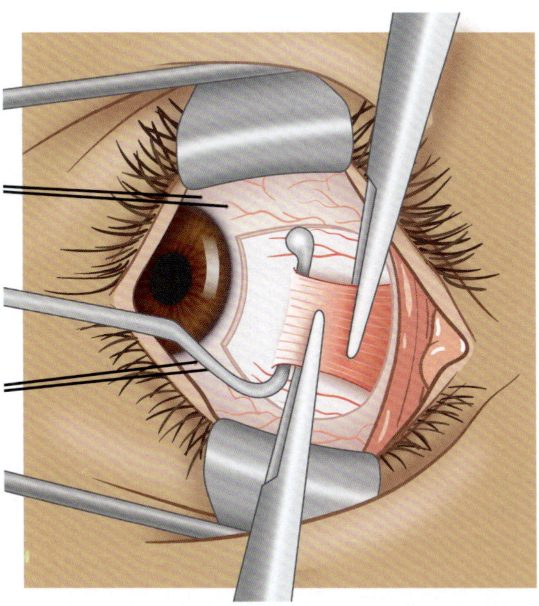

FIGURE 44.7. Placement of hemostats for marginal myotomy.

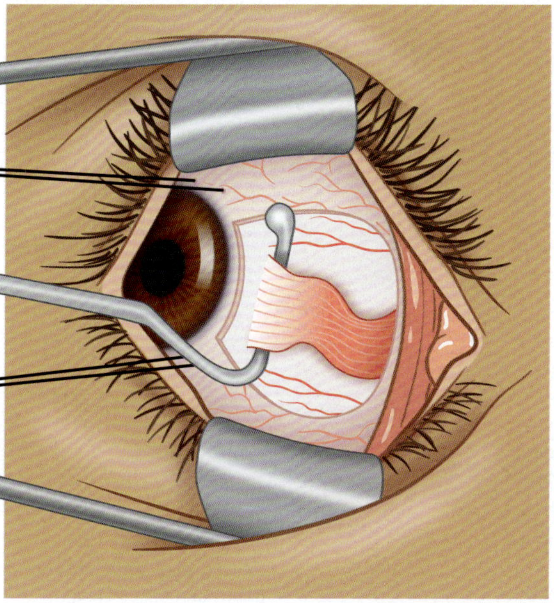

FIGURE 44.8. Muscle elongation following marginal myotomies (Z-myotomy).

If the eye is hyperdeviated, make the proximal cut on the horizontal muscle from above to effectively shift the insertion inferiorly (ie, more recession effect superiorly). If the eye is hypodeviated, make the proximal cut from below to effectively shift the insertion superiorly. Use this approach similarly for horizontally shifting vertical rectus muscle insertions.

- Remove both hemostats and use Westcott scissors to cut the muscle in the crushed areas (Fig. 44.8).
- Bleeding can be controlled with pressure from a Q-tip.

Avoid cautery and do not pull excessively on the muscle to avoid further loss of muscle fibers.

- Close the conjunctiva (see Chapter 43).

POSTOPERATIVE CONSIDERATIONS

- Excessive recession may produce undesirable results, such as limited duction, widened palpebral fissure, muscle slippage, or lower lid ptosis.[1-5]
- A slipped muscle is usually apparent 7-10 days after surgery. It typically manifests as muscle weakness with significant limitation of rotation in the muscle's field of action. Prompt surgery is needed to retrieve and attach the muscle (see Chapter 59).[1,4]

Moderate to large recessions of the superior and inferior rectus muscles may lead to eyelid retraction due to the fascial attachments between these muscles and the levator muscle and lower lid retractors, respectively. Carefully dissect these attachments prior to the recession.

References

1. Buckley EG, Freedman S, Shields MB, et al. *Atlas of Ophthalmic Surgery. Volume III, Strabismus and Glaucoma*. 1st ed. St. Louis, MO: Mosby; 1995.
2. Wright KW, Strube YNJ. *Color Atlas of Strabismus Surgery: Strategies and Techniques*. 4th ed. New York, NY: Springer; 2015.
3. Helveston EM. *Surgical Management of Strabismus*. 5th ed. Wayenborgh; Belgium; 2005.

4. Lambert SR, Lyons CJ. *Taylor & Hoyt's Pediatric Ophthalmology and Strabismus*. 5th ed. Edinburgh; New York: Elsevier; 2017. https://getitatduke.library.duke.edu/?sid=sersol&SS_jc=TC0001791178&title=Taylor%20%26%20Hoyt%27s%20pediatric%20ophthalmology%20and%20strabismus
5. American Academy of Ophthalmology. *Basic and Clinical Science Course, Section 6: Pediatric Ophthalmology and Strabismus*. San Francisco, CA: American Academy of Ophthalmology; 2014.
6. Helveston EM, Cofield DD. Indications for marginal myotomy and technique. *Am J Ophthalmol.* 1970;70:574.

CHAPTER 45

Strengthening Rectus Muscles

Jagger C. Koerner, MD, MBA

INTRODUCTION

There are four procedures to strengthen a rectus muscle: resection, plication ("muscle tuck"), advancement, and injection of bupivacaine (see Chapter 55). This chapter will describe resection, plication, and advancement.[1]

PREOPERATIVE SURGICAL PLANNING

- Perform forced duction testing to determine if a muscle is restricted prior to or at the start of surgery (see Chapter 42). Consider an alternative procedure if the opposing muscle is tight or inelastic (eg, thyroid eye disease, Duane syndrome).
- If the patient has had prior eye muscle surgery, consider anterior segment blood supply. Plication can preserve anterior segment perfusion.[2] In general, do not operate on more than two rectus muscles simultaneously or more than three in total.
- If resecting 5 mm or less, consider plication. Use the same surgical amounts for plication as for resection (see Chapter 42).
- If operating on a patient with thin conjunctiva (typically older patients; ie, 60 years of age or older) or prior scarring, consider a limbal incision (see Chapter 43).
- If operating on a young patient without scarring, consider a fornix incision (see Chapter 43).
- If using an adjustable suture (see Chapter 48) with a resection procedure, consider resection combined with a hang back. For example, a 6-mm resection hung back 2 mm from the insertion could be left in place for a net effect of 4-mm resection, advanced to the insertion for a 6-mm resection, or hung back further for a smaller resection effect.
- If operating on a vertical rectus muscle, counsel the patient about possible postoperative lid changes. Minimize these changes by disinserting the lid retractors from the rectus muscles as completely as possible during surgery. Lid changes are most commonly seen with inferior rectus resections >5 mm and superior rectus resections of 8 mm or more.

RECTUS RESECTION (VIDEO 45.1)

- Isolate the rectus muscle on a Jameson muscle hook after creating the incision of choice (see Chapter 43). When isolating the superior rectus muscle, avoid incorporating the superior oblique. Similarly, when isolating the lateral rectus muscle, avoid incorporating the inferior oblique. Pass the muscle hooks just posterior to the insertion, hugging the sclera. Avoid large blind hooking movements.
- Once the muscle is isolated, clean the muscle from its fascial attachments with sharp and blunt dissection. This is generally done more extensively for resection procedures compared with recessions. Have your assistant elevate the conjunctiva and put Tenon capsule on tension to facilitate dissection. Carry this dissection as far posterior as possible over the inferior and superior rectus muscle to help disinsert lid retractors. Avoid dissection into the orbital fat. Firmly rubbing a dry cotton tip applicator from anterior to posterior on the surface of the muscle can be helpful.
- Once the muscle is cleaned and isolated, place a second large muscle hook (often a square hook) behind the first. The muscle should be under gentle tension and slightly elevated off the sclera. Using calipers, measure the amount of muscle to be resected and place a double-armed 6-0 Vicryl (or Polysorb) suture at this location in the typical fashion (see Chapter 43). Do not shift the suture anteriorly or posteriorly in the muscle tissue as the knots are tightened. If carrying out a large resection, consider placing a central "security" knot as the muscle will be under considerable tension once secured to the insertion (Figs. 45.1-45.5).
- Place a small straight hemostat anterior to Vicryl suture, taking care to not incorporate suture into the hemostat. Cut flush across the anterior surface of the hemostat with a Westcott scissor. Cauterize the exposed muscle in the hemostat and then remove the hemostat. Check the muscle to be sure it is secure and that the sutures were not cut or cauterized.
- Trim the resected muscle leaving a small muscle "stump" at the ends to help grasp the insertion site.
- Stabilize the insertion with two locking Moody forceps or a single Castro Viejo forceps. The side of the forceps with two teeth should be on the more posterior edge of the insertion for extra stability.
- Check to ensure that the muscle has not been twisted or "flipped." Pass the needle on each end of the double-armed Vicryl suture through the original insertion. Do not pass the needles through the thin tissue behind the insertion, but rather into the ridge at the insertion. Often a needle at the correct depth will NOT be visible as it

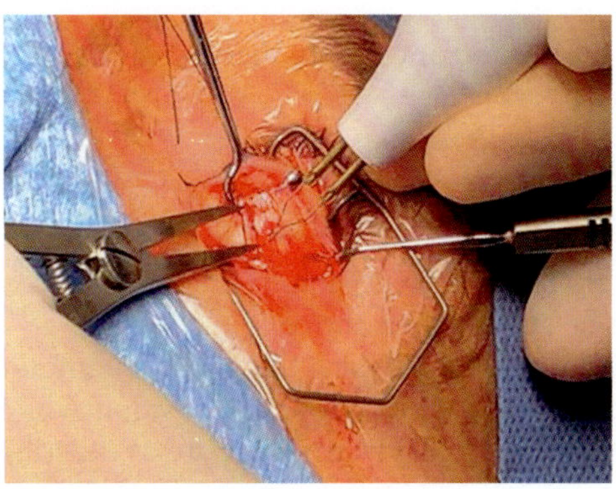

FIGURE 45.1. After isolating the muscle, the amount of resection is measured with a caliper. Light cautery is applied to help with hemostasis and mark the location for placing sutures.

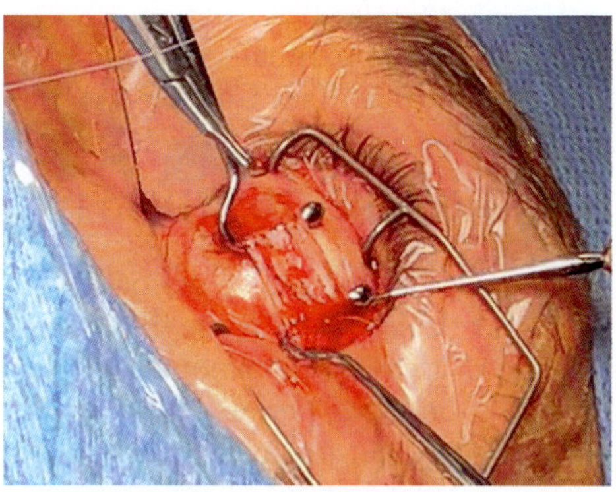

FIGURE 45.2. A second large hook provides gentle counter traction and elevates the muscle to facilitate suturing, measuring, and cautery.

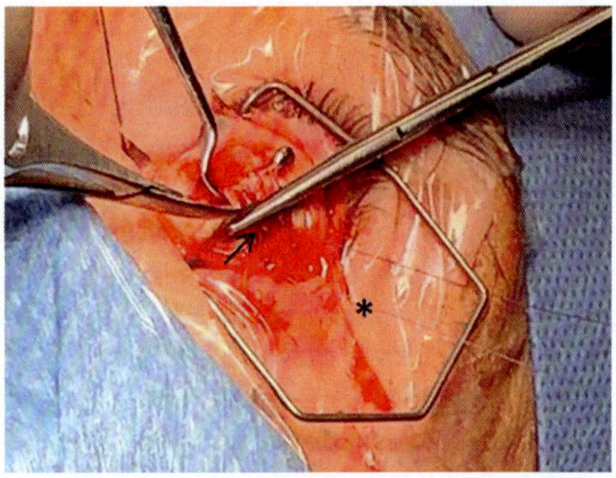

FIGURE 45.3. The hemostat is placed just limbal/anterior to the previously placed sutures (*arrow*) that are kept out of the way (*asterisk*) while the muscle is transected with Westcott scissors.

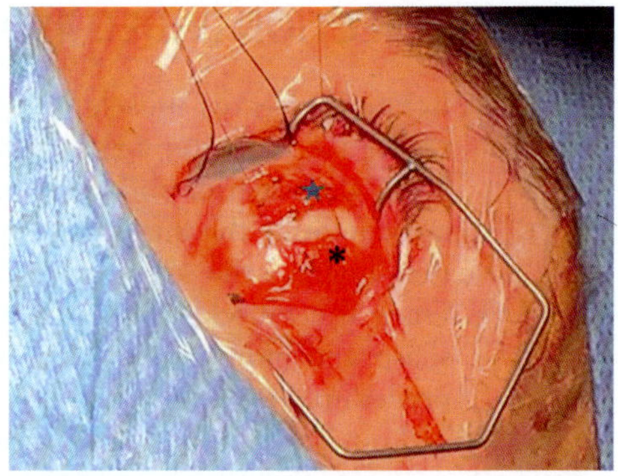

FIGURE 45.4. The sutures in the muscle (*asterisk*) are passed through the original insertion. Excess muscle was trimmed from this area leaving a small "stump" to suture into (*star*).

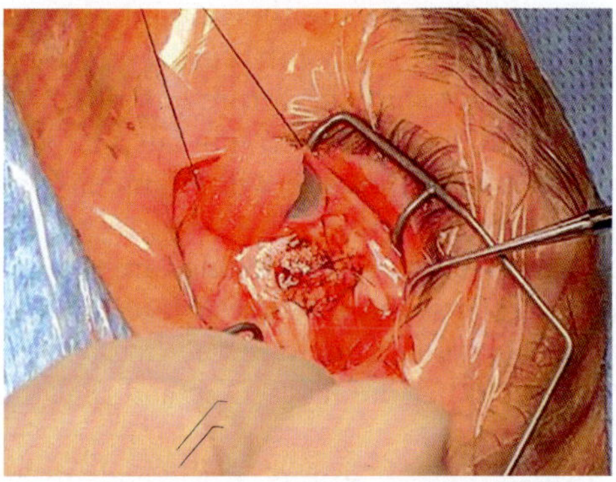

FIGURE 45.5. The resected muscle is then secured firmly to the original insertion and tied down.

passes through the insertion. Some sclera should be incorporated in the pass. Avoid only suturing to the muscle stump. Maintain the width of the muscle insertion so that the muscle is not sagging or bunched.

- Remove any traction on the eye prior to pulling the eye toward the resected muscle. After tightening the first throw, hold the knot in place using a needle holder to prevent the muscle from slipping while preparing for the second throw. Visualize that both poles of the muscle have been pulled up completely with no connective tissue in the needle tracks before performing additional throws and securing the Vicryl suture. Some surgeons leave the suture ends a bit long and tuck the ends under the muscle edge.
- Reapproximate the conjunctiva with interrupted 8-0 Vicryl sutures in the usual manner (see Chapter 43).

PLICATION (RECTUS TUCK) (VIDEO 45.2)

- Plication can be performed via limbal or fornix incision.
- Isolate and expose the rectus muscle as described above.
- Measure the amount of plication with calipers. Mark the plication amount with a marking pen or by holding the calipers at the appropriate position while placing the suture. Avoid heavy cautery. Place the double-armed suture as described above avoiding the ciliary arteries.

Using loupes or an operating microscope for magnification may be helpful to visualize the arteries. Occasionally, it can be easier to avoid the ciliary arteries by using two single-armed Vicryl sutures.

- Remove one of the muscle hooks and use the other hook to hold and manipulate the eye.
- Secure the preplaced sutures to the sclera with partial-thickness bites that enter at the edge of the muscle insertion and run almost parallel to the insertion and slightly anterior to the insertion. A "crossed swords" technique can be used but is not necessary. It is often helpful to pass one of the bites back-handed, or shift positions to avoid using the nondominant hand for one of the scleral passes.
- After making both scleral passes, the muscle hook is removed and the muscle is advanced toward the insertion site causing it to bunch up on top (easier) or fold under itself (more difficult). Next, the suture is tied as described above for resections, and the conjunctiva is reapproximated with several interrupted 8-0 Vicryl sutures (see Chapter 43).

RECTUS ADVANCEMENT

A rectus muscle can be advanced in its entirety, selectively (eg, inferior fibers), after previous recession, or as an initial operation. This section describes advancing a previously recessed muscle to correct a consecutive deviation.

- Review the expected position of the muscle to plan the initial dissection. Consider using a limbal incision and traction suture to facilitate exposure.
- Identify the muscle insertion with a small muscle hook. Locate the insertion prior to carrying the dissection posteriorly so that the muscle is not disinserted inadvertently. Dissect bluntly with a Westcott scissors *under* the muscle belly to free adhesions and facilitate hooking the muscle. Hook the muscle with a large muscle hook; Katena muscle hooks are thin gauge and can be helpful in situations with scarring.
- After identifying the insertion and placing it on gentle traction with the muscle hook, clean the muscle as described previously. Check the muscle carefully for stretched scar (see Chapters 54 and 59). If a stretched scar is identified, the sutures should be placed posterior to the stretched scar ensuring muscle fibers are incorporated into the sutures. Use two single-armed, or one double-armed, 6-0 Vicryl suture to secure the muscle as described in Chapter 43. When exposure is difficult, use two single-armed sutures. A grooved (Wright) muscle hook protects the sclera and facilitates suturing when exposure is difficult.
- Measure where the muscle attaches to sclera and compare this with the expected location of the muscle. Consider marking the sclera at the center of the muscle insertion with a marking pen for reference prior to disinsertion of the muscle. Disinsert the muscle with Westcott scissors.
- Determine the location to reattach the muscle. The standard tables are a starting point, though advancement is a "strong" procedure and reduction of the surgical amount should be considered, especially for large deviations.[3] Consider "on the table adjustment" and/or adjustable sutures.
- Mark the location to reinsert the muscle with a caliper and secure the preplaced sutures to the sclera with partial-thickness bites. Ensure that the muscle has not twisted or "flipped" and that the insertion is not bunched up.
- Remove any traction on the eye prior to pulling the eye toward the muscle. After tightening the first throw, hold the knot in place using a needle holder to prevent the muscle from slipping while preparing for the second throw. Visualize that both poles of the muscle have been pulled up completely with no connective tissue in the needle tracks before performing additional throws and securing the Vicryl suture.
- Reapproximate the conjunctiva with interrupted 8-0 Vicryl sutures in the usual manner (see Chapter 43).

POSTOPERATIVE CONSIDERATIONS

- The typical postmedications, patient instruction, and restrictions are used after resection procedures (see Chapter 42).
- In addition to the potential complications (see Chapter 54) after all eye muscle surgeries, patients who have had resection procedures should be monitored for:
  - Dellen formation: This is most common after medial rectus procedures as the conjunctiva, tenons, and muscle stump can be particularly bulky in this area. Redundant conjunctiva may need to be carefully trimmed after muscle strengthening procedures using limbal incisions. Excessive conjunctival and subconjunctival bulk may be more common after plication procedures. Limiting plication to 4 mm of the medial rectus muscle can help prevent this, as can excising the rectus muscle still attached to the insertion completely in resection procedures. While these problems typically improve over time, a prolonged steroid/antibiotic course and lubrication may be needed.
  - Lid fissure abnormalities: The palpebral fissure can be narrowed with vertical muscle strengthening procedures, even when taking care to disinsert the lid retractors.
  - Ocular rotation limitation: Restriction of ocular rotation in the field opposite of the operated muscle can occur. If not desirable, an "on the table adjustment" can be performed by temporarily tying the muscle suture and performing forced ductions to titrate the amount of resection appropriately (see Chapter 48).

Postoperatively over-corrected muscles can be "stretched" in the office under topical anesthesia by grasping the conjunctiva at the limbus and asking the patient to slowly and firmly pull in the direction of the over-corrected muscle (eg, for a tight medial, grasp and stabilize the eye at the temporal limbus and ask the patient to adduct the eye). Patients can also be prescribed "stretching exercises" to do at home in the hopes of encouraging a tight muscle to loosen. The patient is asked to move the eye both toward and away from the tight muscle as far as possible and hold in each position for a count of 10 before releasing. Several "sets" several times/day can be prescribed. These maneuvers are most likely to be successful in the early (first few weeks) postoperative period before the muscle has firmly attached to the globe.

  - Late under correction: After plication or resection procedures, the muscle can stretch and loosen over time, weakening the resection effect. This can be minimized by ensuring adequate tissue is incorporated into the locking bites and sclera is incorporated into the passes by the insertion.[4]

References

1. Buckley EG, Freedman SF, Shields BM. *Atlas of Ophthalmic Surgery*. Vol. III. St. Louis: Mosby; 1995;68-74.
2. Oltra EZ, et al. The effect of rectus muscle recession, resection and plication on anterior segment circulation in humans. *Br J Ophthalmol*. 2015;99(4):556-560.
3. Kim BH, et al. Surgical dose-effect relationship in single muscle advancement in the treatment of consecutive strabismus. *J Pediatr Ophthalmol Strabismus*. 2014;51(2):93-99.
4. Alkharashi M, Hunter DG. Reduced surgical success rate of rectus muscle plication compared to resection. *J AAPOS*. 2017;21(3):201-204.

CHAPTER 46

Inferior Oblique Procedures

Yasmin Poustchi Mali, MD

WEAKENING OF THE INFERIOR OBLIQUE: MYECTOMY, RECESSION, ANTERIORIZATION, AND EXTIRPATION

Preoperative Considerations

- Unilateral superior oblique palsy:
  - Perform preoperative strabismus measurements and intraoperative forced duction testing, specifically the superior oblique traction test (see chapter 42), which may influence the surgical plan. Specifically, consider the following factors when determining the surgical plan:
    - Magnitude of the hypertropia.
    - Pattern of the hypertropia.
    - Presence of superior oblique laxity.
  - Weakening of the inferior oblique muscle is preferred if:
    - The hypertropia is worse on adduction and contralateral upgaze.
    - The tropia is <15-20 prism diopters in primary gaze.
    - There is no superior oblique laxity on forced duction testing.
  - Either inferior oblique recession or myectomy have been found to be successful to weaken the inferior oblique muscle function.
  - In cases of large hypertropia in primary position or in downgaze, operation on 2 or 3 muscles may be necessary and almost always includes inferior oblique weakening. The patient is at higher risk for overcorrection when simultaneous surgery is performed.
  - Always consider the possibility of bilateral superior oblique palsy prior to operation as unilateral inferior oblique weakening may unmask superior oblique palsy on the other side.[1]
- "V"-pattern strabismus (see Chapter 51):
  - Perform careful and detailed preoperative strabismus measurements and assessment of extraocular muscles. When developing a surgical plan, consider the following factors:
    - The prism diopter difference between upgaze and downgaze.
    - The presence of inferior oblique overaction.
    - The presence of hypertropia in side gaze.

- Weakening of the inferior oblique muscles is preferred if there is significant inferior oblique overaction, a V-pattern strabismus with a difference between upgaze and downgaze of at least 15 prism diopters, and hypertropia documented in side gaze.
- Inferior oblique weakening procedures have little effect on horizontal strabismus correction. Therefore, surgery to correct the horizontal strabismus is performed concomitantly.

- Dissociated vertical deviation (DVD):
    - Frequently seen in conjunction with inferior oblique overaction.
    - Inferior oblique recession and anteriorization (also called "inferior oblique anteriorization" or "inferior oblique anterior transposition") weakens the inferior oblique and can be used for the same indications as other inferior oblique weakening procedures. This procedure has the added benefit of holding the eye down and can be particularly useful in the setting of dissociated vertical deviation (DVD) with inferior oblique overaction.
    - When the inferior oblique insertion is transposed from beneath the lateral rectus to the lateral border of the inferior rectus insertion, the inferior oblique will function to mechanically hold the eye down. The neurovascular bundle of the inferior oblique along the lateral border of the inferior rectus becomes the effective origin for the distal portion of the inferior oblique.
    - Inferior oblique anteriorization, especially if the inferior oblique is placed closer to the limbus than the inferior rectus insertion, may lead to postoperative hypotropia and limitation of elevation, especially in abduction ("antielevation syndrome").[2]

The type of inferior oblique weakening procedure is typically based on surgeon preference as no difference in effectiveness has been found.[1]

Surgical Procedure: Inferior Oblique Exposure and Isolation (Video 46.1)

- Place a traction suture or a Moody locking forceps at the limbus between the inferior and lateral rectus muscles. Expose the inferotemporal quadrant of the eye by pulling the eye superiorly and nasally.
- Use two forceps to elevate the conjunctiva about 8 mm from the limbus.
- Expose the bare sclera by opening the conjunctiva and Tenon capsule with one snip to create an incision parallel with the limbus.
- Use two toothed forceps to grasp the posterior aspect of the opening and then elevate the Tenon capsule out of the incision.

The pinkish-appearing inferior oblique muscle is embedded in the whitish-appearing Tenon capsule. Use a low temperature cautery to maintain good hemostasis as blood staining in the Tenon capsule can make identifying the pink inferior oblique muscle belly difficult.

- Use a hand over hand technique to lift the Tenon capsule until the inferior oblique muscle belly appears in the wound.
- After identifying the inferior oblique, firmly grasp the anterior aspect and carefully elevate it out of the incision using two forceps about 5 mm apart.
- Once you have direct visualization of the posterior aspect of the muscle, use a Stevens tenotomy hook to enter the Tenon capsule under the inferior oblique and elevate the muscle on the hook by aiming the hook superiorly.

Avoid damage to the vortex vein by carefully visualizing it along the temporal border of the inferior rectus muscle, about 10-12 mm posterior to insertion.

- Use two forceps to apply gentle downward pressure to push the point of the hook through the Tenon tissue without splitting the inferior oblique.
- Insert a second muscle hook into the same hole as the first taking care to minimally spread these hooks apart until you are sure that the muscle has not been split.

Avoid blindly passing muscle hooks in the fornix because defects in posterior Tenon can lead to fat prolapse, adhesions, and restriction. Any large defects should be closed with sutures.

- Carefully inspect the inferior border of the inferior oblique to ensure that it has been completely isolated. A completely white triangular-shaped space should be visible when viewing the muscle anteriorly and posteriorly (use a Desmarres retractor for exposure, if necessary). If a pinkish material is seen in the Tenon space under the inferior oblique, remove one of the hooks, place it under the remaining tissue and hook it as described above until the entire inferior oblique is isolated. Forceps may also be used to help place remaining inferior oblique fibers onto the hook.
- Once the entire muscle is on the two small tenotomy hooks, spread them slightly and replace them with 1 or 2 larger hooks (eg, a Jameson and a square hook).

It is surprisingly easy to become disoriented and hook the wrong muscle inadvertently, especially if the muscle has been difficult to isolate or if there is bleeding. For an extra safety step, once the inferior oblique muscle is on the larger hook, use the small tenotomy hook to hook the edge of the inferior rectus and lateral rectus muscles to ensure that the correct muscle, the inferior oblique, has been isolated and no other muscles have been inadvertently incorporated.

Surgical Procedure: Inferior Oblique Myectomy (Video 46.1)

- Isolate the inferior oblique as described previously.
- Use two small straight hemostats to clamp across the entire inferior oblique muscle belly, with one near the insertion and the other 1-5 mm from the first.
- Cut the muscle close to the hemostat on both sides using Westcott scissors. Cauterize the exposed tissue on the end of each hemostat to reduce postoperative lower lid edema and ecchymoses.

Examining the space between the hemostats can ensure that the entire muscle was isolated and cut. Residual fibers can cause persistent post-operative overaction of the muscle.

- After removing the hemostats, position the inferior oblique back in the incision and gently slide the proximal portion of the inferior oblique into the inferior fornix using forceps.
- Reapproximate the conjunctiva by using two forceps to elevate the ends of the incision and allowing the Tenon capsule to retract.
- Close the conjunctival incision with interrupted 8-0 Vicryl or 6-0 plain gut sutures.

Postoperative Considerations

Inferior oblique surgery can also be associated with postoperative periorbital ecchymosis and pain; consider discussing this during preoperative consent process. Also consider instillation of bupivacaine in the sub-Tenon space at the end of the case to treat postoperative pain.

Surgical Procedure: Inferior Oblique Recession

- Isolate the inferior oblique as described above.
- After placing a large hook (eg, Jameson hook) under the inferior oblique, pass another large hook (eg, square hook) under the lateral rectus.

- Expose the insertion of the inferior oblique by retracting the conjunctiva and lateral rectus with a small Stevens tenotomy hook or forceps.
- Place a hemostat as close as possible to the insertion making certain to incorporate the entire inferior oblique muscle.
- Disinsert the inferior oblique by cutting along the hemostat between the muscle and sclera with Westcott scissors.
- Cauterize the cut end of the muscle on the hemostat.
- Just behind the hemostat, place a 6-0 double-armed Vicryl suture with a locking knot at both ends (see Chapter 42).
- Remove the hemostat.

Excessive pulling or tugging of the muscle can lead to hemorrhage due to breakage of the vein along the under surface of the inferior oblique. Excessive pulling of the muscle can rarely cause damage to the ciliary ganglion with resulting mydriasis and loss of accommodation.

- Expose the lateral border of the inferior rectus by placing a Jameson muscle hook under the inferior rectus and a Desmarres lid retractor into the conjunctival opening.
- Elevate the lateral border of the inferior rectus with a small Stevens tenotomy hook to facilitate exposure of the vortex vein which is located about 10-12 mm posterior to the lateral insertion of the inferior rectus.
- Reattach the inferior oblique to the sclera by placing the posterior suture anterior to the vortex vein and the anterior suture 3-4 mm closer to the limbus and parallel to the lateral border of the inferior rectus (Fig. 46.1).
- Tie the suture ends together.

The location of reattachment can be used to vary the degree of recession. The above location is considered a 10-mm recession. Postoperative hypotropia may be noted if the inferior oblique is reattached in a more anterior (closer to the limbus) position (see "anti-elevation" below).

- Reapproximate the conjunctiva by using forceps to elevate the two conjunctival ends and allowing Tenon capsule tissue to retract.
- Close conjunctival incision with interrupted 8-0 Vicryl sutures.

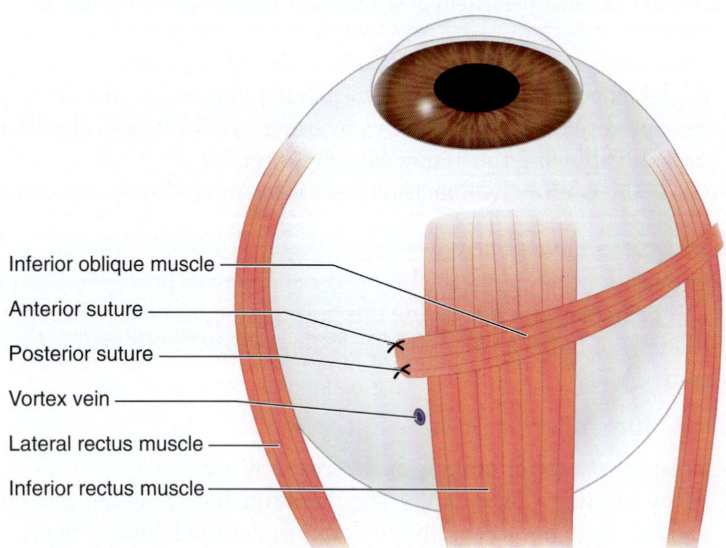

FIGURE 46.1. Inferior oblique recession.

Surgical Procedure: Inferior Oblique Recession and Anteriorization

- Isolate, expose, and disinsert the inferior oblique on a hemostat at the inferior oblique insertion as described above.
- Just behind the hemostat, place a 6-0 double-armed Vicryl suture with a locking knot at both ends (See Chapter 42).
- Remove the hemostat.
- Reattach the inferior oblique to the sclera by placing the anterior suture adjacent to the lateral insertion of the inferior rectus and the posterior suture at a point along a line that would be an extension of the inferior rectus insertion (Fig. 46.2).

Placing the posterior suture 1-2 mm more anteriorly than the inferior rectus insertion can further augment the degree of anteriorization, but carries a risk of hypotropia and antielevation syndrome. To avoid significant antielevation, place the sutures very close together (~1 mm apart), bunching the inferior oblique muscle, and no closer to the limbus than the inferior rectus insertion.

- Tie the suture ends together.
- Reapproximate the conjunctiva by using forceps to elevate the two conjunctival ends and allowing Tenon capsule tissue to retract.
- Close conjunctival incision with interrupted 8-0 Vicryl sutures.

Postoperative Considerations

Antielevation syndrome can occur after inferior oblique anteriorization. Patients will have characteristic bulging of lower lid on upgaze, significant fundus excyclotorsion, and limitation of elevation in abduction. This complication can be particularly noticeable with unilateral surgery and can make the inferior oblique in the opposite eye appear to overact postoperatively (because of fixation duress in the operative eye in abduction).[4]

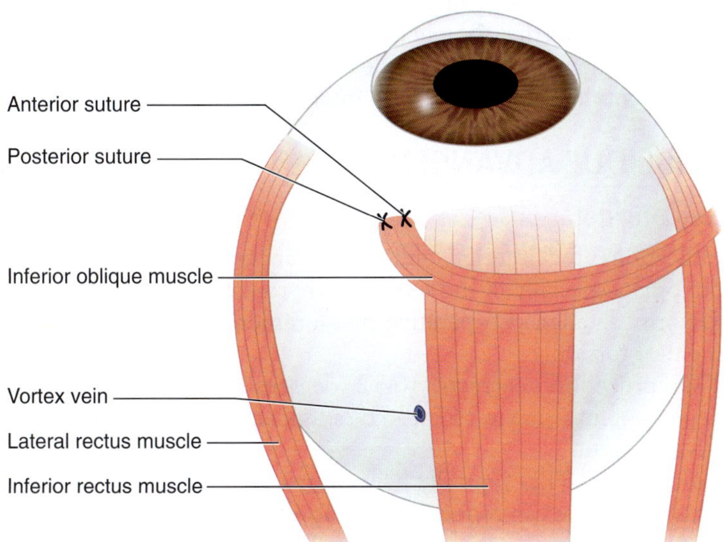

FIGURE 46.2. Inferior oblique recession and anteriorization.

Inferior Oblique Extirpation

Preoperative Considerations

- Indications for inferior oblique extirpation include persistent overaction after an inferior oblique recession or myectomy or as a primary procedure with significantly overacting inferior oblique muscles in the setting of "V"-pattern strabismus or unilateral superior oblique palsy. Persistent overaction of the inferior oblique after a weakening procedure can occur because some of the muscle fibers were missed at the first surgery, insufficient recession, or scarring. Particularly after a myectomy, it is possible for the cut end of the muscle to reattach to sclera in an unfavorable location.[3]

Surgical Procedure: Inferior Oblique Extirpation

- Isolate, expose, and disinsert the inferior oblique on a hemostat at the inferior oblique insertion as described above.
- After placing a Jameson muscle hook under the inferior rectus insertion, increase exposure by placing a Stevens tenotomy hook under the lateral border of the inferior rectus posteriorly.
- Stretch the inferior oblique laterally and identify the whitish bulge (site of inferior oblique nerve insertion) in the inferior oblique along its posterior border and underneath the inferior rectus.
- Clamp about 7-8 mm of this tissue with a straight hemostat.
- Extensively cauterize this area and if possible, the blood vessel located in that tissue.
- Cut the cauterized tissue with Westcott scissors. The inferior oblique will appear longer after the nerve is transected.
- Use a second hemostat to clamp across the entire inferior oblique muscle as close as possible to the lateral border of the inferior rectus.
- Cut the section of the inferior oblique between the two hemostats with Westcott scissors.
- Cauterize the stump of the inferior oblique on the remaining hemostat.
- Remove the hemostat and allow the inferior oblique to retract.
- Reapproximate the conjunctiva by using forceps to elevate the two conjunctival ends and allowing Tenon capsule tissue to retract.
- Close conjunctival incision with interrupted 8-0 Vicryl sutures.

INFERIOR OBLIQUE ADVANCEMENT

Preoperative Considerations

- Indications for inferior oblique advancement include intorsion and torsional diplopia, especially in the setting of thyroid eye disease (TED) (see Chapter 59).
- Perform detailed preoperative measurements including double Maddox measurement of torsion.
- This procedure corrects 10-12 degrees of intorsion per eye. Large (20-30) degrees of intorsion in TED can be surgically corrected with bilateral inferior oblique advancement.
- Patients with TED typically have intorsion in the setting of an A-pattern exotropia. This procedure can reduce the A-pattern as well.[3]

VIDEO Surgical Procedure: Inferior Oblique Advancement (Video 59.1)

- Isolate, expose, and imbricate the inferior oblique as described previously for recession or anteriorization.
- Hook the entire lateral rectus muscle on a large muscle hook.
- Pass the two sutures attached to the inferior oblique under the lateral rectus muscle (ie, between the muscle and sclera).

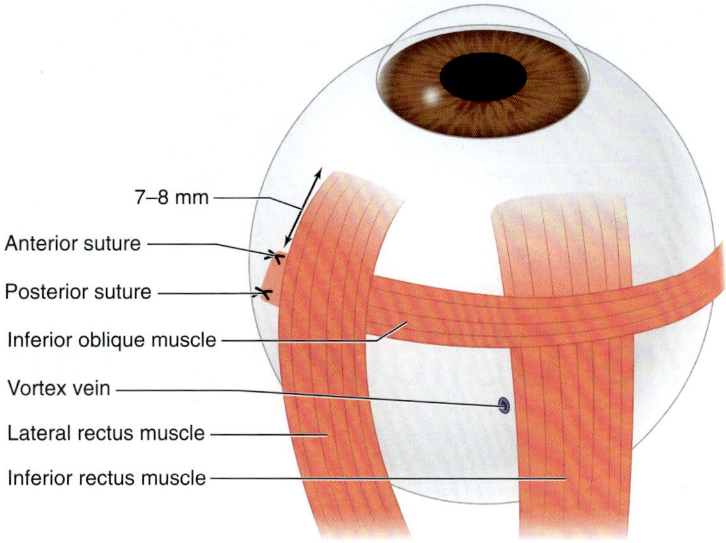

FIGURE 46.3. Inferior oblique advancement.

- Keep the eye in straight adduction while marking a point on the sclera 8 mm posterior to the insertion of the lateral rectus.
- Reattach the inferior oblique muscle by placing the posterior suture 2-3 mm posterior to the mark and the anterior suture 2-3 mm anterior to the mark so that the center of the inferior oblique is at 8 mm posterior to the lateral rectus insertion (Fig. 46.3).
- Reapproximate the conjunctiva by using forceps to elevate the two conjunctival ends and allowing Tenon capsule tissue to retract.
- Close conjunctival incision with interrupted 8-0 Vicryl sutures.

Postoperative Considerations

If the patient is under corrected, it is possible to return the patient to surgery to resect and reattach 5 mm of the advanced inferior oblique muscle.

References

1. Traboulsi EI, Utz VM. *Practical Management of Pediatric Ocular Disorders and Strabismus. A Case-Based Approach*. New York, NY: Springer; 2016.
2. Buckley EG, Shields MB. "Inferior oblique procedures." In: Buckley EG, Shields MB, Freedman S, eds. *Atlas of Ophthalmic Surgery. Volume III: Strabismus and Glaucoma*. St. Louis, Missouri: Mosby; 1991:86-103.
3. Del Monte MA. "2001 - An ocular odyssey: lessons learned from 25 years of surgical treatment for graves eye disease." *Am Orthopt J*. 2002;52:40-57.
4. Kushner BJ. "The effect of anterior transposition of the inferior oblique muscle on the palpebral fissure." *Arch Ophthalmol*. 2000;118:1542-1546.

CHAPTER 47

Superior Oblique Procedures

HongVan Le, MD

SUPERIOR OBLIQUE MUSCLE

The superior oblique (SO) intorts, depresses, and abducts the eye (see Chapter 42). Patients with a SO palsy will typically demonstrate a hypertropia that increases in adduction of the affected eye, as well as extorsion. Subjects with a SO palsy may have normal-appearing versions, and the Parks-Bielschowsky three-step test can be helpful to make the diagnosis. The three-step test has a 70% sensitivity[1] and 50% specificity.[2] Bilateral SO palsies often cause increased extorsion and a large V-pattern esotropia. In some instances, a strengthening procedure such as a SO tuck can help to address vertical and torsional alignment issues due to a SO palsy. The Harada-Ito procedure is used to address excyclotorsion (without much vertical misalignment) by advancing the anterior portion of the SO (forwards and laterally) so that the axis around which the SO rotates the globe is closer to the anterior-posterior axis. Other surgical options for SO palsy may include weakening the ipsilateral antagonist (the inferior oblique, see Chapter 46) or weakening the yoke muscle (the contralateral inferior rectus). In contrast, SO overaction can result in an A-pattern strabismus (see Chapter 51). In these cases, SO weakening procedures such as tenotomy, partial tenotomy with or without a spacer can be helpful. Brown syndrome (SO tendon sheath syndrome) may also require SO weakening procedures. Caution should be taken in performing SO procedures in fusing patients as torsional issues can arise.

SUPERIOR OBLIQUE EXPOSURE

- Positioning:
  - The patient's head should be angled with the chin up so that the forehead is level with the operating table, and the superior orbital rim is perpendicular to the operating table.
  - The surgeon should sit so that the dominant hand has good access to the superior fornix. Often sitting on the same side of the patient as the dominant hand works well. Alternatively, the surgeon may want to sit opposite the eye operated.
- Nasal approach to SO tendon (Fig. 47.1):
  - Place a single 6-0 silk traction suture or locking Moody forceps at the 12 o'clock limbus and rotate the eye downward.
  - Make an opening through the conjunctiva and Tenon capsule just nasal to the border of the superior rectus (SR) and extend posteriorly for several millimeters using the Westcott scissors (Fig. 47.1A).

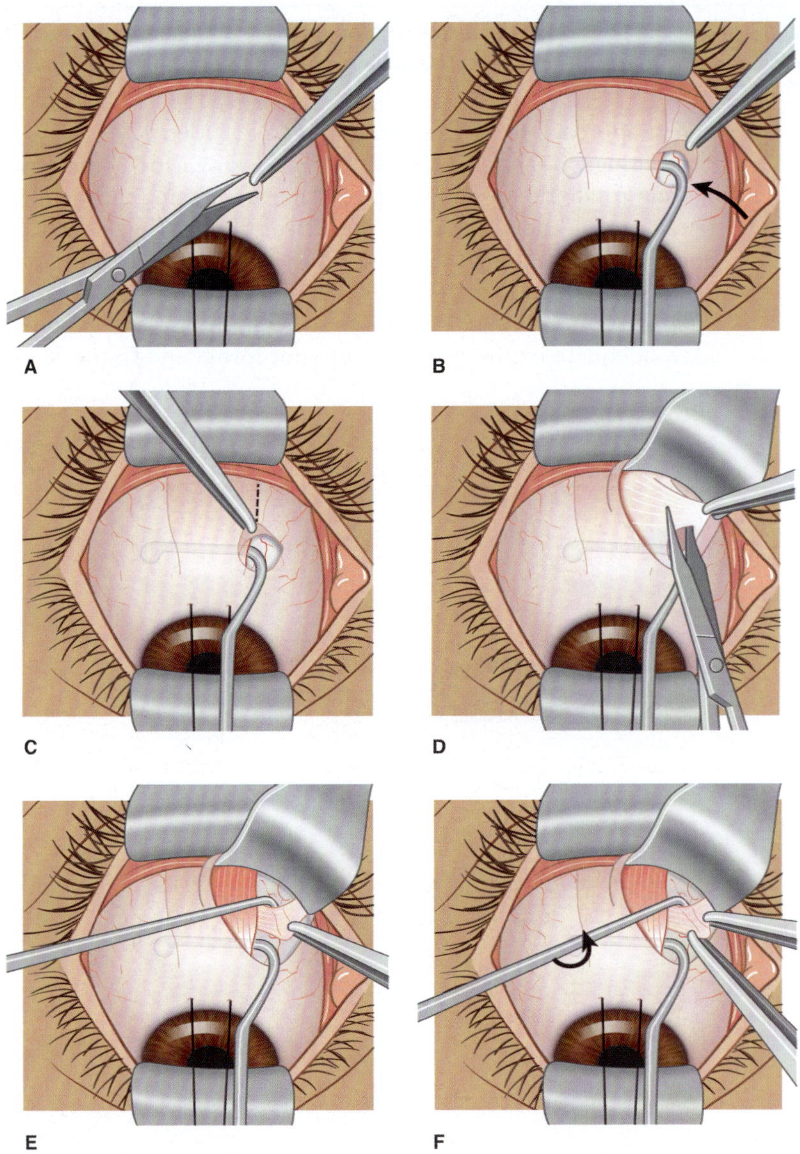

FIGURE 47.1. Nasal approach to superior oblique exposure.

- Hook the SR muscle, taking care to not pass the hook too far posteriorly to avoid hooking the SO tendon (Fig. 47.1B).
- Once the SR muscle is hooked, the incision can be enlarged along the border of the SR muscle (Fig. 47.1C). Insert a small Desmarres or Fison retractor into the conjunctival and Tenon capsule opening to allow for adequate exposure.
- Use sharp and blunt dissection to identify the SO tendon. Be careful when dissecting tissues between the SR and sclera so that the SO is not inadvertently injured (Fig. 47.1D). The SO fibers can be identified as silvery, white and running from underneath the SR muscle and coursing nasally.
- Place a small Stevens tenotomy hook underneath the SO tendon making sure to rotate the point of the tenotomy hook upward to secure the tendon on the hook (Fig. 47.1E).
- Gently remove any intermuscular septum still adherent to the tendon by grasping the tissue with forceps on either side and forcing the blunt end of the tenotomy hook up through the tissue (Fig. 47.1F).
- Pass a second Stevens tenotomy hook through the opening created on either side of the SO tendon and then gently spread the hooks.

To confirm that the tissue isolated is the SO tendon, place a finger on the trochlea and pull on the tendon gently with the muscle hook. The pulling on the tendon should be felt at the trochlea.

VIDEO

- Temporal approach to SO tendon (Fig. 47.2) (Video 47.1):
  - Place a single 6-0 silk traction suture or locking Moody forceps at 12 o'clock limbus and rotate the eye downward. Make an opening through the conjunctiva and Tenon capsule along the lateral border of the SR. (Fig. 47.2A).
  - Isolate and hook the SR muscle near its insertion taking care to not pass the hook too far posteriorly, which may inadvertently engage SO fibers (Fig. 47.2B). Insert a Desmarres or Fison retractor into the conjunctiva and Tenon capsule opening to allow adequate exposure to the superior fornix and to the SO tendon insertion.

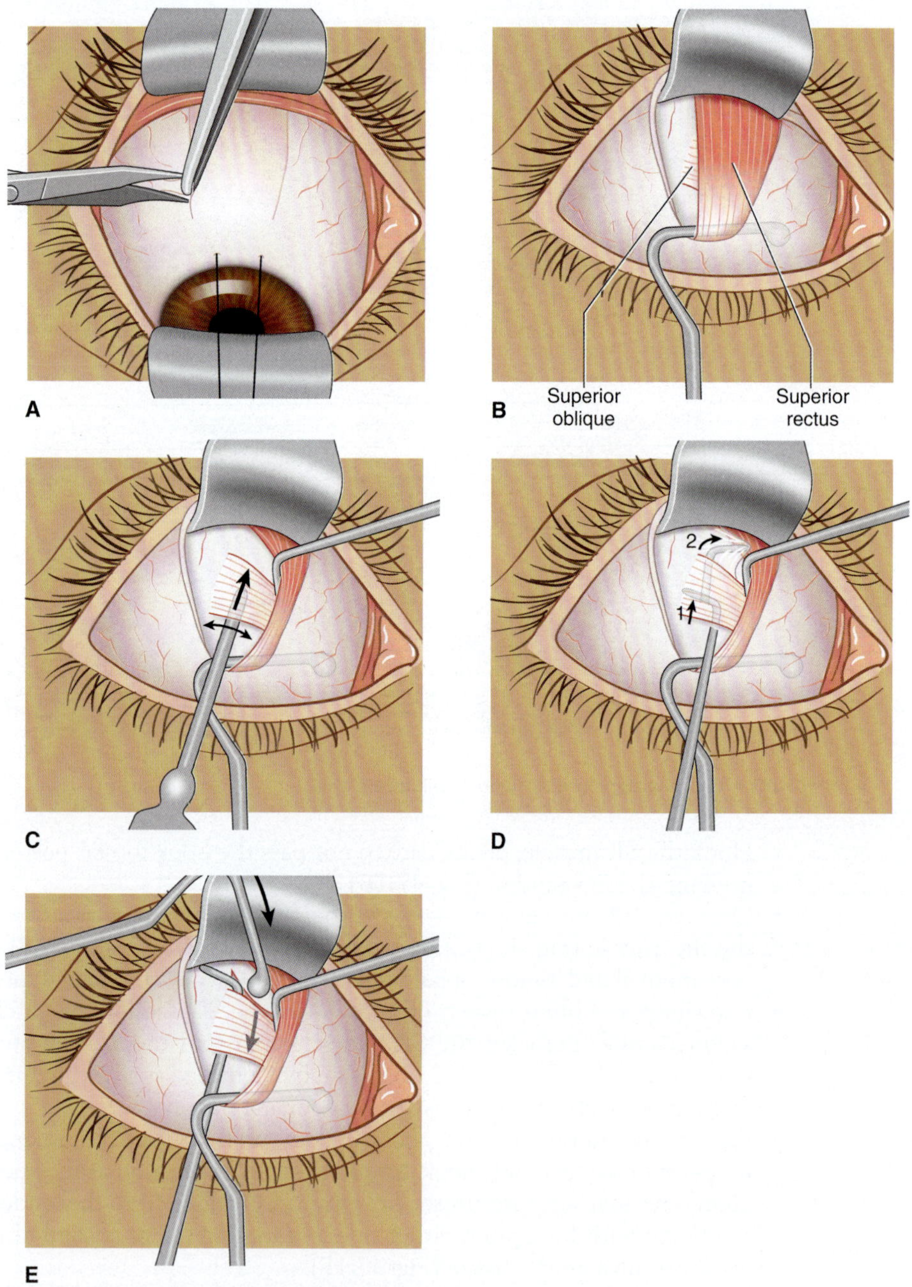

FIGURE 47.2. Temporal approach to superior oblique exposure.

- While retracting the SR nasally, use an iris spatula (tiny malleable ribbon retractor) or a smooth forcep to gently dissect and elevate the fine, silvery fibers of the SO tendon from the sclera by gently moving the instrument side to side and pushing the tip posteriorly (Fig. 47.2C). If the SO tendon is not obvious, start more anteriorly, close to the SR insertion for this maneuver. If the SO still is not apparent, pull the superior rectus more nasally to look for the insertion. Be aware that the anatomy may be abnormal in cases that require SO surgery.

The SO tendon can almost always be identified on the temporal side using the above-described maneuvers. If it cannot be identified on the temporal side, it may be easier to find the tendon on the nasal side of the SR then follow the SO tendon under the SR to the SO insertion.

- Place a Stevens tenotomy hook underneath the SO tendon insertion until the posterior border is reached. When the tip is beyond the posterior edge of the tendon, rotate the hook end superiorly (Fig. 47.2D). Use forceps to gently remove the fibers of the intramuscular septum. Care should be taken during this step to avoid damaging the superior temporal vortex vein, which lies just posterior to the insertion of the SO tendon.
- Once the SO tendon is isolated on a Stevens tenotomy hook, pass a larger Jameson muscle hook underneath the insertion to encompass the entire tendon (Fig. 47.2E).

SO WEAKENING PROCEDURES

VIDEO Tenotomy (Video 47.1)

- Isolate the SO from a nasal approach or temporal approach. The nasal tenotomy is preferred for a "complete" tenotomy (eg, Brown syndrome), while the temporal approach may address A-pattern without completely crippling the SO function, and may be a more "gentle" approach to consider, especially in a fusing patient to potentially avoid inducing torsion.[3,4]
- If on the temporal side, separate any attachments of the SR to the underlying SO tendon. Running the large muscle hook back and forth between the SO and overlying SR can be helpful to separate the connections.
- Leave the two Stevens muscle hooks in place and gently spread the hooks far enough apart to enable Westcott scissors to make a cut through the tendon. A modification includes a posterior tenotomy (up to 7/8 width of the tendon) so that the anterior torsional fibers are spared. This procedure can be titrated intraoperatively based on the forced duction test. Forced duction testing can also be used to confirm complete tenotomy. Take care to not convert a partial tenotomy into a total tenotomy with aggressive forced duction testing.

Spacer (Fig. 47.3)

- Isolate the SO from a nasal approach (Fig. 47.1).
- Place a double-armed Dacron suture through the tendon just nasal to the SR border and secure the suture in the tendon. Place a second double-armed 5-0 Dacron suture ~3 mm nasal to the first (Fig. 47.3A).
- Cut the SO tendon between the preplaced sutures (Fig. 47.3B).

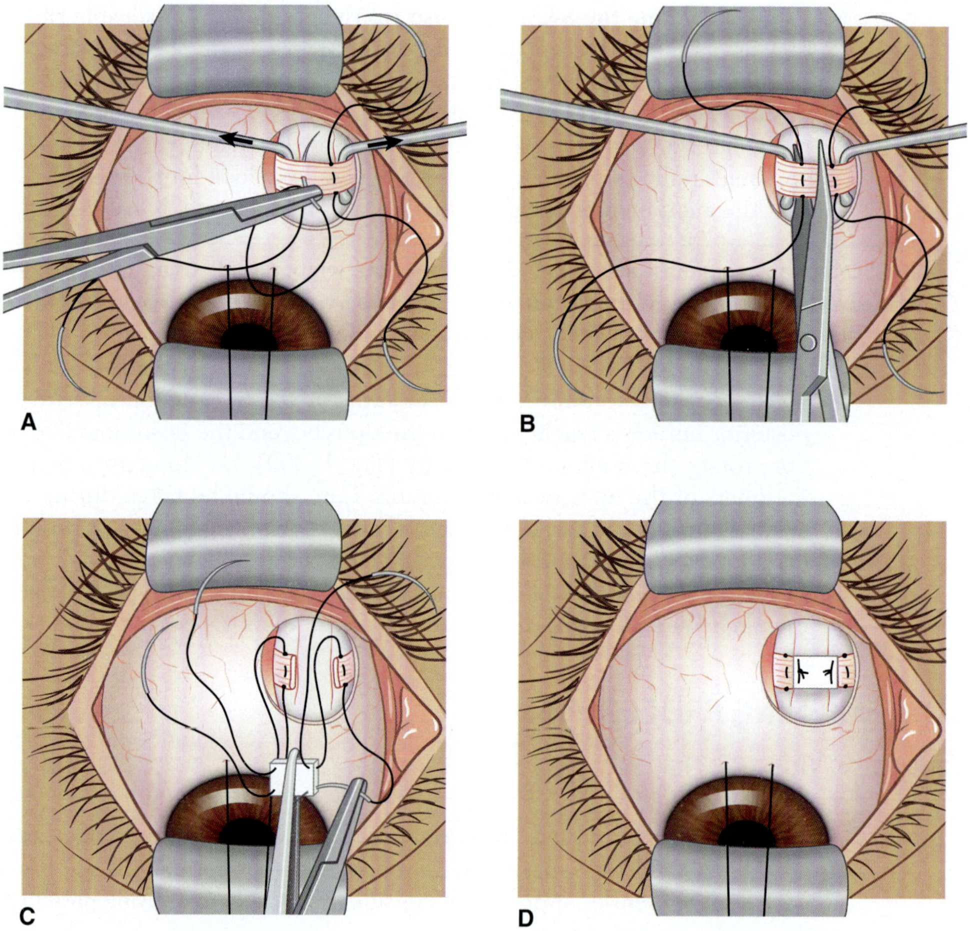

FIGURE 47.3. Superior oblique spacer.

- Reattach the cut ends of the SO tendon to a 240 silicone band (the same material used for scleral buckling surgery) (Fig. 47.3C). The length of the band can range from 4 to 7 mm depending on the amount of desired weakening or overaction of the SO. Place the double-armed sutures into each end of the band extending ~1 mm from the edge. Pull the suture ends until the tendon is adjacent to the silicone band.[5]
- Tie the two ends of each double-armed Dacron suture together. Position the band into the superior nasal fornix (Fig. 47.3D). One potential complication of this procedure is that the expander can extrude through the conjunctiva over time.

Instead of a silicone expander, an adjustable suture expander technique can be utilized. Two double-armed 6-0 polyester sutures are used to secure the SO tendon and are placed 4 mm apart (Fig. 47.4A). The SO tendon is transected between the preplaced sutures (Fig. 47.4A). The two suture pairs are then tied to each other using a bowtie style slipknot, leaving a 2-8 mm gap between the cut ends of the tendon (Fig. 47.4B). Adjustment can be made intraoperatively depending on traction testing and fundus torsion. Once adjustment is completed, the slipknot can be converted to a square knot by cutting one of the pairs of sutures and pulling the ends through to the other side (Fig. 47.4C).[6]

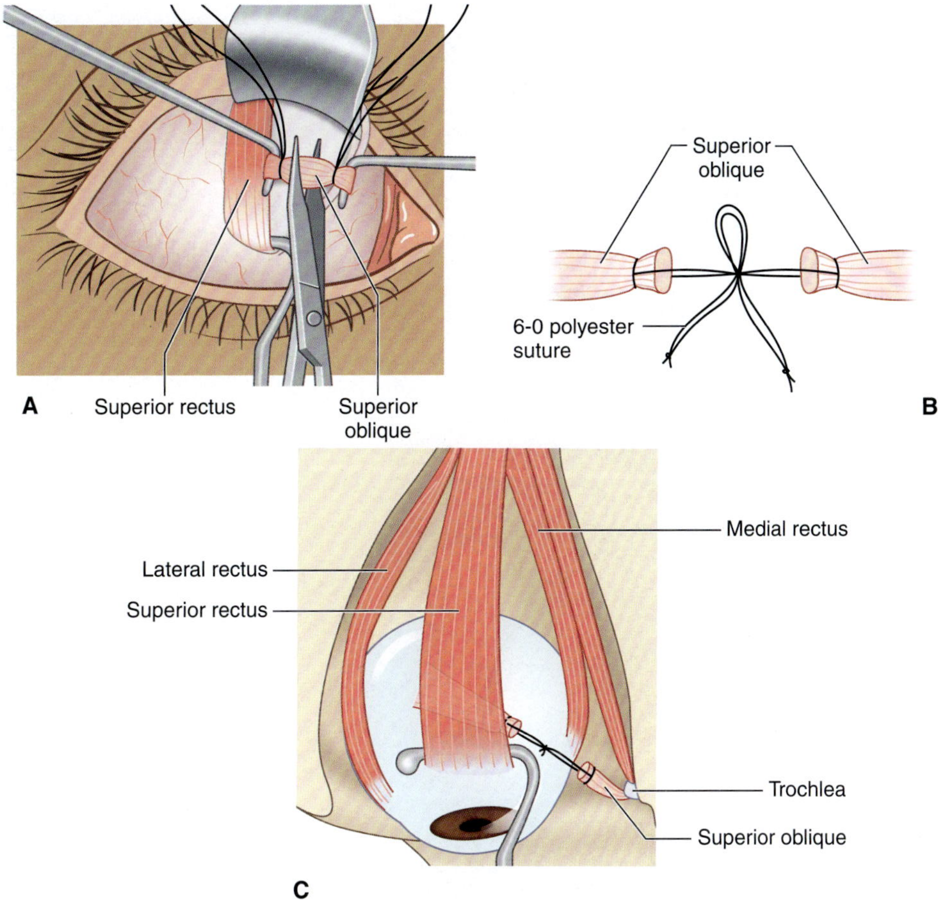

FIGURE 47.4. Superior oblique adjustable suture expander.

SO STRENGTHENING PROCEDURES

Tuck (Fig. 47.5)[7]

- Isolate the SO tendon from a temporal approach (Fig. 47.2).
- Measure and mark with a surgical marking pen the desired amount of SO tendon tuck. The amount to tuck depends on the laxity of the tendon (Fig. 47.5A).
- Use a nonabsorbable, double-armed suture (5-0 Dacron, 5-0 Mersilene) and pass the suture through the previously marked sites. These can be placed as two single-armed sutures, one on each side (Fig. 47.5B-D, Fig. 47.5F), or as a single double-armed suture through the middle of the tendon (Fig. 47.5F).
- Pass both ends of the needles through the insertion of the SO, making sure to incorporate approximately one-quarter of the tendon width (Fig. 47.5C).

> **Alternatively, a tendon tucker can be used to place the suture.**

- Temporarily tie the suture to itself with a slip knot, forming a fold or tuck in the tendon (Fig. 47.5D).
- Perform a forced duction test (Fig. 47.5E). During the forced duction testing, the eye should be capable of elevating past the midline while in adduction. If the tendon is tucked excessively and significant restriction is met during forced duction testing, the amount of SO tuck should be reduced to avoid an iatrogenic Brown syndrome. Repeat forced duction testing until the eye can be elevated above midline in the adduction.

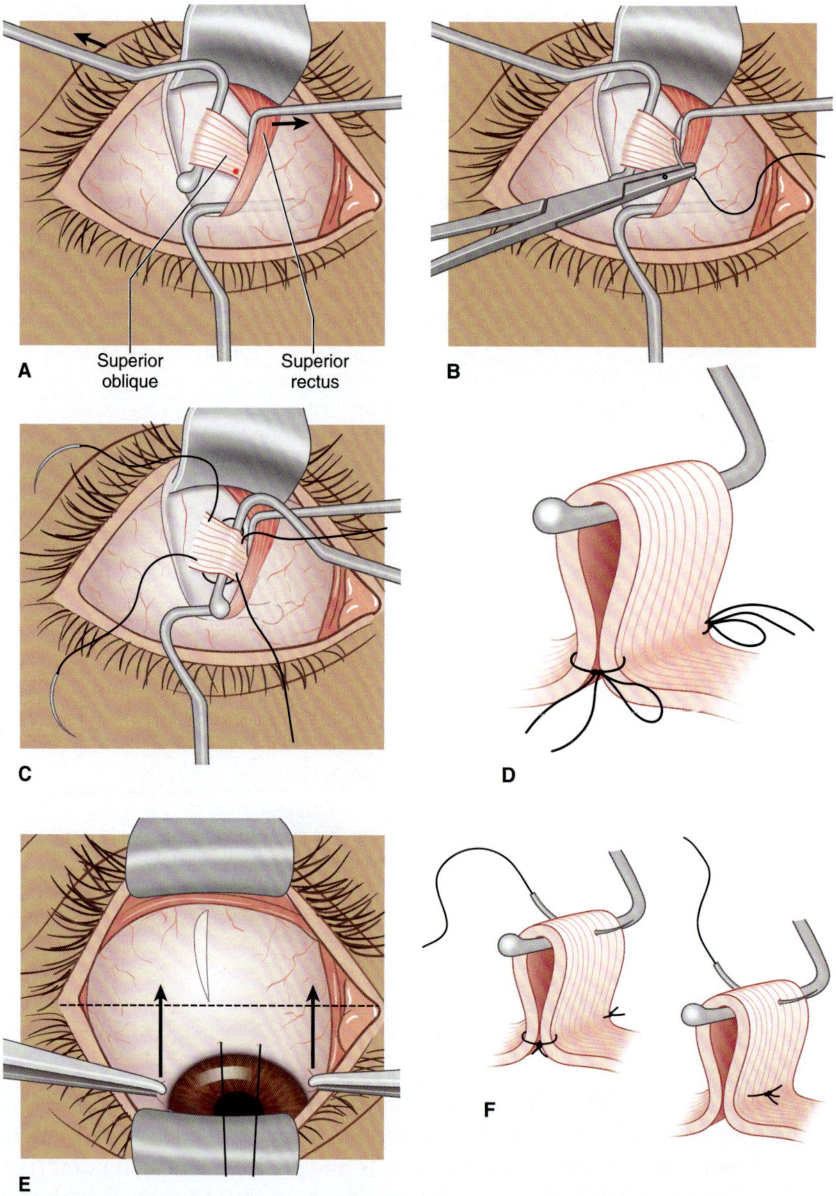

FIGURE 47.5. Superior oblique tuck.

- Permanently tie the suture once an acceptable forced duction test has been accomplished. Measure and record the final amount of tuck, which will be double the distance from the suture to the top of the folded tendon.
- Optional: Place an additional suture through the top end of the tuck to loosely secure the excess SO tendon to the sclera. Record the location of this suture to locate the SO tendon if a reoperation is necessary (Fig. 47.5F).

HARADA-ITO PROCEDURE[8,9]

There are two methods of performing the Harada-Ito (HI) procedure (Fig. 47.6). In the original method, a suture is placed around the anterior 1/4-1/3 of the SO fibers and both arms of the suture are passed through the sclera 7-8 mm posterior to the LR insertion (Fig. 47.6A). The tightness of the suture is adjusted intraoperatively to induce the appropriate amount of incyclotorsion. In the Fell's modification of the HI procedure,

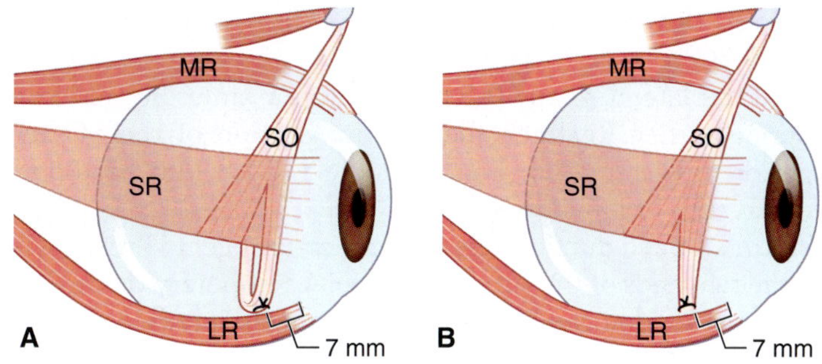

FIGURE 47.6. Harada-Ito procedure **(A)** and Fell's Modification of Harada-Ito procedure **(B)**.

the suture is placed in the anterior 1/4-1/3 of the SO tendon insertion. The sutured portion of the SO tendon insertion is disinserted and reattached just superior to the superior border of the LR, 7-8 mm posterior to the LR insertion (Fig. 47.6B).

Harada-Ito Fell's Modification (Figs. 47.6B and 47.7)

- Isolate the SO from the temporal approach (Fig. 47.2).
- Split the anterior fibers of the SO tendon (approximately 1/4 of the total fibers) using a tenotomy hook and lengthen the split by moving the tenotomy hook back and forth. Westcott scissors can also be used to extend this division nasally (Fig. 47.7A).
- Place a nonabsorbable suture (5-0 Dacron) into the anterior portion of the isolated SO tendon and secure it (Fig. 47.7B). It may also be helpful to wrap the suture around the tendon and tie it to itself, as the tendon is often very thin and friable.

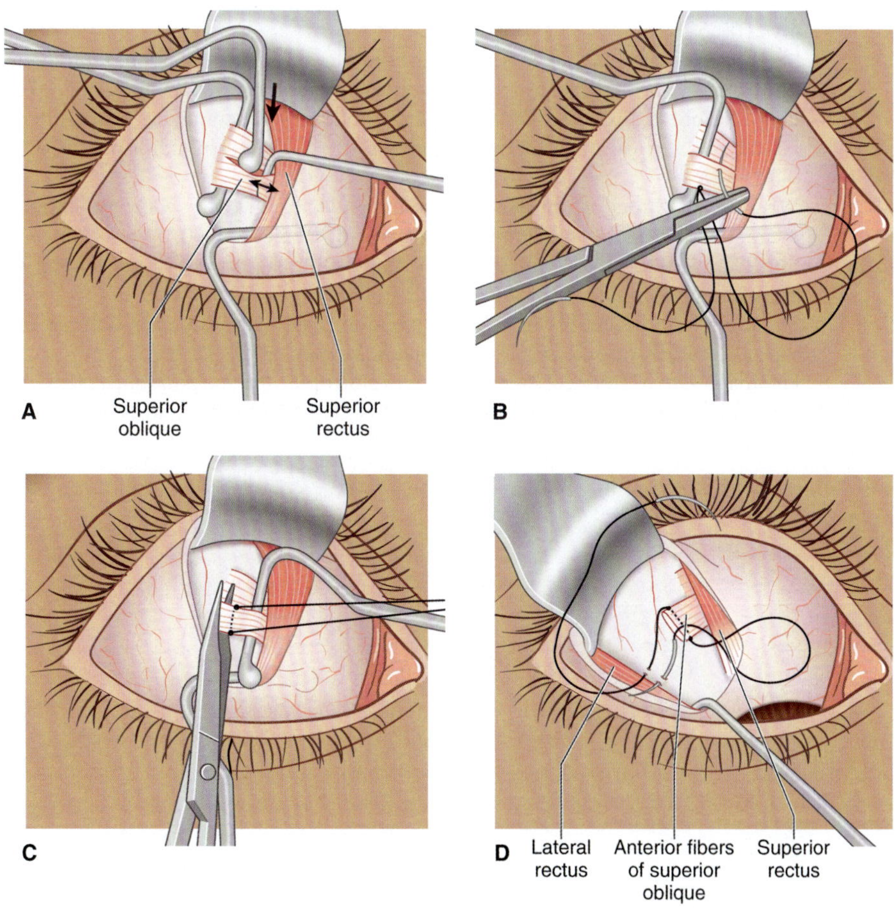

FIGURE 47.7. Fell's Modification of Harada-Ito procedure.

- Disinsert this portion of the tendon from the sclera using Westcott scissors (Fig. 47.7C).
- Isolate the lateral rectus (LR) muscle on a Jameson muscle hook and expose the superior border. Reattach the anterior portion of the SO tendon to an area just superior to the superior border of the LR, ~8 mm posterior to the LR insertion (Fig. 47.7D).
- Perform a forced duction test to avoid an iatrogenic Brown syndrome.
- Tie the two ends of the suture together. A temporary tie can be placed, and the position of the tendon can be adjusted postoperatively (see Chapter 48).

It may be helpful to mark the superior limbus preoperatively to judge the amount of torsional rotation achieved intraoperatively from the Harada-Ito procedure.

If an iatrogenic Brown syndrome is noted postoperatively, then the tendon has been advanced too far laterally or too much of the SO tendon has been incorporated in the advancement and corrective action is recommended at that time. If torsional diplopia from an overcorrection is noted in the immediate postoperative period, observation may be sufficient as the situation usually improves in 2-4 weeks.

References

1. Manchandia AM, Demer JL. Sensitivity of the three-step test in diagnosis of superior oblique palsy. *J AAPOS*. 2014;18(6):567-571. doi: 10.1016/j.jaapos.2014.08.007.
2. Demer JL, Kung J, Clark RA. Functional imaging of human extraocular muscles in head tilt dependent hypertropia. *Invest Ophthalmol Vis Sci*. 2011;52(6):3023-3031. doi: 10.1167/iovs.10-6596.
3. Velez FG, Velez G, Thacker N. Superior oblique posterior tenectomy in patients with Brown syndrome with small deviations in the primary position. *J AAPOS*. 2006;10:214-219.
4. Ung T, Raoof N, Burke J. Effect of superior oblique weakening on vertical alignment and horizontal and vertical incomitance in patients with A-pattern strabismus. *J AAPOS*. 2011;15:9-13.
5. Wright KW. Superior oblique silicone expander for Brown syndrome and superior oblique overaction. *J Pediatr Ophthalmol Strabismus*. 1991;28:101-107.
6. Suh DW, Guyton DL, Hunter DG. An adjustable superior oblique tendon spacer with the use of nonabsorbable suture. *J AAPOS*. 2001;5(3):164-171.
7. Saunders RA. Treatment of superior oblique palsy with superior oblique tendon tuck and inferior oblique muscle myectomy. *Ophthalmology*. 1986;93:1023.
8. Harada M, Ito Y. Surgical correction of cyclotropia. *Jpn J Ophthalmol*. 1964;8:88-96.
9. Fells P. Management of paralytic strabismus. *Br J Ophthalmol*. 1974;58:255-265.

CHAPTER 48

Adjustable Sutures in Strabismus Surgery

Federico G. Velez, MD

PREOPERATIVE CONSIDERATIONS

- Indications:
  - Patient selection:
    - Any patient undergoing eye muscle surgery who can tolerate adjustment under topical anesthesia (pediatric patients if the surgery center or hospital allows short sedation in the recovery room). Preoperatively, the conjunctiva can be manipulated with cotton swabs to get an idea of the patient's ability to cooperate with adjustment.
    - Adjustable sutures can be especially helpful in conditions in which the results of surgery may be unpredictable (eg, thyroid eye disease, reoperations) or in situations in which the patient does not have a large range of fusion or suppression, and results must be exact to avoid diplopia.
  - Indications/conditions:
    - Diplopia.
    - Reoperations.
    - Restrictive strabismus.
    - Harada-Ito procedure (see Chapter 47).
    - Adjustable "Faden" operation (see chapter 49).
    - Hang-back technique.
      - Thin sclera (ie, high myopia).
      - Surgery secondary to retinal detachment or glaucoma devices (see chapter 59).
- Surgical procedures in which adjustable sutures may be used:
  - Rectus muscle recessions.[1]
  - Rectus muscle resections.[1]
  - Rectus muscle plication.[3]
  - Rectus muscle tenotomy and miniplication.[4]
  - Superior oblique Harada-Ito.[2]

INTRAOPERATIVE CONSIDERATIONS

Keep the cornea moist and protected to reduce post-operative blur. Consider using apraclonidine for vasoconstriction rather than phenylephrine to reduce pupillary dilation that may interfere with postoperative adjustment.

- Anesthesia (see chapter 1):
  - Topical.
    - Potential indications:
      - First time surgery.
      - Recession, plication, and resection.
      - Risk for general anesthesia.
    - Technique:
      - Start with topical anesthetic eye drops in both eyes.
      - Place lidocaine 3.5% ophthalmic gel on the surgical eye.
      - Prep and expose both eyes for patient comfort, keeping in mind that the patient will need to sit up during surgery.
      - Use sterile strips on eyelashes, rather than sticky plastic adhesives.
      - Evaluate the alignment intraoperatively. Sit the patient up and do a cover test while the patient is fixing at a target placed as far away as possible. Keep all drapes and equipment sterile in case additional surgery is needed.
      - Complete the adjustment in the operating room or perform a same day or delayed adjustment in the recovery room or clinic.
  - Peribulbar or retrobulbar block:
    - Typically only considered for unilateral surgery.
    - Limits immediate and early postoperative adjustment because there must be adequate time for the anesthetic to reverse prior to adjustment.

Do not use bupivacaine (Marcaine) in the block if same day adjustment is planned. Consider avoiding dilating drops because pupil reactivity can be one indication of anesthetic reversal.

  - General anesthesia:
    - Preferred in patients who are uncooperative or anxious.
    - Preferred in patients needing extensive dissection such as glaucoma shunt, scleral buckle, severe scarring, oblique muscle surgery.
    - Use with caution in patients with medical comorbidities.
- Incision (see chapter 43):
  - Fornix.
    - Advantages:
      - Less scarring.
      - Less postoperative irritation.
      - Preservation of limbal vessels.
      - Single incision allows surgery on two adjacent rectus muscles.
      - Covered sutures.
    - Disadvantages:
      - Limited exposure.
      - Reduced elasticity of adult conjunctiva.
      - More complex adjustment due to the oblique perpendicular relation between the sutures and the muscle path.
      - Not ideal for topical anesthesia.

- Para limbal.
  - Advantages:
    - Great exposure.
    - Preservation of limbal vessels.
    - Ideal technique for topical anesthesia.
    - Allows complete conjunctival closure.
  - Disadvantages:
    - Persistent redness.
    - Irritation.
    - Risk of cutting the insertion when making incision.
- Limbal.
  - Advantages:
    - Great exposure.
    - Less bleeding.
  - Disadvantages:
    - Persistent redness.
    - Irritation.
    - Requires conjunctival recession to expose the adjustable sutures or post-adjustment conjunctival closure.

The limbal incision can be closed with a flap of the conjunctiva that can fold back to expose the sutures then fold toward the limbus to close (Fig. 48.1).

SURGICAL PROCEDURE: ADJUSTABLE SUTURE (VIDEO 48.1)

- Attaching the muscle: After performing the standard eye muscle surgery technique, reinsert the muscle on the sclera with partial-thickness scleral passes at the desired position (ie, the original insertional stump). Alternatively, in patients undergoing resections, reinsert the muscle anterior to the original insertion to allow for both postoperative advancement (anterior to the original insertion) as well as recession.

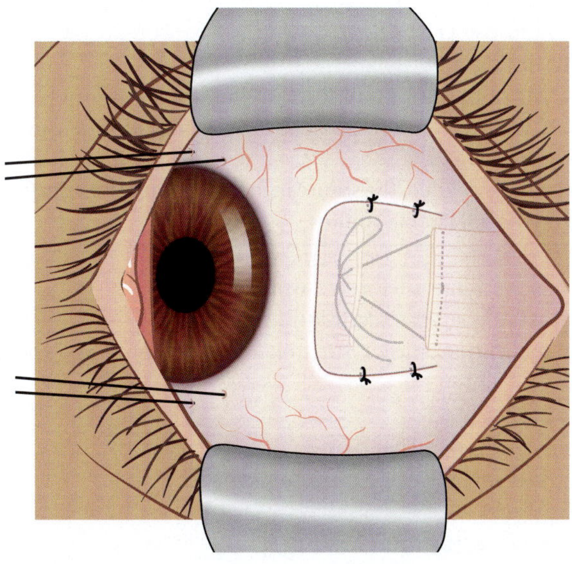

FIGURE 48.1. Conjunctival flap to cover the adjustable knot with a limbal incision.
The conjunctiva is pulled up as if closing the wound normally; sutures are placed along the wings of the limbal incision at the level or just anterior to the level of the adjustable knot instead of at the limbus, leaving a flap of the conjunctiva to cover the knot. If the wing is long, it may be helpful to place a second suture posteriorly along the wing. This also gives added security in case the proximal suture tears during adjustment.

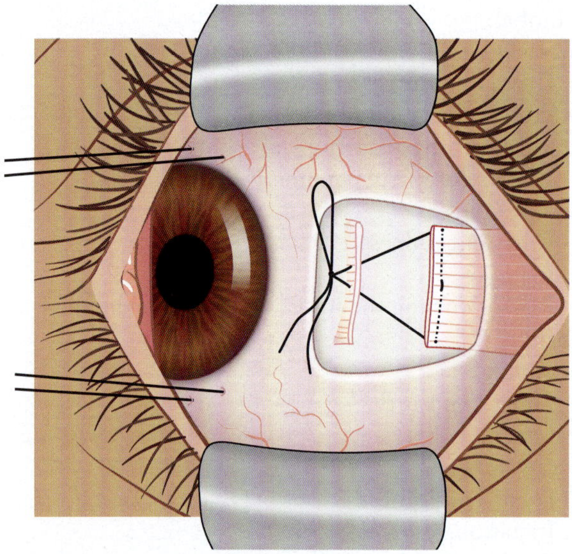

FIGURE 48.2. Slip knot (½ bow tie) adjustable suture technique.
The first knot is a double throw surgeon's knot. Once this is in place, then the next knot is thrown, but the suture is pulled through only partially, leaving a loop. The ends are trimmed to ~3 cm (leave ends long enough to tie at the time of adjustment). It is helpful to leave suture that forms the loop a little shorter, so it is obvious which suture to pull to release the loop. At the time of adjustment, the shorter end can be pulled to untie the loop and adjust the muscle. If the muscle is in the proper place, the loop can be pulled through to convert the knot to a permanent knot. Another option if the muscle does not need to be adjusted is to leave the slip knot in place (assuming all suture is tucked in under the conjunctiva). This avoids unnecessary adjustment, but is not as secure as tying the knot permanently and leaves extra suture behind, which will cause a bit more inflammation during healing.

- Adjustable knot options:
  - Slip knot (half-bow tie technique) (Fig. 48.2).
    - Advantage—Simple technique.
    - Disadvantage—Not possible to determine the final position of the muscle after adjustment.
  - Sliding noose (Fig. 48.3).
    - Advantages:
      - More precise final position based on millimeters.
      - Complete coverage of sutures under the conjunctiva.

In case an adjustment is needed, the sutures can be externalized using a preplaced ripcord or bucket-handle secured on the adjustable sutures.

    - Disadvantage—More complex.
- Semiadjustable suture technique (Fig. 48.4).
  - This technique allows further advancement, but the amount of re-recession is limited.
  - Advantages:
    - Less postoperative drift.
    - Lower incidence of muscle slippage.
  - Indications:
    - Medial rectus muscle surgery.
    - Inferior rectus muscle surgery.
  - Technique (originally described by Kushner.[5])
    - Imbricate each muscle corner with a single-armed absorbable or nonabsorbable suture. Reinsert the muscle at the desired recession position using the preplaced

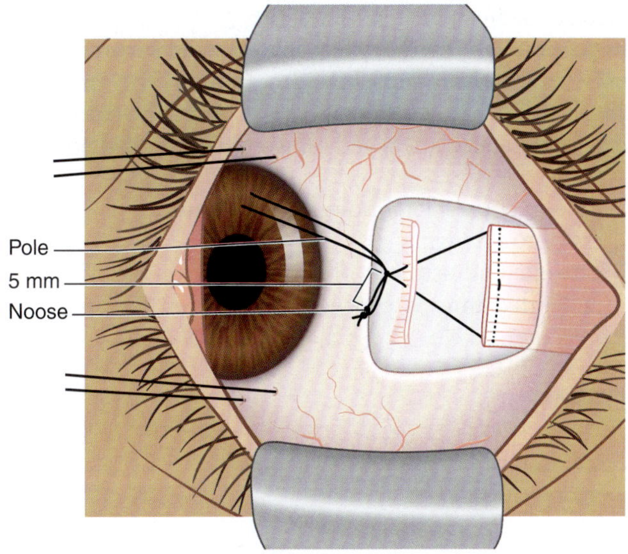

FIGURE 48.3. Sliding noose adjustable suture technique.[6]
The needles should be passed so that the two sutures exit the sclera close to one another. The two muscle sutures are called the pole sutures and are pulled up and clamped 7-8 cm from the insertion. A square knot is tied abutting the clamp. A separate piece of 6-0 Vicryl suture (the noose) is wrapped around the pole sutures once or twice and tied tightly with a square knot. The ends of the noose suture are tied together at about 5 mm to provide a "bucket-handle" for manipulation of the noose during adjustment. The noose is adjusted to achieve the desired hang-back. The pole sutures can then be trimmed to about 5 mm and the pole and noose both tucked in for later adjustment if needed (and left as is if no adjustment needed). Alternatively, the pole sutures can be left a bit longer and tied permanently to one another then trimmed once the desired alignment is obtained.

single-armed suture. The width (separation between the scleral insertion) should be less than the muscle width to allow a central muscle sagging.

- Preplace a double-armed absorbable suture imbricating the central two-thirds of the muscle width. Place the central double-armed sutures at the original insertion for later adjustment.

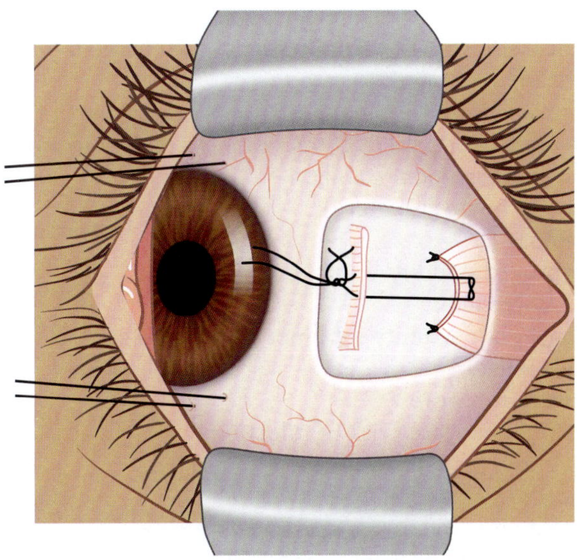

FIGURE 48.4. Semiadjustable suture technique.
The two poles are secured to the sclera closer together than the muscle width to allow central sag of the muscle. An additional suture is passed through the center of the muscle and attached to the insertion with an adjustable suture (slip knot or sliding noose) to allow a limited adjustment of the muscle.

- Modified semiadjustable:
  - Using a double-armed or two single-armed sutures, imbricate each corner of the muscle or the entire muscle width. Reinsert the muscle on the sclera at the original insertion with two scleral bites. One of the sutures is again passed to capture the central muscle fibers and reinserted on central portion of the muscle insertion.
  - Advantages:
    - Three fixation scleral points for the muscle.
    - Less central sagging.
    - Controlled adjustment of the central muscle fibers or one-half of the muscle if a slanted muscle procedure is desired for vertical, horizontal, or torsional correction.

ADJUSTMENT TIMING

Allow several minutes of binocular vision prior to assessment regardless of when adjustment is performed.

- Intraoperative.
  - Advantages:
    - Can easily do more surgery if needed.
    - Less theoretical risk of infection because no suture exposure.
    - Finish adjustment before patient is transferred to recovery.
  - Disadvantages:
    - Blurred vision.
    - Can not correct patient refractive error while in the operating room.
    - Limited evaluation in different gaze position.
    - Requires special surgical bed that allows the patient to sit up.
    - Lack of alignment stability.
- Immediate (1-6 hours postoperative).
  - Advantages:
    - Same day as surgery.
    - Possible decreased risk of infection.
    - Can do in recovery room with nursing support and IV drugs in case of vagal response.
    - Finish adjustment before patient is discharged.
  - Disadvantages:
    - Blurred vision (pupillary dilation, corneal dryness, bloody tears).
    - Possibly poor patient cooperation secondary to anesthesia effect.
    - Lack of alignment stability.
- Delayed (24 hours and more).
  - Advantage:
    - Improved stability.
    - Less blurriness.
    - Longer opportunity for binocular vision (several hours-days).
  - Disadvantages:
    - Suture exposure.
    - Possible increased risk of infection.
    - Potential for vagal response in office.
    - Bleeding.
    - Irritation.
    - May be more difficult to move the muscle.

POSTOPERATIVE MANAGEMENT

- Consider use of antibiotic and/or steroid postoperatively.
- Use of ointment in the immediate postoperative period may make the adjustment more difficult due to vision blurriness and suture slippage.
- Place and cover the tails of the adjustable sutures under the conjunctiva to decrease inflammation, irritation, and prevent suture bacterial colonization.

POTENTIAL COMPLICATIONS

- Suture exposure.
- Infection.
- Granuloma.
- Persistent redness.
- Conjunctival scarring.
- Muscle slippage.
- Creeping forward of the muscle after large recessions.

To prevent the muscle from creeping forward, an alternative technique includes a semi-hang back technique where two scleral fixation points are placed posterior to the muscle insertion and anterior to the desired final muscle position. This can help to prevent the muscle from creeping forward, but it limits the amount of advancement during the adjustment.

References

1. Siegel L, Lozano MJ, Santiago AP, Rosenbaum AL. Adjustable and nonadjustable recession and resection techniques. In: Rosenbaum AL, Santiago AP, eds. *Clinical Strabismus Management Principles and Surgical Techniques*. 1st ed. Philadelphia, PA: W.B. Saunders; 1999: 435-448.
2. Metz HS, Lerner H. The adjustable Harada-Ito procedure. *Arch Ophthalmol*. 1981;99:624.
3. Velez FG, Demer JL, Pihlblad MS, Pineles SL. Rectus muscle plication using an adjustable suture technique. *J AAPOS*. 2013;17(5):480-483.
4. Chang MY, Pineles SL, Velez FG. Adjustable small-incision elective tenotomy and plication for correction of incomitant vertical strabismus and torsion. *J AAPOS*. 2015;19(5):410-416.
5. Kushner BJ. An evaluation of the semi adjustable suture strabismus surgical procedure. *J AAPOS*. 2004;8(5):481-487. Erratum in: *J AAPOS*. 2005;9(2):204.
6. Nihalani BR, Whitman MC, Salgado CM, et al. Short tag noose technique for optional and late suture adjustment in strabismus surgery. *Arch Ophthalmol*. 2009;127(12):1584-1590.

CHAPTER 49

Posterior Fixation Sutures

Charles J. Bock Jr, MD

PREOPERATIVE CONSIDERATIONS

In strabismus where a strengthening procedure is contraindicated or not possible, weakening of the contralateral yoke muscle may be considered. Posterior fixation employs four mechanisms of action: (1) limiting maximal ocular rotation of the operated muscle, (2) decreasing total strength of the operated muscle by effectively shortening the muscle, (3) increasing innervation to the weak (paired yoke) muscle by Herring's Law of Equal Innervation, and similarly, (4) increasing relaxation of the contralateral antagonist via Sherrington's Law of Reciprocal Innervation.

Greater surgical effect is generally possible on the medial and inferior rectus muscles due to the shorter arc of contact of these muscles with the globe compared to the lateral rectus muscle; therefore, it is easier to achieve more weakening effect on the medial and inferior rectus muscles without being as far posterior. Care must be taken when considering surgery on the superior rectus muscle due to the presence of the superior oblique tendon in the field of operation.

- Indications for posterior fixation in incomitant strabismus:
  - Paretic:
    - Sixth nerve palsy.
    - Internuclear ophthalmoplegia.
  - Restrictive:
    - Orbital fracture or other trauma.
    - Prior surgery with orbital hardware: scleral buckle, glaucoma implant.
  - Potentially combined etiology:
    - Duane syndrome.
    - Monocular elevation deficiency.
  - Esotropia:
    - High AC/A resistant to weaning bifocal.
    - Convergence excess.
  - Other potential indications:
    - Dissociated vertical deviation.
    - Nystagmus with head position.

SURGICAL PROCEDURE

Adequate exposure is critical. The fixation suture is generally placed 15-20 mm posterior to the limbus. Suture selection is important.

While 6-0 Mersilene on an S-28 needle (Ethicon) or 5-0 Mersilene on an S-14 needle (Ethicon) can be used, a shorter spatulated needle is preferred, due to exposure concerns. The 5-0 polyester suture on an R-5 needle (Alcon) is excellent for this, though the suture material often drags Tenon tissue. Another choice is the CV-8 Gore-Tex, TTc-9 needle (Gore Medical); this needle is tapered, rather than spatulated, but short and easily maneuvered.

Posterior Fixation without Recession

With the muscle on the muscle hook, the sutures are placed on an equal distance posterior to the limbus. Retract orbital tissue with a Desmarres or Fison retractor, using a neurosurgical sponge if necessary. Use a small hook to gently lift the edge of the muscle so that the suture pass through the sclera is at the muscle edge. Incorporate 1/4-1/3 of the muscle in the pass. Repeat on the opposite side, and tie both sutures securely (Figs. 49.1 and 49.2).

Posterior Fixation with Recession

Once the muscle has been disinserted from the globe, retract it gently with orbital tissue. Here, there are two options: (1) place two sutures through the sclera at locations corresponding to the edges of the muscle as above, reattach the muscle, then pass the needles through the edge of the muscle (Figs. 49.3 and 49.4), or (2) pass a single double-armed suture through the sclera at a position corresponding to the center of the muscle, reattach the muscle, and then bring each needle up through the muscle and tie on top and in the center of the muscle (Figs. 49.5 and 49.6).

Adjustable Fadenoperation (Figs. 49.7 and 49.8)

So named because it achieves the posterior fixation effect without permanent posterior fixation sutures (ie, adjustment is possible); this procedure is technically combined resection and recession of a single rectus muscle. Resect a portion of the rectus muscle, then recess it an equal or greater amount; posterior fixation effect alone is

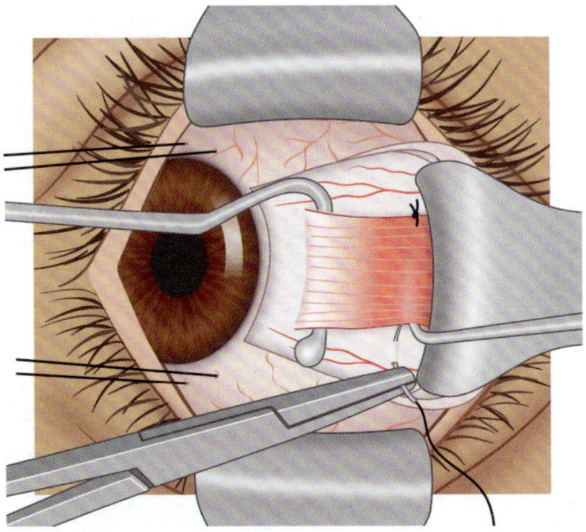

FIGURE 49.1. Fadenoperation without recession, showing placement of posterior fixation suture.

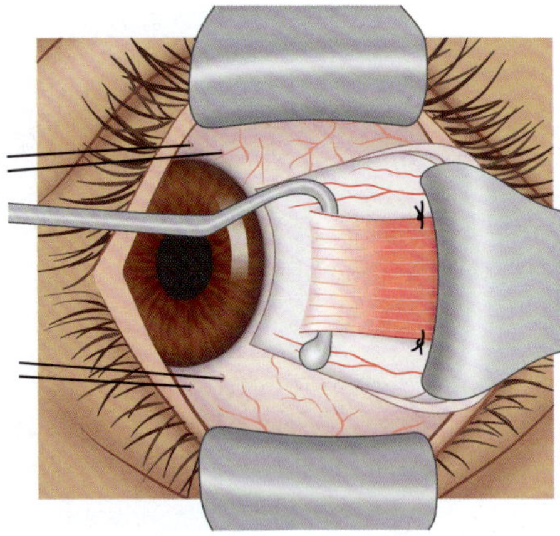

FIGURE 49.2. Completed Fadenoperation without recession, with symmetric placement of both posterior fixation sutures.

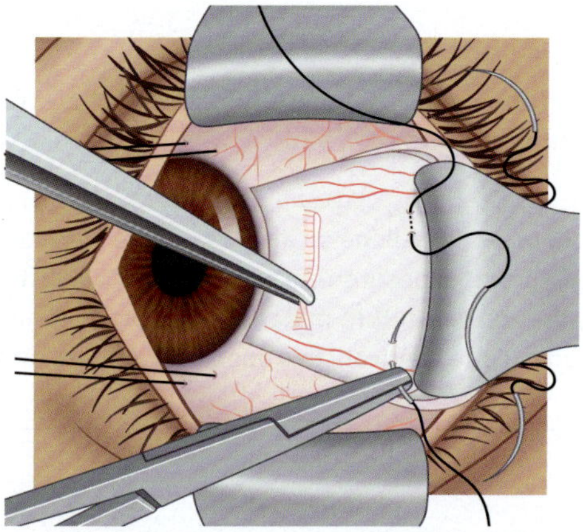

FIGURE 49.3. Fadenoperation with recession, showing placement of two posterior fixation sutures.

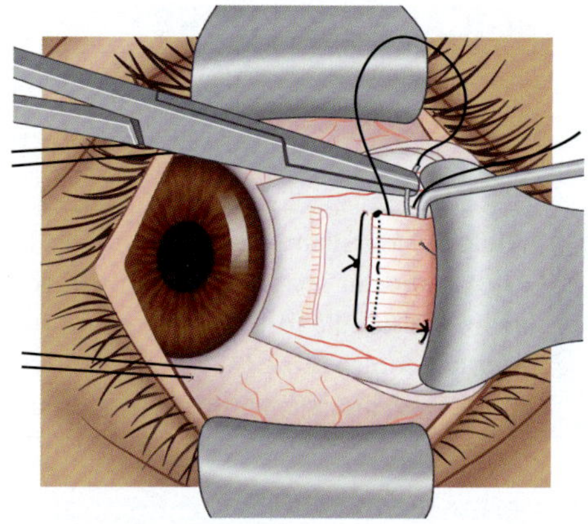

FIGURE 49.4. Completion of Fadenoperation with recession; sutures must be placed symmetrically.

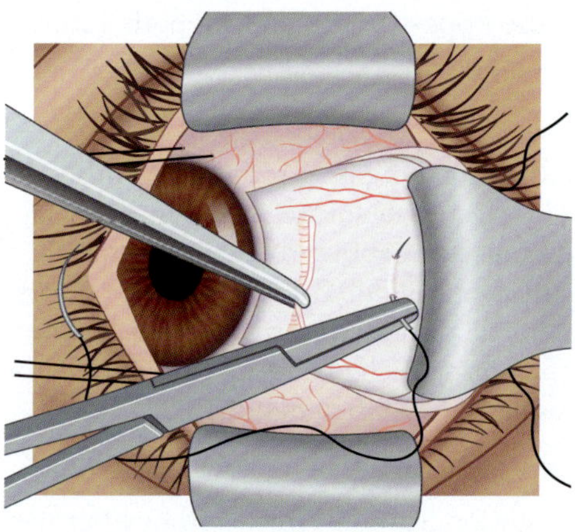

FIGURE 49.5. Fadenoperation with recession, showing placement of one, central posterior fixation suture.

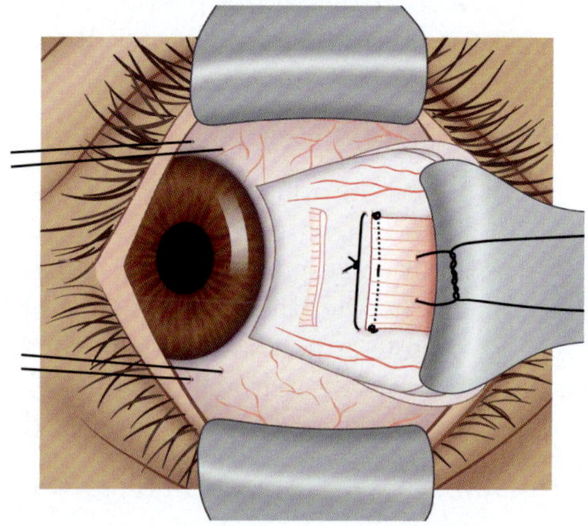

FIGURE 49.6. Completion of Fadenoperation with recession and a single posterior fixation suture; the posterior fixation suture may be brought through the muscle either before or after reattaching the muscle to the globe.

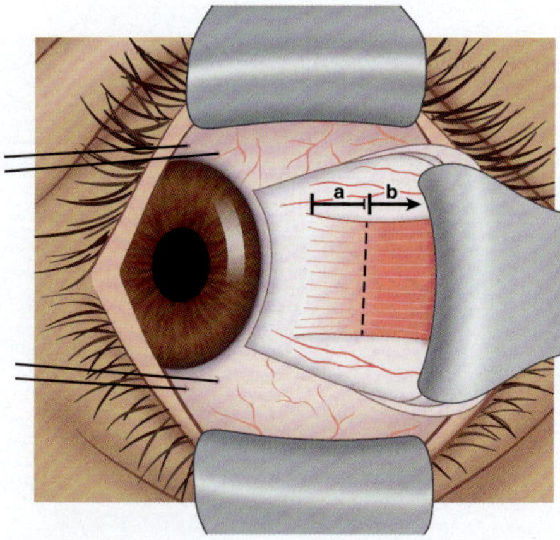

FIGURE 49.7. Adjustable Fadenoperation, where (*a*) represents the amount of intended resection. The suture is placed at this site, and the muscle is recessed (*b*).

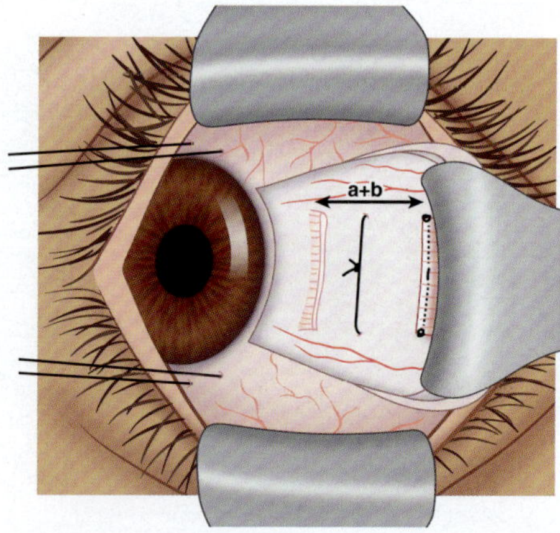

FIGURE 49.8. Finished adjustable Fadenoperation, where $a + b$ represents the total distance (*a*, resected amount, and *b*, amount of additional recession) that the new muscle insertion is placed from the original insertion.

achieved for a recession equal to the amount of resection. Additional recession of the cut muscle end adds a recession effect. The muscle can then be sutured directly to the globe or placed on an adjustable suture. Only small case series exist for this procedure, so consult the suggested readings for additional information and guidance. In general, a resection of 40%-60% of the planned recession (eg, 3- to 4-mm resection with a 7-mm recession) can collapse incomitance and provide the needed recession effect. Resection and recession amounts are often smaller than one might expect; the lateral rectus often requires a larger surgical dose, due to its longer arc of contact with the globe.

Augmented Transposition

Posterior fixation sutures can also be used to increase the effect of transposition procedures (see Chapter 50), as in the Foster modification of full tendon transposition for esotropic ("Type I") Duane syndrome or sixth nerve palsy. Here, the edges of the transposed superior and inferior rectus muscles are sutured through sclera (and in subsequent refinements through the corresponding edge of the lateral rectus muscle) to bring the vertical muscle to the edge of the lateral rectus muscle ~16 mm posterior to the limbus to increase the surgical dose.

POSTOPERATIVE CONSIDERATIONS

- Induced tropias can result if the sutures are not symmetrically placed or if one of the sutures loosens.
- Overcorrection is more likely in some situations, such as when posterior fixation is used to augment a transposition (Foster modification of full tendon transposition). This is especially true in Duane syndrome, since the ipsilateral medial rectus muscle is weak.
- Reoperation is difficult in many cases. By 6 weeks postoperatively, many patients will have complete fibrosis of the muscle anterior to the posterior fixation suture(s). Early reoperation should be considered if there are signs of overcorrection. If the muscle is fibrosed, it is not active; the functional insertion is the site of the posterior fixation suture, and the muscle may need to be resected at this point to avoid additional complications, such as intraoperative pulled-in-two syndrome or postoperative muscle slippage or loss.

Suggested Readings

Bock CJ Jr, Buckley EG, Freedman SF. Combined resection and recession of a single rectus muscle for treatment of incomitant strabismus. *J AAPOS*. 1999;3(5):263-268.

Buckley EG. Posterior fixation suture (Fadenoperation). In: Buckley EG, Shields MB, Freedman SF, eds. *Atlas of Ophthalmic Surgery: Volume III Strabismus and Glaucoma*. St. Louis, MO: Mosby; 1995:126-137.

Buckley EG. Fadenoperation (posterior fixation suture). In: Rosenbaum AL, Santiago AP, eds. *Clinical Strabismus Management, Principles and Surgical Techniques*. Philadelphia, PA: WB Saunders Co.; 1999:491-505.

Foster RS. Vertical muscle transposition augmented with lateral fixation. *J AAPOS*. 1997;1(1):20-30.

Roper-Hall G, Cruz OA. Results of combined resection-recession on a single rectus muscle for incomitant deviation—an alternative to the posterior fixation suture. *J AAPOS*. 2017;21(2):89-93.

Scott AB. Posterior fixation: adjustable and without posterior fixation sutures. In: Lennerstrand G, ed. *Update on Strabismus and Pediatric Ophthalmology, Proceedings of the Joint Congress, Vancouver, Canada*. Boca Raton, FL: CRC Press; 1994:399-402.

CHAPTER 50

Paralytic Strabismus

Jared E. Duncan, MD

PREOPERATIVE CONSIDERATIONS

Paralytic strabismus refers to a group of eye muscle impairments that results from innervation interruption to the third, fourth, and/or sixth cranial nerves. Common causes include motor nerve palsies and disorders of the neuromuscular junction (eg, ocular myasthenia gravis [MG]). Important preoperative considerations include determination of the goals of surgery and the appropriate workup of acute insults to the cranial nerves. Elucidation of these factors is facilitated by a thorough preoperative examination that focuses on more than just motility patterns.

Important Historical Elements to Consider

- Visual symptoms: Is the patient diplopic? Is the diplopia monocular or binocular? Is it horizontal, vertical, or torsional?
- Timing: Are the patient's symptoms acute? Are they fatigable? Worse at end of the day?
- Other symptoms: Does the patient have associated symptoms like headaches, scalp pain/tenderness, nausea/vomiting, or other motor/sensory deficits?

Eye Examination Pearls in the Patient With Paralytic Strabismus

- Look carefully for pupillary changes (afferent pupillary defect, anisocoria), deficits in confrontational visual fields (indicative of possible postchiasmal pathology), and eyelid ptosis. The presence of one or more of these will usually necessitate the need for further workup.
- Perform a thorough yet focused sensorimotor examination.
  - Diagnosis will usually require cover testing in primary gaze, horizontal gazes, vertical gazes, and head tilts. Another measurement in primary gaze with near fixation is also helpful. Surgical planning may require the use of cover testing in all nine positions of gaze and head tilts. The presence of *incomitance* is highly suggestive of muscle paresis or restriction.
  - Carefully evaluate versions and ductions

- Look carefully at force generations (see Chapter 42): indicates residual function of paralytic muscle and guides surgical planning. Force generations can be graded on a scale of mild (>50% function), moderate (25%-50% function), or severe (<25% function to none at all).[1]

Role of Imaging and Neurologic Workup in Patients With Paralytic Strabismus (See Chapter 57)

- The most important factors for determining the need for workup in a patient with paralytic strabismus are timing (acute vs. chronic), age, associated symptoms, and to a lesser extent, past medical history (particularly, a history of cancer).
- When indicated workup should include neuroimaging, with MRI being the preferred modality. Referral to an internist or pediatrician is also imperative, as many patients will have cardiovascular or neurologic risk factors. Blood work for MG may also be indicated.
    - Maintain a high index of suspicion for giant cell arteritis (GCA) in adult patients ≥50 years of age. Erythrocyte sedimentation rate (ESR), C-reactive protein (CRP), and a platelet count are imperative in patients who present with symptoms of GCA.

Features of GCA include: (1) abrupt onset headache, (2) scalp tenderness, (3) jaw and tongue claudication, (4) visual symptoms, (5) constitutional symptoms, (6) polymyalgia symptoms, and (7) limb claudication.

-
    - Blood testing for MG (antiacetylcholine receptor antibody test) is frequently falsely negative. If index of suspicion is high, single-fiber EMG remains the gold standard for diagnosis. A trial of pyridostigmine or oral steroids may also be diagnostic.
    - MG can mimic any form of paralytic strabismus. If in doubt, repeat examination on a different day and/or time may be helpful. Fluctuation in motility measurements may be observed.

Improvement and/or resolution of ptosis and/or diplopia after applying an ice pack to the eyelid for 2 minutes or after a rest period of 15-20 minutes supports a diagnosis of MG.

- Most clinicians prefer to conduct a workup in all patients who present with nontraumatic, acute onset third, fourth, and sixth nerve palsies.[2]
    - A lower threshold for imaging patients includes age <60, presence of associated ocular signs/symptoms (optic disc edema, ptosis, pupillary changes, visual field deficits), and presence of systemic signs/symptoms (headache, weakness, focal neurologic deficits including presence of multiple cranial nerve palsies).

Timing of Surgical Intervention in Patients With Paralytic Strabismus

- Surgery must be delayed in patients who present acutely or who have an unstable medical condition that prevents elective surgery.
- Although opinions vary, it is common to wait a minimum of 6 months before offering surgery in cases of acute-onset paralytic strabismus. In general, patients with vascular or idiopathic etiologies tend to recover more quickly and more frequently than those with traumatic etiologies of acute palsy. Pediatric patients may require earlier intervention to prevent the development of amblyopia in the nonfixating eye. Ensure appropriate penalization (eg, patching) in pediatric cases where surgical management is delayed.

- Interim elimination of diplopia can be achieved with the use of occlusion or temporary (eg, Fresnel) prism (see Chapter 56).
- Consider botulinum toxin injection to the antagonist prior to surgery (see Chapter 55).

In acute sixth nerve palsies secondary to head trauma, botulinum toxin may give temporary relief of diplopia and reduce muscle contractures of the antagonist. It can be particularly helpful in sixth nerve palsies that are severe, bilateral, and/or in children. One disadvantage of botulinum toxin injection is that it may diffuse and cause a vertical deviation that can take longer to resolve than the initial nerve palsy.

Determine Realistic Preoperative Goals for Surgical Repair of Paralytic Strabismus

- The goal of treatment is to produce the largest field of binocular vision possible. Restoration of full muscle function is not typically possible. This goal should be discussed in detail with the patient prior to surgical intervention.

OPERATIVE CONSIDERATIONS

Surgical Planning

- Strengthening the paralytic muscle should only be performed on muscles with mild to moderate function on forced-generation testing.
  - Resect, plicate, or "tuck" the paretic muscle.
  - Strengthening the paralytic muscle often needs to be paired with a weakening procedure of the antagonist muscle.
- Whenever possible look to create a matching deficit in the uninvolved eye.
  - Often helps to satisfy the goal of achieving largest field of binocular vision.
  - Accomplished by weakening yoke muscle of the paretic muscle in uninvolved eye.
  - Example: In a left sixth nerve palsy, weaken the medial rectus muscle of the right eye.
- Long-standing cases of paralytic strabismus may result in contracture of the paralytic muscle's antagonist. Therefore, there may be an additional restrictive component to the strabismus.
  - Perform intraoperative forced ductions to identify restriction (see Chapter 42).

Types of Surgical Procedures to Employ (Where Applicable See Separate Chapters)

- Weakening procedures (recessions, myotomies, myectomies, etc.).
- Strengthening procedures (resections, plications, advancements, tucks, etc.).
- Procedures to address torsion (Harada-Ito).
- Procedures to limit ocular rotation (posterior fixation suture).
- Augmentation procedures (transpositions):
  - Used when ocular rotation in one direction is severely limited, such as in a complete sixth nerve palsy. There are many options to consider.[3]

Full-Tendon Transposition: Entire Rectus Muscle Transposed to a Position Adjacent to Paralytic Muscle

- *Perform conjunctival incision for 270 degrees or 2 fornix incisions*. This allows for exposure of the two adjacent rectus muscles on either side of the paralytic muscle. Example: if performing full-tendon transposition for lateral rectus muscle paresis, you would expose the superior and inferior rectus.
- *Isolate, secure, and remove the muscle to be transposed in the typical manner and suture as for a standard recession procedure (see Chapter 44).*

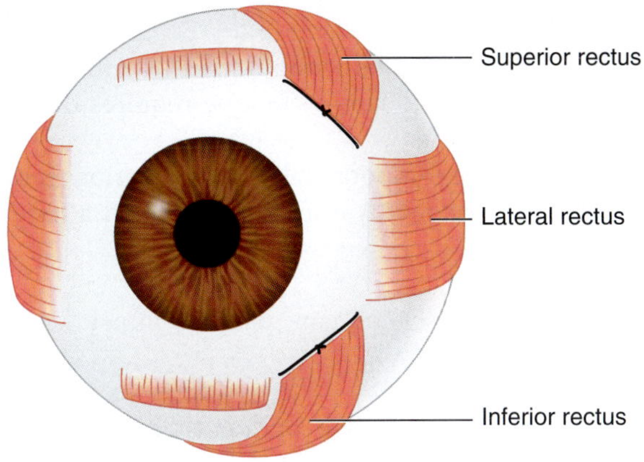

FIGURE 50.1. Example of full-tendon transposition for a complete sixth nerve palsy. The transposed superior rectus and inferior rectus are oriented such that their new insertions are parallel to the corneal limbus. IR, inferior rectus; SR, superior rectus; LR, lateral rectus.

- *Reattach muscles adjacent to paretic muscle using standard scleral passes*. Muscles can be attached with insertions parallel to the limbus (Fig. 50.1) or parallel to the border of the paretic muscle (Fig. 50.2).
- *Close conjunctival incision with interrupted 8-0 absorbable sutures.*
- *Full-tendon transpositions can be augmented using one of several techniques:*
  - Augmentation sutures at the border of transposed muscles to the paretic muscle and/or to the sclera using nonabsorbable suture (see Chapter 49). The author prefers to suture the belly of the transposed muscle directly to the belly of the paralyzed muscle, ~8 mm posterior to the muscle's insertion (Fig. 50.3). Care should be taken to place these sutures evenly to avoid inducing new strabismus (eg, inducing vertical strabismus in a sixth nerve palsy).
  - Injection of botulinum toxin into antagonist muscle (see Chapter 55).
- *Advantages of traditional full-tendon transposition*: predictable, uses familiar techniques, easily reversible.

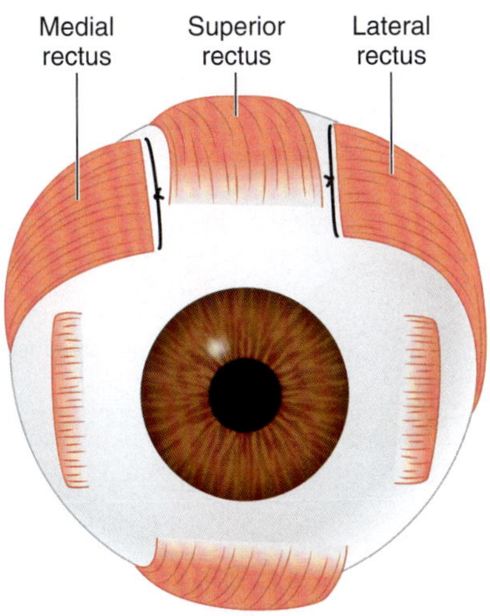

FIGURE 50.2. Example of full-tendon transposition for a patient with double elevator palsy. The transposed lateral rectus and medial rectus are oriented such that their new insertions are parallel to the borders of the superior rectus. MR, medial rectus; LR, lateral rectus; SR, superior rectus.

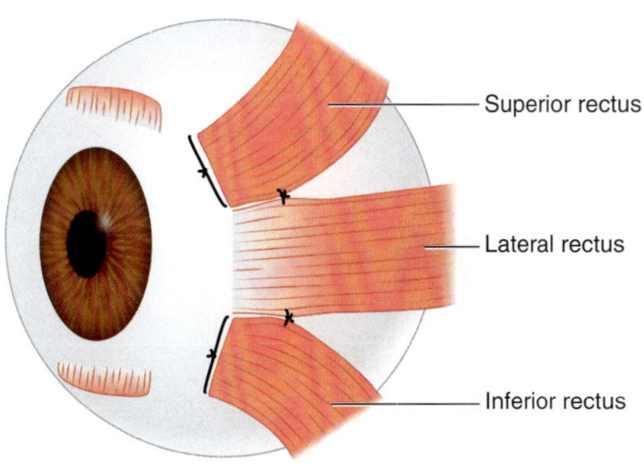

FIGURE 50.3. Example of full-tendon transposition augmented by a nonabsorbable permanent suture. The suture is placed ~8 mm posterior to the paralytic muscle's insertion. The suture is passed directly through each muscle's belly. IR, inferior rectus; SR, superior rectus; LR, lateral rectus.

Alternatives to Full-Tendon Transposition

- *Hummelsheim Procedure:* One half of each functioning rectus muscle is sutured adjacent to the insertion of paretic muscle. This technique requires disinsertion of one half of each functioning rectus muscle.
  - Example: In lateral rectus paresis, the temporal half of the superior rectus muscle and the temporal half of the inferior rectus muscle are sutured adjacent to the lateral rectus muscle (Fig. 50.4).
  - Advantages:
    - Original function of transposed muscle remains partially intact.
    - Preserves anterior ciliary arteries.
  - Disadvantages:
    - May not provide the same amount of ocular rotation that a full-tendon transposition otherwise would.
    - Reoperations are also difficult.
- *Jensen Procedure:* A strip of each functioning rectus muscle is sutured to a strip of the paretic muscle.
  - Example: In lateral rectus paresis, the temporal strip of the superior rectus muscle and the temporal strip of the inferior rectus muscle are sutured directly to the belly of the lateral rectus muscle. A nonabsorbable suture (eg, Dacron) is typically used. Unlike the Hummelsheim procedure, this technique does not require disinsertion of any rectus muscles (Fig. 50.5).
  - Advantages:
    - Original function of transposed muscle remains partially intact.
    - Preserves anterior ciliary arteries.
  - Disadvantages:
    - May not provide the same amount of ocular rotation that a full-tendon transposition otherwise would.
    - Reoperations are difficult.
- *Nishida procedure*[4]: A nonabsorbable (6-0 polypropylene monofilament or 5-0 polyester) suture is secured through the temporal 1/3 of each vertical rectus muscle 8-10 mm posterior to the muscle insertion, taking care to avoid large vessels to reduce the risk of anterior segment ischemia. These sutures are secured to the sclera

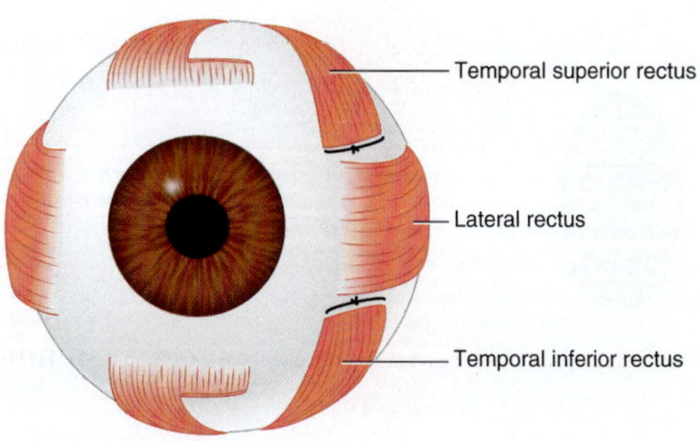

FIGURE 50.4. Illustration of the eye after Hummelsheim procedure for a complete sixth nerve palsy. TIR, temporal inferior rectus; TSR, temporal superior rectus; LR, lateral rectus.

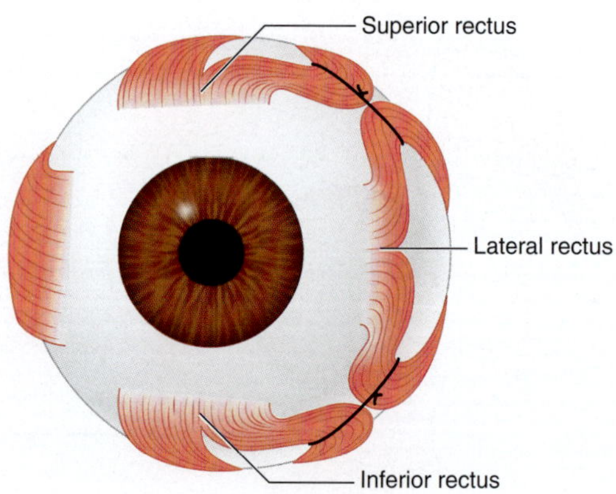

FIGURE 50.5. Illustration of the eye after Jensen procedure for a complete sixth nerve palsy. IR, inferior rectus; SR, superior rectus; LR, lateral rectus.

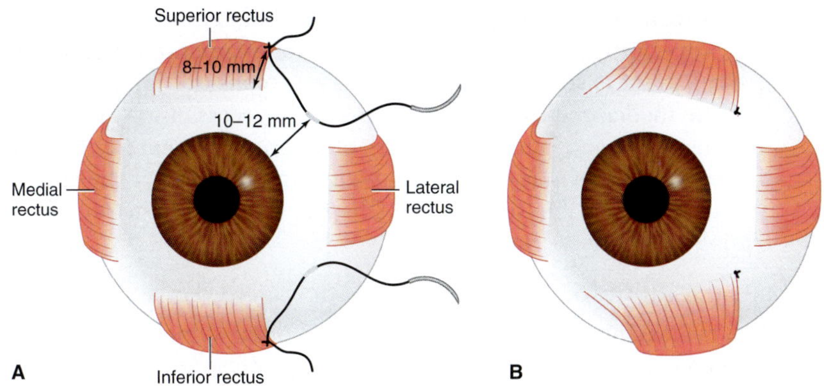

FIGURE 50.6. Illustration of Nishida procedure for sixth nerve palsy. IR, inferior rectus; SR, superior rectus; LR, lateral rectus.

in the superotemporal and inferotemporal quadrants, 10-12 mm posterior to the limbus and 4-5 mm from the edge of the lateral rectus. Care should be taken to keep these bites symmetric to avoid vertical deviations and/or torsion (Fig. 50.6).

> **It is possible to do these sutures as adjustable sutures. It is also possible to place an additional suture posterior to the first to achieve more effect.**

- Advantages:
  - Original function of transposed muscle remains partially intact.
  - Preserves anterior ciliary arteries.
  - Powerful procedure.

Surgical Considerations in the Impairment Management of Sixth Nerve Palsy

- Assign ocular rotation into three general classes: mild, moderate, and severe.
  - *Mild* usually indicates relatively good function of involved lateral rectus and minimal ipsilateral medial rectus contracture.
    - Options including recessing ipsilateral medial rectus (eg, antagonist) or contralateral medial rectus (eg, yoke). This may be combined with a resection of the involved lateral rectus muscle if the amount of eye misalignment is large.
    - Decision to operate on antagonist or yoke medial rectus is determined by adherence to the goal of providing the patient with the largest field of binocular vision. In other words, operate so as to avoid creating an exotropia on contralateral gaze.
  - *Moderate* usually indicates some function of involved lateral rectus with or without ipsilateral medial rectus contracture.
    - Will unequivocally require a combination surgery.
    - Strengthen the involved lateral rectus muscle and combine with medial rectus recession as for the *mild* category described above. Important caveat: if significant ipsilateral medial rectus contracture on forced ductions, the patient will require weakening of ipsilateral medial rectus.
    - An exotropia in side gaze may be unavoidable. If this occurs, a weakening procedure of the contralateral lateral rectus may be needed.
  - *Severe* usually indicates no function of involved lateral rectus with or without ipsilateral medial rectus contracture.
    - Will require muscle transposition surgery combined with ipsilateral and/or contralateral medial rectus recession.

- A common approach is to perform an isolated full-tendon transposition of the superior rectus muscle with a posterior augmentation ("Foster") suture.[5]
- If the patient is still esotropic after surgery, consider injection of botulinum toxin into the medial rectus muscle. Alternatively, recession of the medial rectus muscle may be performed, but there is a risk of anterior segment ischemia (see Chapter 54) if there was a previous full-tendon width transposition of the verticals.
- The use of adjustable sutures (see Chapter 48) may be helpful when surgically correcting a sixth nerve palsy.

Surgical Considerations for the Management of Fourth Nerve Palsy

- The management of fourth nerve palsy is often subjective and varies according to surgeon preference. The choice of procedure often depends on surgeon comfort, but a few key principles can be applied.
  - Determine if chronic or acute. If chronic, look carefully for muscle contracture and spread of comitance.
  - The presence of moderate-severe excyclotorsion (>10 degrees) may require a separate procedure to address torsion (eg, Harado-Ito). Keep in mind that higher degrees of torsion may indicate bilateral fourth nerve palsy. This may be inadvertently unmasked if only performing surgery for a unilateral palsy.
  - Check versions carefully for ipsilateral oblique overaction, ipsilateral superior oblique underaction, and contralateral superior oblique overaction.
  - Intraoperatively check forced ductions for superior oblique laxity (see Chapter 42).
  - Avoid overcorrections. Undercorrections are usually tolerable, especially in patients with large fusional amplitudes. A staged approach for superior oblique palsy helps to avoid overcorrections, which are usually intolerable for the patient.
- Measure the patient's eye misalignment in primary position.
  - If <15Δ, one muscle surgery will probably work.
    - Inferior oblique overaction: Weaken inferior oblique (myectomy or recession).
    - Significant superior oblique laxity on forced ductions: Consider superior oblique tuck.
    - Superior rectus tightness on forced ductions: weaken ipsilateral superior rectus.
  - If >15Δ, two muscle surgery may be needed.
    - Use above principles, but also consider contralateral inferior rectus recession.
    - If proceeding with two muscle surgery, placing one on an adjustable surgery is recommended to avoid overcorrection.
- If significant torsion (>10 degrees) is present, consider Harada-Ito procedure.
- Management of bilateral superior oblique palsy:
  - If no deviation in primary and significant excyclotorsion, consider bilateral Harada-Ito procedures.
  - Alternatives include pairing bilateral superior oblique tucks with inferior rectus recessions and/or medial rectus recessions, bilateral inferior rectus recessions, and bilateral inferior oblique weakening.

Surgical Considerations for the Management of Third Nerve Palsy

- Partial (incomplete) third nerve palsy: Deficit will dictate the appropriate choice of procedure. This will vary according to which muscle(s) are paretic, in addition to the remaining function of that muscle.
- Complete third nerve palsy (see Chapter 59):
  - Involved eye will be exotropic and slightly hypotropic.
  - Surgical goal is to realign the eye in primary position. This can be accomplished in several ways.

- Large recession of functioning lateral rectus muscle. Options include suturing the muscle extremely posterior to the insertion, complete disinsertion of the lateral rectus muscle, or suturing of the lateral rectus muscle to the periosteum of the orbital wall.[6]
- Resect paretic medial rectus muscle. This must be combined with lateral rectus weakening as described above.
- If the patient has significant incyclotorsion from a functioning superior oblique muscle, the above procedures may be combined with a superior oblique tenotomy.
- Nasal transposition of split lateral rectus muscle on adjustable suture.[7]

- Concurrent eyelid ptosis as a result of a total third nerve palsy should be addressed after eye muscle surgery.

POSTOPERATIVE CONSIDERATIONS

- Postoperative antibiotics and anti-inflammatories should be used according to the discretion of the treating surgeon.
- Diplopia and other postoperative sensorimotor concerns may be treated with the use of occlusion, prisms, or orthoptic exercises (see Chapter 56).
- Ensure appropriate continuity of care for patients whose deficits were caused by medical, cardiac, and neurologic insults.

References

1. Buckley EG. Paralytic strabismus. In: Plager DA, ed. *Strabismus Surgery: Basic and Advanced Strategies*. 1st ed. New York, NY: Oxford University Press; 2004:83-116.
2. Tamhankar MA, Biousse V, Ying GS, et al. Isolated third, fourth, and sixth cranial nerve palsies from presumed microvascular versus other causes: a prospective study. *Ophthalmology*. 2013;120(11):2264-2269.
3. Gunton KB. Vertical rectus transpositions in sixth nerve palsies. *Curr Opin Ophthalmol*. 2015;26(5):366-370.
4. Nishida Y, Hayashi O, Oda S, et al. A simple muscle transposition procedure for abducens palsy without tenotomy or splitting muscles. *Jpn J Ophthalmol*. 2005;49:179-180.
5. Foster RS. Vertical muscle transposition augmented with lateral fixation. *J AAPOS*. 1997;1(1):20-30.
6. Morad Y, Kowal L, Scott AB. Lateral rectus muscle disinsertion and reattachment to the lateral orbital wall. *Br J Ophthalmol*. 2005;89:983-985.
7. Shah AS, Prabhu SP, Sadiq MA, et al. Adjustable nasal transposition of split lateral rectus muscle for third nerve palsy. *JAMA Ophthalmol*. 2014;132(8):963-969.

CHAPTER 51

Pattern Strabismus

Michelle S. Go, MD • Laura B. Enyedi, MD

PREOPERATIVE CONSIDERATIONS

Clinical evaluation should include measurement of deviation in multiple positions of gaze with particular attention to the difference in deviation between primary gaze, downgaze (35 degrees chin elevation), and upgaze (25 degrees chin depression). Look for abnormal head position, overelevation or overdepression in adduction, and vertical deviations on lateral gazes. Assessment of fundus torsion can be performed by ophthalmoscopy or fundus photography (Fig. 51.1). Atypical location of muscle insertions may be seen by slit lamp examination or on MRI.

Anomalous head positions often indicate binocularity in that head position. Anomalous head positions can sometimes interfere with motor development in an infant and can cause neck muscular changes and/or neck pain in older children or adults.

Torsion may be a more reliable indicator of oblique overaction than versions.[1] The normal fovea lines up with the lower 1/3 of the disc (upper 1/3 in the indirect view). The fovea will be lower (higher in the indirect view) with extorsion and higher (lower in the indirect view) with intorsion (Fig. 51.1).

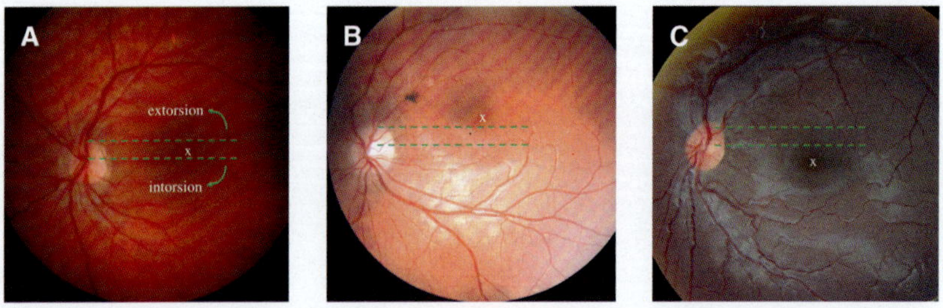

FIGURE 51.1. **A. Indirect view** of normal right fundus showing normal position of the fovea (white x) relative to the optic disc (within green dashed lines) and the location of the fovea with increasing amounts of intorsion or extorsion. **B. Indirect view** of right fundus with extorsion. **C. Indirect view** of right fundus with intorsion.

- Pattern Strabismus Etiologies[1]:
  - Oblique muscle dysfunction.
  - Anomalous orbits.
  - Heterotopy of muscle pulleys.
  - Neural mechanisms.

Types of Patterns[1,2]:

- V-pattern:
  - Difference >15 prism diopters between upgaze and downgaze.
  - May be associated with inferior oblique overaction.
    - Examination findings:
      - Overelevation in adduction.
      - Left hypertropia on right gaze and right hypertropia on left gaze.
      - Fundus extorsion (Fig. 51.1B).
  - Abnormal head positions may be seen:
    - Chin up for V-pattern exotropia.
    - Chin down for V-pattern esotropia.
  - Associations include infantile esotropia, craniofacial anomalies, bilateral superior oblique palsy, Duane retraction syndrome, and Brown syndrome.
- Y-pattern (subtype of V-pattern):
  - Divergence measures greater in upgaze, and there is a minimal change in deviation between primary and downgaze.
  - Examination may reveal bilateral inferior oblique overaction or pseudo-inferior oblique overaction (see sidebar).
  - Associations include Duane retraction syndrome and Brown syndrome.

Pseudo-inferior oblique overaction may present as V- or Y-pattern strabismus. It is thought to result from superior rectus and lateral rectus pulley instability vs cocontraction of the lateral rectus muscles as the eyes elevate in adduction. In pseudo-inferior oblique overaction, there is no hypertropia on direct side gaze, no difference in deviation with right vs left head tilt, and no torsion. Lateral rectus recession with superior transposition (or superior and lateral rectus transposition against the direction of instability) can be effective in normalizing the pattern.[3-5] Inferior oblique weakening procedures are generally not successful.

- Arrow pattern (subtype of V-pattern):
  - Greatest convergence occurs between primary gaze and downgaze (eg, ortho in upgaze, esotropia 5 prism diopters in primary position, and esotropia 20 prism diopters in downgaze).
  - May be associated with bilateral superior oblique palsy, especially when there is also extorsion on downgaze.
- A-pattern:
  - Difference >10 prism diopters between upgaze and downgaze.
  - May be associated with superior oblique overaction.
    - Examination findings:
      - Overdepression in adduction.
      - Right hypertropia on right gaze and left hypertropia on left gaze.
      - Fundus intorsion (Fig. 51.1C).
  - Abnormal head positions may be seen:
    - Chin up for A-pattern esotropia.
    - Chin down for A-pattern exotropia.
  - Associations include bilateral Duane retraction syndrome, craniofacial anomalies, trisomy 21, and spinal column defects.

- λ-Pattern (subtype of A-pattern):
  - Divergence measures greater in downgaze, and there is a minimal change in deviation between primary and upgaze.
  - Examination reveals overdepression on adduction.
  - May be associated with bilateral superior oblique overaction or inferior rectus underaction.
- X-pattern:
  - Divergence increased in upgaze and downgaze compared to primary position.
  - Examination shows overelevation and overdepression on adduction.
  - Associated with longstanding exotropia and Duane retraction syndrome.
  - Possibly due to tight lateral rectus causing a leash effect or overaction of all four oblique muscles.
- Surgery (Table 51.1)[1,6,7]:
  - Inferior oblique weakening for V-pattern deviation with inferior oblique overaction (see Chapter 46):
    - Myectomy.
    - Recession.
    - Anterior transposition—helpful in presence of dissociated vertical deviation or very severe overaction.
    - For pseudo-inferior oblique overaction, see sidebar under Y-pattern.
  - Superior oblique weakening for A- and λ-pattern deviation with superior oblique overaction (see Chapter 47):
    - Traditional superior oblique weakening procedures.
    - In a fusing patient, consider posterior tenotomy to preserve anterior fibers responsible for torsion.
  - V- and A-pattern without oblique overaction:
    - Vertical transposition of horizontal muscles—move horizontal muscle in the direction where you want its effect decreased (or away from where you want its effect increased).
      - Move medial rectus muscles inferiorly in V-pattern and superiorly in A-pattern (Fig. 51.2).
      - Move lateral rectus muscles superiorly in V-pattern and inferiorly in A-pattern (Fig. 51.2).

The direction of horizontal muscle transposition can be remembered by the mnemonic *MALE*. Move the *M*edials to the *A*pex and the *L*aterals to the *E*mpty space.

TABLE 51.1. Pattern Strabismus and Possible Surgeries

Pattern	Surgery
V esotropia/exotropia with IOOA	Horizontal muscle surgery with IO weakening
A esotropia/exotropia with SOOA	Horizontal muscle surgery with SO weakening
V esotropia without IOOA	Bimedial recession with downshift Bimedial slanted recession (inferior > superior poles)
V exotropia without IOOA	Bilateral lateral rectus recession with upshift
A esotropia without SOOA	Bimedial recession with upshift Bimedial slanted recession (superior > inferior poles)
A exotropia without SOOA	Bilateral lateral rectus recession with downshift

IO, inferior oblique; SO, superior oblique; IOOA, inferior oblique overaction; SOOA, superior oblique overaction.
Modified from Kekunnaya R, Mendonca T, Sachdeva V. Pattern strabismus and torsion needs special surgical attention. Eye. 2015;29(2):184-190.

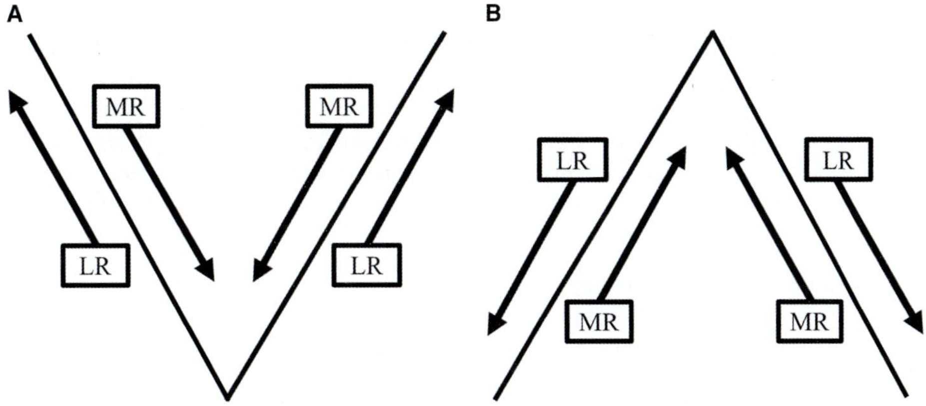

FIGURE 51.2. A. Transpose both medial rectus muscles inferiorly or both lateral rectus muscles superiorly in V-pattern strabismus. **B.** Transpose both medial rectus muscles superiorly or both lateral rectus muscles inferiorly in A-pattern strabismus. (Modified from Kekunnaya R, Mendonca T, Sachdeva V. Pattern strabismus and torsion needs special surgical attention. *Eye*. 2015;29(2):184-190.)

- Muscles can be transposed up to a full-tendon width.
  - One full-tendon width can correct up to 30 prism diopters of A- or V-pattern; this amount seems effective for any clinically significant pattern.[6]
  - Smaller transpositions can also be performed.[7]
    - ¼ tendon width for 10 prism diopters.
    - ½ tendon width for 15 prism diopters.
    - ¾ tendon width for 20 prism diopters.
- Transposition of horizontal muscles does not affect the primary position and can be performed alone or with recessions or resections.

Monocular recess/resection with vertical transposition may worsen or create new torsion, particularly in patients with good binocularity and stereopsis.[1,6]

- Procedure Pearls
  - Can use limbal or fornix incision. If using a fornix incision, consider the transposition direction when planning the placement of the surgical wound. For example, if transposing the lateral upward, make the incision in the superotemporal fornix.
  - Attach the pole of the muscle nearest the insertion first. For example, if transposing the lateral upward, attach the inferior pole of the muscle first.
  - Measure recessions carefully. The first pole (ie, pole nearest insertion) is attached to the sclera at the desired recessed location, measured from the insertion. The pole farther from the insertion is measured from the limbus (insertion distance plus recession distance).
  - Adjustable sutures can be used, but hang back recessions will reduce the amount of transposition effect achieved.
- Insertion slanting procedures:
  - For V-pattern esotropia, recess the inferior poles of both medial rectus muscles a greater amount than the superior poles.
  - For A-pattern esotropia, recess the superior poles of both medial rectus muscles a greater amount than the inferior poles.
  - Recess superior poles for the amount of esotropia in upgaze; recess inferior poles for the amount in downgaze.
- Horizontal transposition of vertical muscles—may worsen existing torsion and requires operation on additional muscles; thus, it is not a popular technique.

Craniosynostosis and Pattern Strabismus

Patients with craniosynostosis syndromes (eg, Apert, Crouzon, Pfeiffer syndromes) can have multiple ophthalmic problems including exposure keratopathy, optic atrophy, refractive errors, and amblyopia. Strabismus is common, often complex, and incomitant with horizontal, vertical, and torsional components. V-pattern exotropia is particularly common, and esotropias (common) and A-patterns (less common) also are typical. Results of strabismus surgery can be unpredictable. Normalizing head position and improved alignment in primary gaze and downgaze are reasonable surgical goals.

- Etiology of strabismus[8,9]:
  - Absent or anomalous rectus muscles:
    - Abnormal insertion.
    - Bifid.
    - Atrophic.
    - Hypertrophic.
  - Abnormalities or absence of the superior oblique tendon and/or displacement of the trochlea.
  - Shallow and excyclo-rotated orbits:
    - Rotation of the origins and/or insertions of the rectus muscles which can contribute to elevation in adduction and depression in abductions as well as the V-pattern (Fig. 51.3). Note: This can mimic severe inferior oblique overaction and superior oblique underaction.
      - Transposing all four horizontal rectus muscles can help the V-pattern and normalize the positions of the muscles, reducing the verticals in side gaze.
    - Abnormal positions of the origins and/or insertions of the oblique muscles, which alter their actions and may cause an imbalance of their actions.
      - Inferior oblique overaction:
        - Weakening the inferior obliques alone often has little effect on the V-pattern or the over elevation in adduction, but is sometimes combined with other procedures.
      - Superior oblique underaction:
        - May be due to abnormalities or absence of the superior oblique or to the abnormal positions and actions of the rectus muscles.[10]
        - Superior oblique tucks (see Chapter 47) can be considered for the extorsion and V-pattern.
    - Abnormalities of the connective tissue pulleys.
- Strabismus surgery: There are many different approaches (indicating the complexity and difficulty of correcting the strabismus), and surgery should be tailored to the specific needs of the patient. Results are unpredictable, and patients often need more than one surgery. Orbital and mid-face surgeries can impact strabismus[8-9].

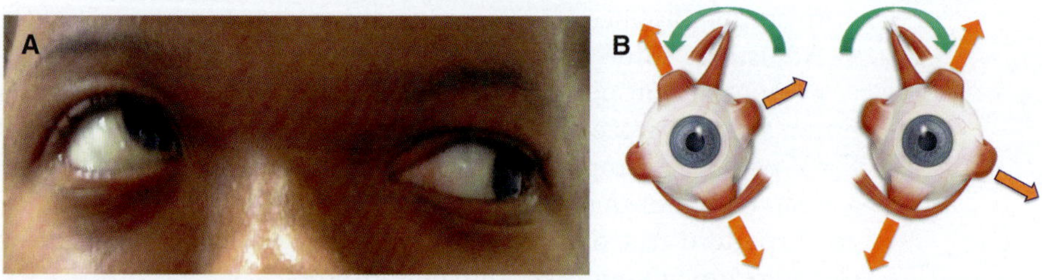

FIGURE 51.3. A. Child with Apert syndrome in left gaze. Note the downslanting orbits with excyclo-rotation of the orbits. There is significant elevation of the right eye in adduction and depression of the left eye in abduction. This was associated with V-pattern exotropia, which improved with transposition of all four horizontal rectus muscles (medials transposed inferiorly and laterals transposed superiorly). **B.** Typical excyclorotation of the orbits in Apert syndrome rotates the rectus muscles into positions that contribute to V-patterns and to elevation in adduction and depression in abduction.

- General considerations[8,9]:
  - Timing of surgery: Studies of effects of craniofacial surgery on strabismus have varied results.
    - Early surgery (prior to craniofacial surgery) may be more likely to result in binocularity, but more strabismus surgery may be required if strabismus recurs after craniofacial surgery.
    - Later surgery (at least 6 months after orbital or midface surgery) accounts for changes in strabismus (for better or worse) that can occur as a result of the craniofacial repair.
  - Be prepared for abnormalities of the muscles and make several potential surgical plans.
  - Preoperative orbital imaging may give information about anatomic variants and guide the surgical approach.
  - Consider limbal incisions that will give better exposure for abnormal anatomy.
  - Patients often have problems with corneal exposure and may have limited Bell's response. Protect and hydrate the cornea during surgery.
- Procedures to consider[8,10]:
  - Transpositions of the rectus muscles to normalize the positions (eg, transpose medials down, laterals up, verticals toward midline):
    - Addresses V-pattern.
    - Addresses torsion.
    - Addresses upshoots/downshoots in sidegaze.
    - Can be combined with recessions and/or resections.
    - Often need to move all four horizontal rectus muscles.
  - Posterior fixation sutures (see Chapter 49) to normalize muscle positions:
    - Can be combined with recessions, resections, and/or transpositions.
  - Inferior oblique weakening (myectomy, recession, anteriorization, denervation/extirpation)[10] (see Chapter 46).
  - Superior oblique strengthening (tucks or advance) (see Chapter 47).

References

1. Kekunnaya R, Mendonca T, Sachdeva V. Pattern strabismus and torsion needs special surgical attention. *Eye*. 2015;29(2):184-190.
2. Pattern strabismus. In: Hered RW, ed. *Basic and Clinical Science Course (BCSC) Section 6: Pediatric Ophthalmology and Strabismus*. San Francisco, CA: American Academy of Ophthalmology (AAO); 2017:112-116.
3. Kushner BJ. Pseudo inferior oblique overaction associated with Y and V patterns. *Ophthalmology*. 1991;98(10):1500-1505.
4. Akbari M, Salabati M, Mahmoudzadeh R, Mirmohammadsadeghi A. Pseudo inferior oblique overaction, clinical findings, mechanism, and surgical outcomes. *Graefes Arch Clin Exp Ophthalmol*. 2019;257(9):2043-2047.
5. Heo H, Lee SH, Yoon KC, Park YG, Park SW. Rectus pulley instability as a cause of Y-pattern exotropia revealed by magnetic resonance imaging. *Arch Ophthalmol*. 2008;126(12):1776-1778.
6. Del Monte MA. *Atlas of Pediatric Ophthalmology and Strabismus Surgery*. New York, NY: American Academy of Ophthalmology; 1993.
7. Buckley EG, Parks MM, Plager DA, Repka MX, Konstantin VNG, Wilson ME. *Strabismus Surgery: Basic and Advanced Strategies*. Oxford: Oxford University Press in cooperation with the American Academy of Opthalmology; 2004.
8. Rosenberg JB, Tepper OM, Medow NB. Strabismus in craniosynostosis. *J Pediatr Ophthalmol Strabismus*. 2013;50(3):140-148.
9. Ron Y, Dagi LR. The etiology of V pattern strabismus in patients with craniosynostosis. *Int Ophthalmol Clin*. 2008;48(2):215-223.
10. Coats DK, Paysse EA, Stager DR. Surgical management of V-pattern strabismus and oblique dysfunction in craniofacial dysostosis. *J AAPOS*. 2000;4(6):338-342.

CHAPTER 52

Duane Retraction Syndrome

Tanya Glaser, MD • Laura B. Enyedi, MD

PREOPERATIVE CONSIDERATIONS

Duane retraction syndrome (DRS) is a spectrum of eye motility disorders caused by misinnervation of the lateral rectus muscle leading to co-contraction of the medial and lateral rectus muscles on attempted adduction with associated globe retraction. Imaging and histopathological studies have demonstrated an absent or hypoplastic 6th cranial nerve nucleus with aberrant innervation by the 3rd cranial nerve.[1,2] DRS can occur in isolation but can also be associated with systemic conditions such as Goldenhar syndrome (oculo-auriculo-vertebral spectrum) or Wildervanck syndrome.

Recognizing the systemic associations is important for surgical planning purposes because they can complicate anesthesia. Specifically, the mandibular hypoplasia, cleft lip, and/or palate and cranio-vertebral anomalies seen in Goldenhar syndrome and the fused cervical vertebrae seen in Wildervanck syndrome can make airway management challenging.

DRS CLASSIFICATION

- DRS Type 1:
  - Poor abduction.
  - Esotropia in primary position.
  - Most common form of DRS (78%).[3]
- DRS Type 2:
  - Poor adduction.
  - Exotropia in primary position.
  - Least common form (7%).[3]
- DRS Type 3:
  - Limited abduction and adduction.
  - Esodeviation, exodeviation, or no deviation in primary position.[4]
  - Uncommon (15%).[3]

- DRS Type 4 (Synergistic Divergence):
  - Proposed additional form of DRS.
  - Abduction of the affected eye on attempted adduction.[5]
- Laterality:
  - Unilateral DRS more commonly affects the left eye.
  - DRS can occur bilaterally.
  - Different types can occur in each eye.

CLASSIC FINDINGS IN DRS

- Limitation (complete or partial) of abduction of the affected eye.
- Limitation of adduction (partial, rarely complete) of the affected eye.
- Retraction and partial closure of the eyelids of the affected eye on adduction.
- Oblique movements of the affected eye (up and in or down and in) on adduction, known as "upshoots" and "downshoots."

Overshoots seen in DRS are thought to be due to a leash phenomenon caused by a tight lateral rectus muscle that slips up or down the globe when the eye adducts.

- Deficiency of convergence in the affected eye.
- Compensatory abnormal head posture is common:
  - Occurs when there is a deviation in primary gaze.
    - With an eso-deviation, the head turn will be toward the side of the affected eye.
    - With an exo-deviation, the head turn will be away from the affected eye.
  - Allows for binocular single vision:
    - Usually allows for binocularity and fusion.
    - Usually prevents strabismic amblyopia.
- Strabismic, anisometropic, or mixed-type amblyopia occurs in about 14% of patients.[6]
- Features of DRS that help to differentiate DRS from a sixth nerve palsy[7]:
  - Globe retraction and lid fissure narrowing on adduction.
  - Small or no eso-deviation in primary gaze despite significant limitation in abduction.
  - Abduction deficit is often less on elevation and depression.
  - Exo-deviation in extreme adduction because of the limitation in both adduction and abduction.

SURGICAL PLANNING IN DRS (FIG. 52.1)

- Perform a complete eye examination:
  - Careful attention should be paid to the angle of deviation, anomalous head position, overshoots, and globe retraction as these findings will dictate the surgical plan.
- Indications for surgical intervention:
  - Significant deviation in primary position.
  - Large face turn (>15 degrees).
  - Severe globe retraction.
  - Large overshoots.[8]

As with paralytic strabismus, it is unlikely that strabismus surgery can restore normal ocular motility. The goal instead is to bring the patient's area of single binocular vision to primary gaze and eliminate or reduce anomalous head positions. Secondary goals include reducing the globe retraction and improving ductions if possible. Surgery on the unaffected eye is often needed for best results, and surgery may need to be staged.

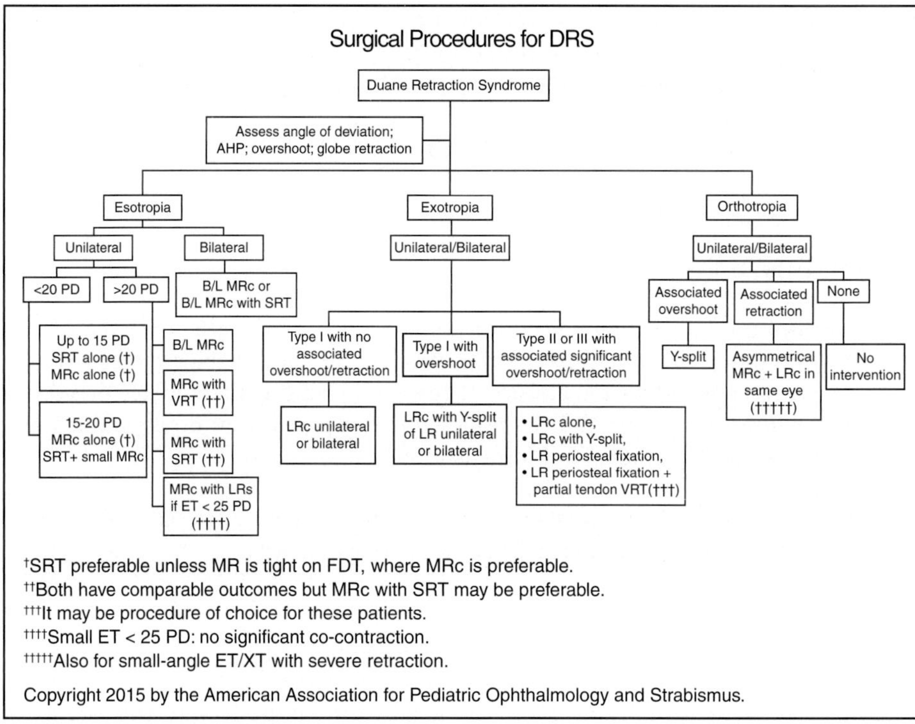

FIGURE 52.1. Flowchart for determining surgical procedure for DRS. AHP, abnormal head posture; B/L, bilateral; LRs, lateral rectus resection; LRc, lateral rectus recession; MRc, medial rectus recession; SRT, superior rectus transposition; U/L, unilateral; VRT, vertical rectus transposition. (Reproduced with permission from Kekunnaya R, Kraft S, Rao VB, Velez FG, Sachdeva V, Hunter DG. Surgical management of strabismus in Duane retraction syndrome. *J AAPOS*. 2015;19(1):63-69.)

UNILATERAL ESOTROPIC DRS

- Isolated unilateral medial rectus (MR) recession when:
  - Deviation is < 20 PD.
  - The MR is tight on forced duction testing.
  - There is at least some degree of abduction in the eye with DRS.
  - Minimal globe retraction and no significant overshoots.
  - The amount of MR recession should be no more than 5-6 mm in order to decrease the risk of an adduction deficit and worsening of an exo-deviation in contralateral gaze.
- Unilateral MR recession can be combined with other procedures to address issues of globe retraction and overshoots.

Recession of the ipsilateral MR can make the exotropia in opposite gaze worse. Comitance can be improved by recession of the contralateral LR (to mitigate the exotropia in opposite gaze) combined with recession and posterior fixation (see Chapter 49) of the contralateral MR (to improve the esotropia in gaze to the side of the DRS).

- Bilateral MR recession when:
  - Larger angle esotropias (> 20 PD).
  - Severe globe retraction.
  - Contracture of the MR in the eye with DRS.
  - The MR recession amount should be no more than 5-6 mm.

In the case of severe globe retraction, the lateral rectus (LR) may also need to be recessed, which can worsen the esotropia in primary gaze. This can be mitigated by a recession of the contralateral MR muscle.

In the case of significant contracture of the MR, large recession (7-8 mm) of the contralateral MR results in postoperative compensatory innervation differences that can decrease the risk of recurrence of the MR contracture in the DRS eye.[9]

- Vertical rectus transposition:
  - The goal of a vertical rectus transposition is to restore abduction:
    - Consider this approach when there is a severe limitation in abduction.[10]
    - If the ipsilateral MR is tight, then weakening of the MR (recession or botulinum toxin) should be considered.
  - The risk of vertical muscle surgery is creating a vertical deviation or torsion.
  - Both vertical muscles can be transposed laterally or only the superior rectus (SR). Surgical approaches are similar to those done for cranial nerve 6 palsy (see Chapter 50).
  - SR–only transposition carries less risk of anterior segment ischemia than superior and inferior rectus transposition.
  - For esodeviations <15 PD, a SR transposition alone, without MR surgery, may be sufficient.
  - For esodeviations >15 PD, a SR transposition can be combined with a MR recession of up to 5 mm.[9]
    - It may be helpful to place the MR on an adjustable suture in these cases (see Chapter 48).

Though resections are generally avoided in DRS (to prevent worsening of globe retraction), in select instances of larger angle esotropias (>20 PD) with only mild globe retraction, limited abduction with clinically normal adduction, and absence of overshoots, a unilateral MR recession and LR resection can be performed. In these cases, the LR should not be resected more than 3.5 mm and the MR not recessed more than 5 mm.[9,11]

BILATERAL ESOTROPIC DRS

- Bilateral MR recession:
  - Most common surgery for bilateral esotropic DRS.
  - The recession amount needed may be greater than what is needed for similar esodeviation in infantile esotropia.[12]
  - Bilateral MR recession can be combined with SR transpositions to the LR (see Chapter 50).

UNILATERAL EXOTROPIC DRS

- Ipsilateral unilateral LR recession:
  - Exotropia < 20 PD
  - Minimal globe retraction and no significant overshoots.
- Bilateral LR recession:
  - Exotropia > 20 PD
  - LR recession can result in further abduction limitation.
  - Recessions should be asymmetric with a larger recession of the contralateral eye, unless the eye with DRS has contracture of the LR muscle.
  - Overshoots are common in exotropic DRS, manage with Y-splitting of the LR muscle (see below).

- Type II DRS with exotropia and significant globe retraction.
    - May require supramaximal recession of the LR or periosteal fixation of the LR (see Chapter 59).
    - Combine vertical rectus transposition laterally with periosteal fixation of the LR to restore some abduction function.

SIGNIFICANT OVERSHOOTS

- Recessions of both ipsilateral horizontal rectus muscles.
- Posterior fixation (Faden operation) of one or both horizontal rectus muscles (see Chapter 49).
- Vertical muscle recession (see text box below).
- Periosteal fixation of the LR (see Chapter 59).
- Y-splitting of the LR muscle (Fig. 52.2)[13]:
    - Very successful for treating overshoot.
    - Can be combined with LR recession(s).

Recession of the SR muscle may be required if there is contracture of the muscle secondary to persistent upshoot of innervational origin. In these cases, contracture leads to hypertropia in all superior fields of gaze and all other characteristics of a SR overaction/contracture syndrome. SR recessions in these cases have to be large. SR recession may also ameliorate globe retraction in some cases.

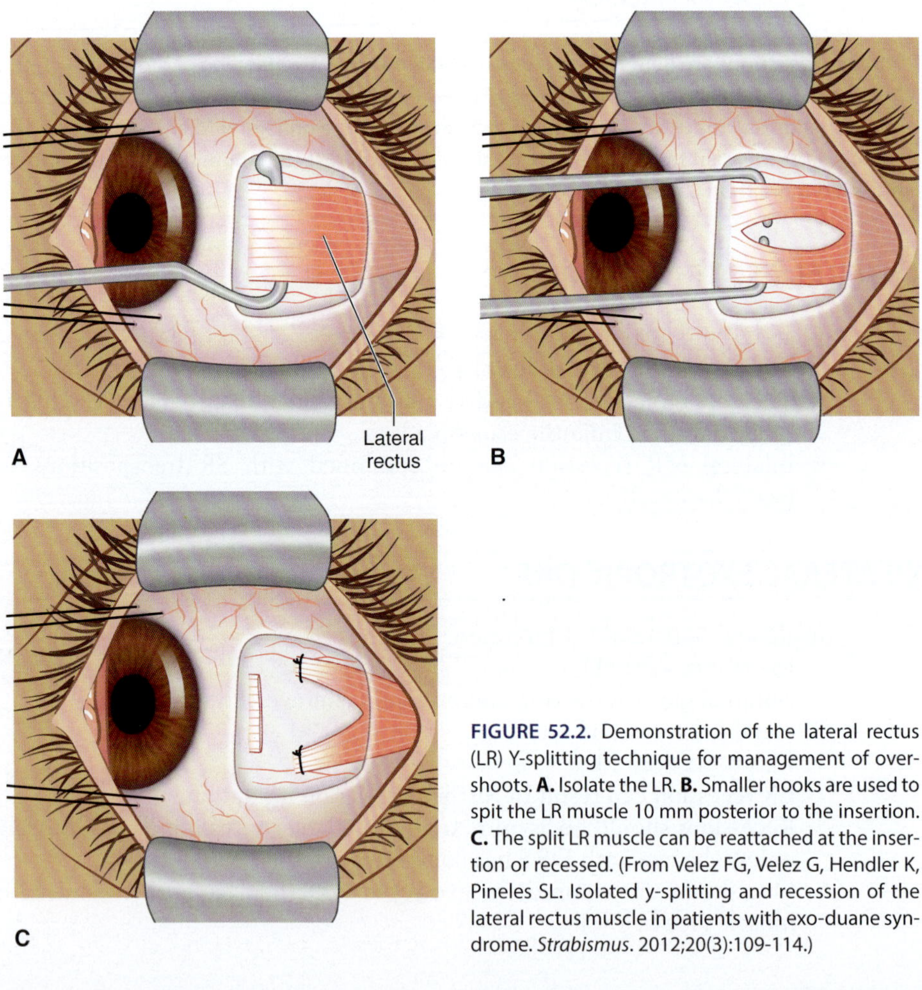

FIGURE 52.2. Demonstration of the lateral rectus (LR) Y-splitting technique for management of overshoots. **A.** Isolate the LR. **B.** Smaller hooks are used to spit the LR muscle 10 mm posterior to the insertion. **C.** The split LR muscle can be reattached at the insertion or recessed. (From Velez FG, Velez G, Hendler K, Pineles SL. Isolated y-splitting and recession of the lateral rectus muscle in patients with exo-duane syndrome. *Strabismus*. 2012;20(3):109-114.)

If the misinnervated LR is causing severe globe retraction or overshoots, consider crippling the muscle with periosteal fixation (see Chapter 59) and then treat the eye as if it has a paralytic sixth nerve palsy by doing a vertical rectus transposition procedure (see Chapter 50).

BILATERAL EXOTROPIC DRS

- Very uncommon.
- Can be treated with either unilateral or bilateral LR recession:
  - If performing a LR recession in an eye with co-contraction, then a small MR recession can also be performed.

SYNERGISTIC DIVERGENCE

- Unfortunately, there is no agreed upon best surgical procedure to treat this rare presentation.

ORTHOTROPIC DRS

- With severe globe retraction:
  - If orthotropic or very small angle eso- or exo-tropia in primary gaze, asymmetric MR and LR recessions can be performed:
    - The LR muscle should be recessed about 1 mm more than the MR muscle.
- With overshoots:
  - Perform a LR Y-splitting procedure (Fig. 52.2).
- No significant globe retraction or overshoots:
  - Observe.

References

1. Hotchkiss MG, Miller NR, Clark AW, Green WR. Bilateral Duane's retraction syndrome. A clinical-pathologic case report. *Arch Ophthalmol*. 1980;98(5):870-874.
2. Kim JH, Hwang JM. Presence of the abducens nerve according to the type of Duane's retraction syndrome. *Ophthalmology*. 2005;112(1):109-113.
3. DeRespinis PA, Caputo AR, Wagner RS, Guo S. Duane's retraction syndrome. *Surv Ophthalmol*. 1993;38(3):257-288.
4. Huber A. Electrophysiology of the retraction syndromes. *Br J Ophthalmol*. 1974;58(3):293-300.
5. Schliesser JA, Sprunger DT, Helveston EM. Type 4 Duane syndrome. *J AAPOS*. 2016;20(4):301-304.
6. Mohan K, Sharma A, Pandav SS. Differences in epidemiological and clinical characteristics between various types of Duane retraction syndrome in 331 patients. *J AAPOS*. 2008;12(6):576-580.
7. Yuksel D, Orban de Xivry JJ, Lefevre P. Review of the major findings about Duane retraction syndrome (DRS) leading to an updated form of classification. *Vision Res*. 2010;50(23):2334-2347.
8. Barbe ME, Scott WE, Kutschke PJ. A simplified approach to the treatment of Duane's syndrome. *Br J Ophthalmol*. 2004;88(1):131-138.
9. Kekunnaya R, Kraft S, Rao VB, Velez FG, Sachdeva V, Hunter DG. Surgical management of strabismus in Duane retraction syndrome. *J AAPOS*. 2015;19(1):63-69.
10. Mehendale RA, Dagi LR, Wu C, Ledoux D, Johnston S, Hunter DG. Superior rectus transposition and medial rectus recession for Duane syndrome and sixth nerve palsy. *Arch Ophthalmol*. 2012;130(2):195-201.
11. Facciani J, Kraft SP. Resecting the lateral rectus in unilateral Duane syndrome. *Binocul Vis Strabolog Q Simms Romano*. 2011;26(4):199-200.
12. Sachdeva V, Kekunnaya R, Gupta A, Bhoompally VR. Surgical management of bilateral esotropic Duane syndrome. *J AAPOS*. 2012;16(5):445-448.
13. Velez FG, Velez G, Hendler K, Pineles SL. Isolated y-splitting and recession of the lateral rectus muscle in patients with exo-duane syndrome. *Strabismus*. 2012;20(3):109-114.

CHAPTER 53

Nystagmus Surgery

Eniolami O. Dosunmu, MD

PREOPERATIVE CONSIDERATIONS

- Indications for surgical intervention:
  - Correct an abnormal head posture (AHP)—a consistent anomalous head turn, tilt, and/or chin position. The goal is to move the null point to primary position.
  - Improve visual function:
    - Studies have demonstrated improvement in visual acuity,[1,2] which allows for better use of binocular function (without the interference of a head position).
    - Even in persons with no AHP, decreasing the frequency of the nystagmus may result in improved visual function.[1,2]
    - In infantile nystagmus, data consistently demonstrates that visual function is improved: recognition time, area of the null zone, and vision in the eccentric gaze.[1]
    - Even if visual acuity does not improve objectively with the AHP and under binocular conditions, many patients report subjective improvement following nystagmus surgery.

Correct all refractive errors first! This can have a significant effect on vision.

  - Dampen nystagmus.
  - Correct other associated strabismus.
- Preoperative assessment:
  - Document observed nystagmus with any AHP (if present) and in all fields of gaze:
    - Direction: Horizontal, vertical, and/or torsional.
    - Description: Jerk or pendular, etc.
    - Frequency.
    - Amplitude.
    - Conjugacy.
  - Determine AHP: Measure the AHP in degrees of turn/chin position/tilt. A goniometer is a useful tool to perform these measurements. The AHP is often most

pronounced when the patient is asked to read the vision chart at the limits of their vision. It is important to observe the patient for more than 5 minutes, preferably longer, to ensure no periodicity.

Be sure to monitor the nystagmus and AHP for a significant period of time (>5 minutes), as detecting periodic alternating nystagmus may require prolonged observation. Review home photographs and videos to ensure that the AHP is consistent and is not changing. Observe the head posture and eye position at various points during the examination including casual conversation, distance and near visual acuity testing, and stereopsis testing.

    - Chin position (vertical).
    - Head tilt.
    - Head turn (horizontal).

The eyeTilt app (see Vision, LLC) is an easy and efficient app that quantifies head tilt in real time.

- Determine if the nystagmus worsens when the head is moved in the opposite direction of the observed AHP.
- Document gaze preference at distance and near. Documenting both gaze and head position can help avoid confusion and errors in surgical planning, as you generally move the eyes toward the AHP.
- Check visual acuity binocularly at distance and near with AHP and in forced fixed primary. Also check monocular visual acuity.

Because an opaque occluder can worsen nystagmus, a Spielmann occluder or fogging with high plus lenses should be used to check monocular visual acuity.

- Determine if there is an associated strabismus that needs to be addressed (see below).
- Remember to consider any previous eye muscle surgery in the surgical plan to avoid anterior segment ischemia (see Chapter 54).
    - If there has been previous eye muscle surgery, in children with no vascular disease, wait at least 6 months between surgeries.
    - In adults, screen for vascular systemic diseases and predispositions to anterior segment ischemia such as smoking, diabetes, and hypertension.

Using video of the patient's eye position and head posture, at distance and near, is also helpful in surgical planning.

- If your patient is able, check fusional amplitudes.

SURGICAL PROCEDURES

Preoperative Assessment

- Manage expectations of parents/caregivers prior to surgery. Emphasize the purpose of the surgery to reduce AHP. The AHP is often not completely resolved, or it may change to a different AHP after surgery. In order to resolve a horizontal or vertical head position, the surgeon will have to create a gaze palsy in the opposite direction (eg, for right head turn/eyes left preference, create a left gaze palsy).
- Write out a surgical plan that includes the current position of eyes and head and post-surgical goals. It is very easy to make a mistake with head position surgery, and it is wise to check yourself at least twice on the surgical plan.

- For horizontal and vertical head positions, think about moving the eyes **TOWARD** the anomalous head position.
- For torsional surgery, think about taking the muscles off, moving the eye the direction you want it to go (intorted or extorted) and then suturing the muscles where they land with the eye in the new position.

- Either fornix or conjunctival incisions can be used. If patient has aniridia or any disease process for which the limbal stem cells need to be spared, a fornix incision is preferred to preserve the limbal stem cells. Ensure excellent conjunctival closure for a good cosmetic outcome. Watch for postoperative dellen formation with large resections.

SURGERIES TO ADDRESS HEAD POSTURES

Horizontal Head Postures[1,3-7]

Determine the appropriate amount of surgery to perform (classic or augmented—see Table 53.1).

If the head turn is significant, only limitation of motility large enough to create a gaze palsy will correct the head turn.

- Right head turn (eyes in left gaze)—move the eyes to the **RIGHT**.
- Left head turn (eyes in right gaze)—move the eyes to the **LEFT**.

Vertical Head Postures[1,7-11,16]

- Chin up (eyes are downward)—move the eyes **UPWARD.**
    - Surgical option 1: Bilateral recessions of the inferior recti (IR) AND bilateral tenectomies (full or posterior 7/8) of the superior oblique (SO) tendons (see Chapter 47). Recommended IR recession amounts vary widely. Consider smaller amounts (4-5 mm) for small head positions (<30 degrees) and larger amounts (7.5-8 mm) for very large (>45 degrees) head positions. Because of the possibility of induced vertical, pattern, or torsional strabismus, some surgeons favor 7/8th tenectomies over full tenectomies of the SO.

TABLE 53.1. Recommended Surgery Doses (mm) for Horizontal Face Turn Surgery in Nystagmus

	Classic	Up to 20 degrees head turn 20% Augmentation	20-40 degrees head turn 40% Augmentation	>40 degrees head turn 60% Augmentation
Right head turn / Left gaze preference (MOVE eyes to the RIGHT)				
RLR resection	8.0	9.5	11	13
RMR recession	5.0	6.0	7.0	8.0
LMR resection	6.0	7.0	8.5	9.5
LLR recession	7.0	8.5	10	11
Left head turn / Right gaze preference (MOVE eyes to the LEFT)				
LLR resection	8.0	9.5	11	13
LMR recession	5.0	6.0	7.0	8.0
RMR resection	6.0	7.0	8.5	9.5
RLR recession	7.0	8.5	10	11

- Surgical option 2: Bilateral recessions of the IR AND bilateral resections of the superior recti (SR). Smaller equal recessions/resections (5/5 mm) for smaller chin positions (<30 degrees), and larger equal recessions/resections (8/8 mm or 10/10 mm) are recommended for larger chin positions.
- Chin down (eyes are upward)—move the eyes **DOWNWARD.**
  - Surgical option 1: Bilateral SR recessions (4-5 mm for small and 7-8 mm for large chin positions) AND bilateral inferior oblique (IO) anterior transposition (see Chapter 46).
  - Surgical option 2: Bilateral recessions of the SR AND bilateral IO myectomies.[1] Note: IO anteriorizations are preferred as myectomies may not be symmetric.
  - Surgical option 3: Bilateral SR recessions (4-5 mm) AND bilateral IR resections (4-5 mm).[6] These numbers may undercorrect large head positions and large resections and recessions (8/8 or 10/10) are often recommended for large head positions (Pediatric Ophthalmology Listserve discussions).

If there is a concomitant horizontal strabismus or a multiplanar head posture, consider operating on one vertical muscle and one oblique muscle to allow simultaneous surgery on the horizontal muscles while reducing the risk of anterior segment ischemia.

Avoid orbital fat in the large recessions and resections. For large resections, be sure the muscle is well imbricated as it will be on significant tension.

In vertical muscle surgeries, carefully dissect the lid retractors to avoid changes in eyelid position.

Head Tilt[1,10-12,15]

Principle: Move the eyes TOWARD the AHP. Example: To correct right head tilt (right eye intorted and left eye extorted)—surgically extort the right eye and intort the left eye. Note: All below surgical examples would be reversed to correct a left head tilt (right eye extorted and left eye intorted).

- Surgical option 1: Vertical transposition of the horizontal muscles.
  Example for right head tilt:
  - Right eye: Transpose the SR nasally by one tendon width (1 TW) placing the muscle the same distance from the limbus it was at its original location, AND the IR (1 TW) temporally, placing the muscle the same distance from the limbus that it was in its original location, to excyclorotate the right eye.
  - Left eye: Transpose the SR temporally (1 TW), placing the muscle the same distance from the limbus that it was in its original location, AND the IR medially (1 TW), placing the muscle the same distance from the limbus that it was in its original location, to incyclorotate the left eye.
- Surgical option 2: Horizontal transposition of the vertical muscles.
  Example for right head tilt:
  - Right eye: Transpose the MR inferiorly. (1 TW) and the LR superiorly (1 TW) to excylorotate the right eye.
  - Left eye: Transpose the MR superiorly (1 TW) and the LR inferiorly (1 TW) to incyclorotate the left eye.

- Surgical option 3: Anterior 7/8 tenectomy on the SO on side of tilt and Harado-Ito on side away from tilt.
  Example for right head tilt:
  - Right eye: Anterior 7/8 SO tenectomy to excylorotate the right eye.
  - Left eye: SO Harada-Ito to incyclorotate the left eye.

MULTIPLANAR HEAD POSTURES[1-13,16]

There are a number of different ways to address a multiplanar head position.

- Correct the most prominent head turn/tilt only and evaluate postoperative results before proceeding with additional surgery. This has the disadvantage of multiple surgeries, and the risk of anterior segment ischemia, but can be useful in certain circumstances, for example, a young child with a significant torticollis that is affecting the child's development.
- Correct the two most prominent turns/tilts.
- Correct all the planes of nystagmus:
  - Example A: Prominent horizontal head turn with a vertical chin position.
    - Correct the head turn by operating on the horizontal recti and transpose the horizontal recti to address the vertical chin position, using the principles discussed above.
  - Example B: Prominent vertical chin position and horizontal head turn.
    - Correct the vertical chin position with an oblique muscle surgery AND one vertical rectus muscle surgery.
    - AND correct the head turn with 10.0 mm recession of the LR of the abducting eye and 7.0 mm recession of the MR of the adducting eye. Note the amount of recession can be based on Table 53.1; however, large numbers are recommended as there is no resection to counterbalance recessions in this scenario.
  - Example C: Horizontal head turn and head tilt.
    - Operate on the horizontal rectus muscles for the head turn and transpose the muscles, using the principles above, to address the tilt.
    - OR operate on the horizontal muscles for the head turn and on the oblique muscles for the tilt.
  - Example D: Horizontal head turn, head tilt, and vertical chin position.
    - Determine if the horizontal or vertical head position is more prominent, and use this to choose which recti muscles to operate.
    - If prominent horizontal head turn, operate on the horizontal recti, transposing them to address the vertical chin position, and operate on the obliques for the tilt.
    - If prominent vertical chin position, operate on the vertical recti, transposing them to address the tilt, and do a large recession of the LR of the abducting eye and 7.0 mm recession of the MR of adducting eye.
- It is important to note that there are several permutations of surgeries that can be used to address a multiplanar head posture. Previous surgery and the degree of the head posture are the determining factors to be used when planning out the surgical procedures.

SURGERY TO INDUCE CONVERGENCE[1,12,16]

- This should only be used in fusing patients, and the nystagmus must dampen with convergence.
- This surgery can be used in patients with and without a head posture.
- Measure fusional amplitudes and prism adapt patient.
  - Place patient in 7 prism diopters (PD) base out (BO), or more, in front of each eye (no Fresnel to avoid blur). Consider prescribing ground in BO prism as a treatment alternative or to confirm improvement in esotropia and nystagmus.
  - Perform bilateral MR recessions.
    - Consider bilateral 3-mm recessions of the MR with tenotomy and reattachment of both LR,[1] if using 7 PD BO prism.
    - If measure larger amplitudes, recommend bilateral recession of the MR 5-7 mm, possibly on an adjustable suture, to help decrease the risk of an overcorrection.[11]

SURGERIES TO DAMPEN NYSTAGMUS

Tenotomy With Reattachment[1,2,14,16]

Performed on the horizontal recti only.

- Imbricate the muscles.
- Detach muscles from the globe.
- Reattach to the globe at the original insertion.

Large Horizontal Recti Recessions[4,15,16]

The muscles are placed posterior to the equator. A recession has more effect on the MR than on the LR. Bilateral recessions of 10-mm on the MR and 12 mm on the LR are recommended.

Tenotomy/reattach and large recessions have been reported to be effective in periodic alternating nystagmus where the null point alternates.

Excision of the Horizontal Recti[17]

Removal of all the horizontal recti muscles. There are limited data available for this procedure, or the results. The surgery needs to be performed with an orbital surgeon.

STRABISMUS AND NYSTAGMUS SURGERY[1,2,14,16,18]

Without Abnormal Head Posture

- Surgical option 1: Bilateral recessions for the strabismus with tenotomy and reattachment of the other horizontal recti muscles.
- Surgical option 2: Recess/resect of the horizontal recti for the total deviation.

With Abnormal Head Posture

- Determine the fixing/preferred eye.
- Use prism over the fixing/preferred eye to correct the head posture.
- Use prism over the nonpreferred eye to correct the strabismus.
- Perform a recess/resect procedure on each eye based on the required prism.

References

1. Hertel RW, Granet DB, Shah V, et al. Audience Directed Workshop: Modern Evaluation and Treatment of Nystagmus. American Association for Pediatric Ophthalmology and Strabismus Annual Meeting, March 2019, Washington, DC.
2. Hertle RW, Dell'Osso LF, FitzGibbon EJ, et al. Horizontal rectus tenotomy in patients with congenital nystagmus: results in 10 adults. *Ophthalmology*. 2003;110(11):2097-2105.
3. Kestenbaum A. Nouvelle operation du Nystagmus. *Bull Soc Ophthalmol Fr*. 1953;6:599-602. [Article in French].
4. Anderson JR. Causes and treatment of congenital eccentric nystagmus. *Br J Ophthalmol*. 1953;37(5):267-281.
5. Mitchell PR, Wheeler MB, Parks MM. Kestenbaum surgical procedure for torticollis secondary to congenital nystagmus. *J Pediatr Ophthalmol Strabismus*. 1987;24(2):87-93.
6. Nelson LB, Ervin-Mulvey LD, Calhoun JH, et al. Surgical management for abnormal head position in nystagmus: the augmented modified Kestenbaum procedure. *Br J Ophthalmol*. 1984;68(11):796-800.
7. Parks MM. Symposium: nystagmus. Congenital nystagmus surgery. *Am Orthopt J*. 1973;23: 35-39.
8. Pierse D. Operation on the vertical muscles in cases of nystagmus. *Br J Ophthalmol*. 1959;43(4):230-233.
9. Roberts EL, Saunders RA, Wilson ME. Surgery for vertical head position in null point nystagmus. *J Pediatr Ophthalmol Strabismus*. 1996;33(4):219-224.
10. Noorden Von GK, Jenkis RH, Rosenbaum AL. Horizontal transposition of the vertical rectus muscles for treatment of ocular torticollis. *J Pediatr Ophthalmol Strabismus*. 1993;30:8-14.
11. Spielman A. Clinical rationale for manifest congenital nystagmus surgery. *J AAPOS*. 2000;4(2):67-74.
12. de Decker W, Conrad HG. Torsionale Umlagerung, Rüstzeug bei komplettem frühkindlichen Schielsyndrom (Torsional shift operation—a tool for management of Lang's early-onset strabismus syndrome). *Klin Monbl Augenheilkd*. 1988;193(6):615-621 [Article in German].
13. de Decker W. Kestenbaum transposition in nystagmus therapy. Transposition in horizontal and torsional plane. *Bull Soc Belge Ophtalmol*. 1987;221-222:107-120.
14. Dell'Osso LF, Hertle RW, Williams RW, et al. A new surgery for congenital nystagmus: effects of tenotomy on an achiasmatic canine and the role of extraocular proprioception. *J AAPOS*. 1999;3(3):166-182.
15. Helveston EM, Ellis FD, Plager DA. Large recession of the horizontal recti for treatment of nystagmus. *Ophthalmology*. 1991;98(8):1302-1305.
16. Hertle RW. Surgical Treatment of Nystagmus: on Whom, When and How to Operate? Pediatric Ophthalmology Subspecialty Day 2016. Knights Templar Eye Foundation Pediatric Ophthalmology Education Center, American Academy of Ophthalmology. https://www.aao.org/annual-meeting-video/surgical-treatment-of-nystagmus-on-whom-when-how-t
17. Sinskey RM, Eshete A. Maximal subtotal extirpation of the horizontal rectus extraocular muscles for the treatment of nystagmus with no null point. A report of four successful human cases. *Binocul Vis Strabismus Q*. 2002;17(4):297-302.
18. Cooper EL, Sandall GS. Surgical treatment of congenital nystagmus. *Arch Ophthalmol*. 1969;81(4):473-480.

CHAPTER 54

Strabismus Surgery Complications

Jill C. Rotruck, MD

INTRODUCTION

All surgeries carry risks and may have unexpected outcomes. Fortunately, severe complications in strabismus surgery are rare. It is important to understand the most common and most severe complications of strabismus surgery in order to provide appropriate preoperative counseling and expeditious management of complications, when they arise.

INFECTION

- Incidence:
  - Any 0.14%.[1]
  - Severe 0.06%.[2]
- Organisms (see Table 54.1)
- Intraoperative contamination
  - Sutures and needles have a 15%[3]-31%[1] colonization rate during routine strabismus surgery, in spite of povidone-iodine prep.

TABLE 54.1. Causative pathogens for poststrabismus surgery infections

Frequency	Organism
More common	• Methicillin-susceptible *Staphylococcus aureus* (MSSA)[a] • *Streptococcus pyogenes*
Less common	• Methicillin-resistant *Staphylococcus aureus* (MRSA) • *Staphylococcus epidermidis* • *Streptococcus pneumoniae*
Rare	• Coagulase-negative *Staphylococcus* • *Haemophilus influenzae* • *Pseudomonas aeruginosa*

[a]MSSA is the most common.

- Risk factors[1]:
  - Poor hygiene.
  - Eye rubbing.
  - Young age.
  - Developmental delay.
  - Trisomy 21.
  - Immunocompromise.
  - Sinusitis.
  - Ear infection.
  - History of MRSA infection or colonization.
- Infection types (see Table 54.2):
  - Conjunctivitis.
  - Preseptal cellulitis.
  - Orbital cellulitis.
  - Subconjunctival and sub-Tenon capsule abscess (Fig. 54.1).
  - Suture abscess.
  - Endophthalmitis.
- Symptoms (usually rapidly progressing):
  - Pain.
  - Photophobia.
  - Red eye.
  - Ocular discharge.
  - Blurring.
  - Fever/fatigue.
- Signs:
  - Decreased visual acuity.
  - Periorbital and eyelid edema.
  - Proptosis.
  - Mucopurulent discharge.
  - Conjunctival injection.
  - Bump or bulge under the conjunctiva or Tenon capsule, especially over the muscle (Fig. 54.1).
  - Chemosis.

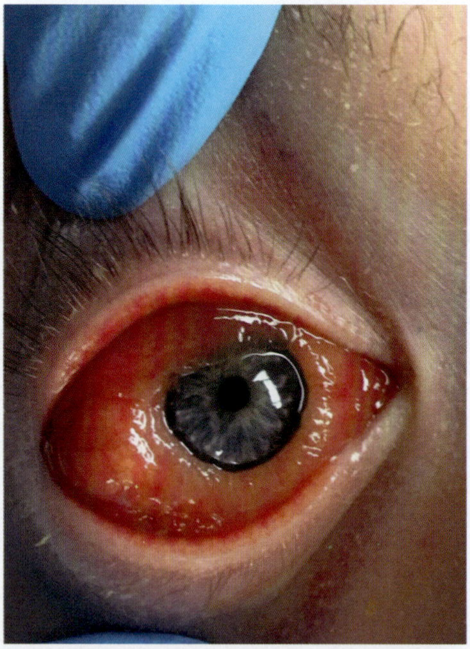

FIGURE 54.1. A lateral rectus abscess with a prominent bulge and opacity over the lateral rectus is seen following strabismus surgery with associated conjunctival chemosis and injection. This was the appearance 5 days after uncomplicated strabismus surgery in a child with Trisomy 21. (Courtesy of Laura B. Enyedi, MD.)

  - Intraocular inflammation—anterior chamber cell and fibrin, hypopyon, vitreous cell, blunting of red reflex.
  - Retinal holes or tears secondary to deep scleral passes, which may allow entry of pathogens into the eye.
  - Optic nerve swelling suggestive of orbital cellulitis.
  - Pain with extraocular movements.
  - Fever.
- Timing:
  - On average, onset of clinical features occurs between 3 and 7 days postoperatively but may present the following day or not until weeks later.[1]
- Evaluation:
  - Vision.
  - Pupils.
  - Color vision.
  - Motility.
  - Intraocular pressure.
  - External.
  - Anterior segment (slit lamp).
  - Posterior segment (dilated fundus examination).
- Diagnosis and management (see Table 54.2).
- Broad-spectrum antibiotics (see Table 54.3).
- Prognosis:
  - When treated in a timely manner, postoperative infections rarely lead to permanent vision loss. Conjunctivitis, preseptal cellulitis, and sub-Tenon capsule abscesses that do not progress to orbital cellulitis generally do not permanently impact vision.
  - Prompt treatment of orbital cellulitis can prevent vision loss; however, vision can be compromised by inflammation or compression of the optic nerve or vasculature. Rarely, orbital cellulitis is complicated by meningitis or brain abscess.[4]
  - Unfortunately, the prognosis following post–strabismus surgery endophthalmitis is poor, with only an estimated 36% retaining normal vision.[5] The prognosis for visual recovery is improved with early treatment within the first postoperative week.[5]
- Prevention:
  - Treat blepharitis and address poor hygiene preoperatively.
  - Prep with povidone-iodine 5% in the fornix prior to surgery to decrease bacterial contamination of sutures and needles.[5] Repeat use of 5% povidone-iodine in the fornix after placement of the speculum to further decrease contamination rates.[5]
  - Isolate eyelids and lashes with an adhesive drape to reduce contamination.[3] (This has not been shown to reduce rates of infection following strabismus surgery.)

3M Tegaderm transparent film is useful to isolate the lashes after prepping with povidone-iodine.

  - Place povidone-iodine 5% in the fornix at the conclusion of the case (noninferior for infection prevention compared to the use of topical antibiotic-steroid combination for 1 week postoperatively[6]).
  - Consider presoaking sutures in 5% povidone-iodine prior to use; this has been shown to reduce bacterial colonization of suture.[7]
  - Consider use of postoperative topical antibiotics. Note, no studies confirm their efficacy in preventing postoperative infections.
  - If known, treat modifiable infection risk factors, such as sinusitis or ear infection, prior to surgery.
  - Consider the use of prophylactic systemic antibiotics in high-risk patients, such as those with Trisomy 21 or immunocompromise.
  - Do not complete a known deep scleral pass and consider removal of sutures with a known deep scleral pass, as contaminated suture may pass into the intraocular space.[3]

TABLE 54.2. Findings and management/treatment of poststrabismus surgery infections

Infection type	Findings	Management/treatment
Conjunctivitis	• Mild to severe conjunctival injection and chemosis • Absence of subconjunctival collection or signs of orbital cellulitis	• Culture conjunctival incision site and/or drainage • Prescribe broad spectrum topical and oral antibiotics, as there is a high risk of orbital cellulitis through the surgical incision. Consider that conjunctivitis may also be due to allergic response to postoperative drops • Use a different drug class than initial antibiotic • Follow-up within 24 hours for signs of developing orbital cellulitis
Preseptal cellulitis	• Eyelid swelling • Normal vision, pupils, motility, and optic nerve • Absence of proptosis	• Culture conjunctival incision site and/or drainage • Prescribe a broad-spectrum oral antibiotic. Clindamycin provides good coverage for the majority of the reported pathogens following strabismus surgery, including community-acquired MRSA. Consider concomitant use of broad-spectrum topical antibiotics, as incision site is the likely entry point of infection • Follow-up within 24 hours for signs of orbital cellulitis
Subconjunctival or sub-Tenon capsule abscess (Figure 54.1)	• Bump or bulge under the conjunctiva or Tenon capsule, often over the muscle • +/– signs of orbital cellulitis	• Obtain CT or MRI imaging to evaluate for extent of infection into the orbit • Drain the abscess promptly and obtain cultures at the time of drainage. Consider involvement of an oculoplastic specialist for abscesses extending into the orbit • Treat with broad spectrum topical and systemic antibiotics • Consider admission for IV antibiotics
Orbital cellulitis	• Eyelid swelling • Proptosis • Chemosis • Conjunctival injection • Limited extraocular movements • Decreased vision • Decreased color vision • Optic disc edema • Elevated intraocular pressure	• Culture conjunctiva incision site and/or drainage • Obtain blood cultures • Obtain CT or MRI imaging to evaluate for orbital abscess. If an abscess is present, refer to an oculoplastic specialist to evaluate for abscess drainage • Admit to the hospital for broad spectrum IV antibiotics, including MRSA coverage
Endophthalmitis	• Eyelid swelling • Conjunctival injection • Chemosis • Intraocular inflammation (anterior chamber cell, fibrin, hypopyon, vitreous cell and haze) • Decreased vision • Possible scleral or retinal penetration with suture visible on retinal examination	• Carefully inspect the incision and muscle reattachment sites for signs of extraocular infection or abscess • Perform a detailed fundus examination to evaluate for evidence of scleral perforation with suture at the site of muscle reattachment, as this may have been the inciting event. Ensure no retinal holes or detachments are present. Consider referral to retinal or uveitis specialist • Perform vitreous aspiration or anterior chamber paracentesis for gram stain and cultures • Inject broad spectrum intravitreal antibiotics • Treat intraocular inflammation with topical steroids and a cycloplegic agent to prevent sequelae • Treat as above for signs of associated cellulitis or extraocular abscess

TABLE 54.3. Common antibiotic regimens for poststrabismus surgery infections

Method of administration	Antibiotic	Coverage	Uses
Topical	Fortified vancomycin 25 mg/mL with either tobramycin 15 mg/mL or gentamicin 15 mg/mL	Broad spectrum coverage of the common causes of poststrabismus surgery infection (Table 54.1)	Severe infections
	Moxifloxacin or gatifloxacin	Good gram-positive and gram-negative coverage, but do not cover MRSA and limited coverage of *P. aeruginosa*	Less severe infections without increased risk of MRSA
	Polymyxin B sulfate-trimethoprim	Covers *P. aeruginosa* and staphylococcal species, including community-acquired MRSA (CA-MRSA); inconsistent coverage against *H. influenzae*, streptococcus species, and gram-negative bacteria	Can combine with a fluoroquinolone to add MRSA coverage
Oral	Clindamycin	Good coverage for most poststrabismus surgery pathogens, including CA-MRSA; however, does not provide coverage for *H. influenzae*, *P. aeruginosa*, or gram-negative bacteria	Consider an additional or alternative agent if noncovered pathogens are of particular concern, such as with concurrent sinusitis or history of pseudomonas infection
Intravenous	Vancomycin and piperacillin-tazobactam combined	Broad spectrum	Orbital cellulitis
Intravitreal	Vancomycin 1 mg/0.1 mL and ceftazidime 2 mg/0.1 mL	Broad spectrum	Endophthalmitis

ANTERIOR SEGMENT ISCHEMIA

- Incidence—0.008%.[8]
- Cause:
  - Tenotomy of the rectus muscles during strabismus surgery severs the anterior ciliary artery in the muscle capsule that serves the anterior segment.
  - More common when three or more muscles are operated but has been reported with disinsertion of only two rectus muscles.[9]
  - The risk is increased for surgery of multiple muscles, even at different time points.[3]
  - The risk is greatest for surgery of the vertical rectus muscles and least for the lateral rectus muscle.[10]
- Risk factors[9,10]:
  - Older age.
  - Atherosclerosis.
  - Diabetes mellitus.
  - Hematologic disorders that increase blood viscosity.
  - Thyroid ophthalmopathy.
  - Scleral buckle placement.
- Signs and symptoms:
  - Mild: pupillary abnormalities, decreased iris perfusion, iris atrophy.[10]
  - Severe: uveitis, keratopathy, corneal edema with possible scarring, cataract,[10] phthisis bulbi.[3]

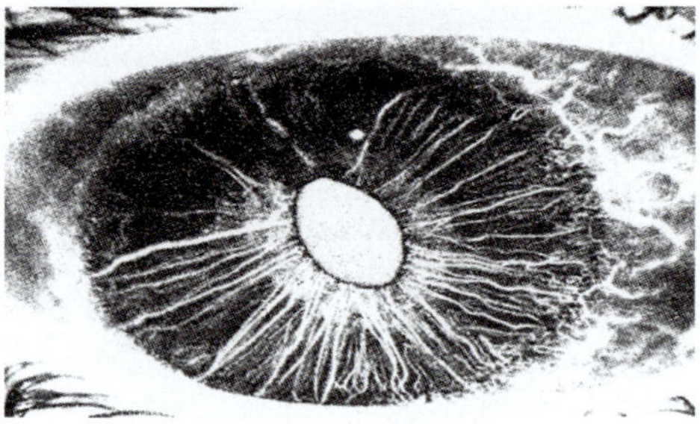

FIGURE 54.2. Iris fluorescein angiography showing poor iris perfusion and pupil irregularity superotemporally consistent with anterior segment ischemia. (Courtesy of Federico Velez, MD.)

- Course:
  - Typical onset occurs 1-2 days after surgery.
  - Most symptoms resolve within 2 weeks, but recovery of iris circulation may take up to 12 weeks in those with more significant ischemia and severe presentation.[10]
  - Iris atrophy is the most common sequelae.
- Evaluation:
  - Perform a complete eye examination to determine the extent of ocular changes and look for infection signs and risk factors. See evaluation under infection section above.
  - Consider fluorescein angiography,[11] indocyanine green angiography,[10] or optical coherence tomography angiography[10,12] to evaluate for iris ischemia (Fig. 54.2).

Patients with anterior segment ischemia show delayed or absent filling of the iris vessels in the affected area.

- Management—Topical and systemic corticosteroids are frequently administered, although the efficacy of this treatment has not been well-studied.[13]
- Prevention:
  - Avoid simultaneous removal of three or more rectus muscles.
  - When appropriate, consider surgical techniques that spare the anterior ciliary vessels, such as plication in place of resection,[9] microvascular dissection of the anterior ciliary vessels,[8] partial transposition procedures,[8] or partial tenotomies.[10]

SCLERAL PERFORATION

- Incidence—0.07%-5.1%.[14]
- Cause—Occurs most commonly due to deep suture pass during reattachment of the muscle to the sclera, but may occur at any time during the case.[3]
- Risk factors:
  - Recessions are more likely to have sclera perforation than resections, presumably due to thinner sclera more posteriorly.[5]
  - Myopia, presumably due to thinner sclera from axial elongation.[15]
- Signs and symptoms:
  - Intraoperative signs.
    - A feeling of giving way during a scleral pass.
    - Uvea or vitreous present on the suture or on the sclera at the site of the pass.
    - Softening of the eye.
    - Vitreous, retinal, and/or subretinal hemorrhage.
    - Retinal hole or subretinal fluid at perforation site.
  - Postoperative.
    - Flashing lights and floaters.
    - Vision changes.

- Management:
  - Passing the suture through and leaving in place may increase risk of endophthalmitis, as needles and sutures are known to have a high rate of contamination.[3]
    - If you believe your pass was deep, but have not completed it, gently grasp the suture behind the needle and pull the suture in order to safely back the needle out of the scleral tunnel. Place the scleral pass at a different location.
    - If you pass the suture through and become aware of signs of a deep pass, stop progressing the suture through. Resuture the muscle. Cut the initial suture near the scleral tunnel and remove. Trim the original suture flush to the muscle. Attach the muscle to the sclera with scleral passes at a different location.
    - Consider use of 5% povidone-iodine or antibiotic drops at the surgical site and oral or IV antibiotic prophylaxis.[3]
  - Perform a dilated examination with scleral depression to evaluate for retinal holes, tears, or detachment. Holes and tears can be treated with laser or cryo-retinopexy.[3] Although children have a formed vitreous and are at low risk of detachment, it may be difficult to examine the peripheral retina while awake. If available, consider laser or cryo-retinopexy at the time of strabismus surgery.
- Prevention:
  - A hang-back technique can decrease the risk of perforation for difficult to place posterior scleral passes.[3]

OVER AND UNDER CORRECTIONS (SEE CHAPTER 59)

Slipped Muscle

- Incidence—0.05%[14]-10%.[8]
- Cause—The muscle capsule, rather than the muscle or tendon, was incorporated into the bites to secure the muscle. The muscle and tendon retract within the muscle capsule, while the capsule remains attached to the sclera.[16]
- Signs and symptoms:
  - Incomitant strabismus with reduced duction and reduced saccadic velocity in the field of action of the affected muscle and widening of the palpebral fissure with movement into the field of action of the affected muscle.[16]
  - Typical onset is around a week after surgery and may progress over months.
- Management:
  - Surgical correction:
    - Consider a limbal incision to improve exposure and limit traction on the muscle capsule attachment.
    - Identify the muscle capsule still attached to the globe and follow posteriorly to find the muscle still attached to the capsule.
    - Measure the location of the muscle relative to the limbus and the current insertion site of the capsule.
    - Place sutures through the muscle belly with locking bites. Detach and resect the empty muscle capsule.
    - Attach the muscle to the sclera at a location based on current strabismus measurements and the amount of posterior slippage of the muscle.
      - Note that the change in angle is about 3 prism diopters for each 1 mm of muscle advancement.[8]
- Prevention:
  - Carefully dissect and remove Tenon capsule directly over the tendon or muscle where sutures are to be passed.
  - Use full-thickness locking bites to ensure the muscle has been incorporated into the bite.[3]

Lost Muscle

- Incidence—0.02%.[8]
- Cause:
  - Muscle and capsule are fully detached from the globe and retracted posteriorly into the orbit.
  - May occur intraoperatively or postoperatively due to issues with suture passes into the muscle or the sclera.
  - Pulled-in-two syndrome (PITS)—the muscle separates from the globe at the tendon or ruptures at the muscle belly due to tension from the muscle hook.
- Signs and symptoms:
  - Large angle strabismus with a large ductional deficit in the field of action of the affected muscle.
  - If occurs postoperatively, generally occurs hours to days following surgery.[8]
- Management:
  - If occurs intraoperatively, recover and reattach the muscle immediately.
  - If occurs postoperatively, perform surgical exploration as soon as possible before muscle contraction and scarring occur.[8]
  - If going for a second surgery, consider preoperative imaging to identify the position of the muscle in the orbit.[8]
  - General principles for finding a lost muscle:
    - Allow for good exposure. Use a limbal incision or convert a fornix incision into a limbal incision.
    - Avoid bleeding. Consider use of phenylephrine drops to help with hemostasis. Cauterize as needed to maintain a clear view. Bayonet style bipolar cautery will make orbital cautery easier.[17] Suction can help to maintain a clear view while cautery is performed.[17] Avoid excessive tissue manipulation, which promotes bleeding.
    - Know the anatomy. The muscle will retract into the muscle capsule within Tenon capsule. In the posterior orbit behind the globe, the rectus muscles will travel along the periorbita next to the orbital wall, rather than adjacent to the globe.[17]
    - Perform an intentional search for the muscle capsule. Do not search blindly, as this will lead to bleeding and fat prolapse, obscuring the view and promoting scarring.
    - Occasionally, the oculocardiac reflex can help identify the muscle (ie, a reduction of heart rate as tissue containing the extraocular muscle is pulled). Ask the anesthesia team to avoid drugs that block the oculocardiac reflex when searching for a lost muscle.
    - Maintain good exposure. Retract the conjunctiva and Tenon capsule to expose the global surface of the Tenon capsule.[3] A broad malleable ribbon retractor can also be used to displace the globe toward the opposite orbital wall.[17]
    - Use fine toothed forceps to carefully inspect the global surface of the Tenon capsule for the opening of the muscle capsule within Tenon capsule.[3]
    - If the muscle is present at the capsule opening, grasp it firmly with toothed forceps and secure on a suture with at least two locking bites.
    - As described by Jordan et al.,[17] if the muscle is not present at the Tenon capsule opening, use a single or double pronged skin hook on each side of the tunnel to open it. Advance the hooks posteriorly one at a time in 3-5 mm increments until the muscle is identified and grasp and secure the muscle, as above.[17]
    - Secure the muscle to the sclera at the desired location.
  - If a lost muscle cannot be found, consider performing a muscle transposition or, if the risk for anterior segment ischemia is too high, tethering the globe in primary position with permanent sutures.[8,18]

- Prevention:
  - Avoid damage to sutures during surgery.
    - Avoid grasping the suture with toothed forceps.[3]
    - Be wary of cautery burning through the suture with direct contact or by creating warm air currents that can attract the suture to the cautery tip.
    - Check that the muscle is secure on the suture after disinsertion from the globe. If it is not secure, take another full-thickness locking bite.
  - Limit dissection of the muscle capsule and check ligaments to prevent far posterior retraction of the muscle capsule.[3]

Scar Remodeling/Stretched Insertion Scar

- Cause—Scar tissue develops at the scleral attachment site of the muscle, which can lengthen over time[3,8] (Fig. 54.3).
- Signs and symptoms—Strabismus occurring a month to years after surgery with minimal under action of the affected muscle.[16]
- Risk factors—Thyroid eye disease, especially with surgery of the inferior rectus.[16]
- Management:
  - Isolate the muscle. Secure the muscle belly on sutures. Excise the scar tissue completely.
  - As with a slipped muscle, attach the muscle to the sclera at a location based on current strabismus measurements and the amount of posterior slippage of the muscle.
    - Note that the change in angle is about 3 prism diopters for each 1 mm of muscle advancement.[8]
- Prevention:
  - Onset around 1 month may be related to Vicryl sutures dissolving. Consider use of permanent sutures for repair or in high-risk patients.[16]

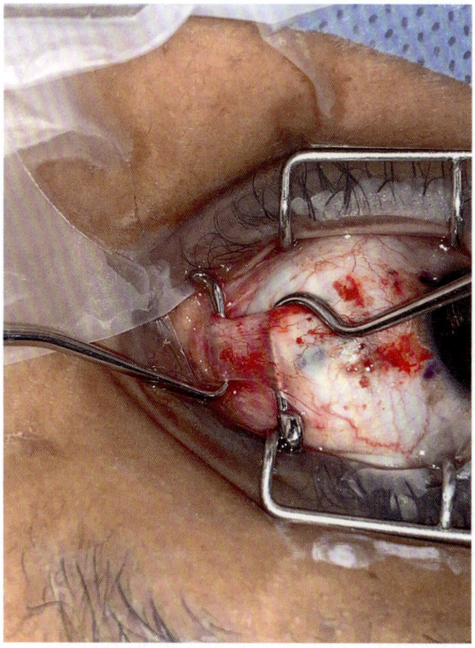

FIGURE 54.3. Stretched scar at the medial rectus insertion in a patient who underwent medial rectus recession 40 years prior and presented with a long-standing large exotropia and mild adduction deficit. (Courtesy of Laura B. Enyedi, MD.)

Fat Adherence Syndrome

- Cause—Violation of posterior Tenon capsule with entry of extraconal fat into the episcleral space leads to scarring of the fat, muscle, orbital connective tissue, and sclera.[3,8] Scarring may be attached to the orbital periosteum.[3]
- Signs and symptoms—Progressive restrictive strabismus presenting weeks to months after surgery.[3,8]
- Risk factors—Disruption of the posterior Tenon capsule frequently occurs during isolation of the inferior oblique muscle.
- Management:
  - Surgical release of adhesions.[3,8]
  - Consider use of amniotic membrane between the conjunctiva and underlying tissues to prevent recurrent adhesions.
- Prevention:
  - Visualize the posterior inferior oblique muscle prior to isolation and avoid incorporating excess posterior Tenon capsule onto hooks during muscle isolation.
  - Suture defects in posterior Tenon capsule that are evident during surgery to prevent fat prolapse.
  - Reposit prolapsed adipose tissue, if possible. For large amounts of prolapsed fat tissue that cannot be reposited, clamp fat flush with the Tenon capsule defect and resect the prolapsed fat. Suture Tenon capsule.

Deviations From Large Surgical Corrections

- Recessions—A large recession can limit duction in the field of action of the muscle, especially if the muscle is placed posterior to the equator.[18]
- Resections—A large resection may lead to restriction and globe retraction opposite the field of action of the operated muscle.[18] For large resections, consider a temporary tie of the suture and perform a forced duction test prior to permanently tying the suture.[18]

CONJUNCTIONAL ABNORMALITIES

Displaced Plica Semilunaris

- Cause:
  - Medial conjunctival scarring with dragging of the plica semilunaris toward the limbus.[19]
  - The plica is mistaken for the conjunctival edge and is incorporated in the conjunctival closure.[19]
- Risk factors:
  - Reoperation, leading to greater scar tissue formation.[19]
  - Large medial rectus resections or advances which drag conjunctival tissue anteriorly and cause conjunctival bunching.
  - Excessive hydration of the conjunctiva during surgery, which can obscure landmarks.
- Signs and symptoms:
  - Poor cosmesis due to plica semilunaris located closer than normal to the limbus.
  - May limit abduction if scarring is significant.
- Management:
  - Incise the conjunctiva anterior to the scarred area or starting at the limbus, depending on the extent of anterior displacement and conjunctival scarring. Carefully mobilize scar tissue and conjunctiva using blunt dissection. Take great care to not to disturb the medial rectus muscle, if recently operated.

    - Allow the plica semilunaris to retract back to its normal position and measure the size of the defect created. This will be larger than the amount of scarred conjunctiva that was resected. Prepare an amniotic membrane or conjunctival autograft[19] the size of the defect.
    - Using fibrin glue or dissolvable sutures, secure the amniotic membrane or a conjunctival autograft to the conjunctival edges of the defect.
- Prevention:
    - For complex procedures, mark the edges of the conjunctival incision edges with a sterile marking pen for easy identification during conjunctival closure.
    - For large medial rectus resections or advances, consider tacking the conjunctiva down to the sclera just anterior to the insertion or to the muscle belly with a double-armed 8-0 Vicryl suture to prevent the plica and other redundant conjunctiva from creeping toward the limbus.

Fibrosis and Adhesions

- Cause—Adherence of the conjunctiva to Tenon capsule, intermuscular membrane, adipose tissue, sclera, and extraocular muscles.[20]
- Risk factors[20]:
    - Bleeding.
    - Excessive cautery.
    - Reaction to dissolvable sutures.
    - Infection.
    - Muscle capsule injury.
    - Multiple procedures in the same region.
- Signs and symptoms:
    - Chronic injection of the conjunctiva.
    - Conjunctival irregularity.
    - Mechanical restriction.
- Management:
    - Dissect adhesions and fibrotic bands between the conjunctiva and underlying structures.[21] Resect conjunctiva with cosmetically objectionable scarring.
    - Cut amniotic membrane or a conjunctival autograft to fit the defect and secure with dissolvable suture or fibrin glue (see Chapter 20). If the defect is small, the conjunctiva can be recessed several millimeters and the sclera left bare.
    - If bulbar and palpebral conjunctiva were affected, consider placing a symblepharon ring.[21]
- Prevention—In high-risk cases, such as reoperation on a patient with a history of fibrosis, consider use of amniotic membrane as a spacer between the conjunctiva and underlying tissues.[20]

POSTOPERATIVE LESIONS

Pyogenic Granuloma (Lobular Capillary Hemangioma) (Fig. 54.4)

- Incidence—2%-4%.[8]
- Cause—Proliferation of fibrovascular tissue in response to trauma.[3]
- Pathology—Mixed acute and chronic inflammation with capillary proliferation in a lobular pattern.[22] It is neither pyogenic, nor a granuloma.
- Signs and symptoms:
    - Pink, fleshy mass with rapid growth typically appearing a few weeks after surgery.[23] May cause irritation and foreign body sensation.

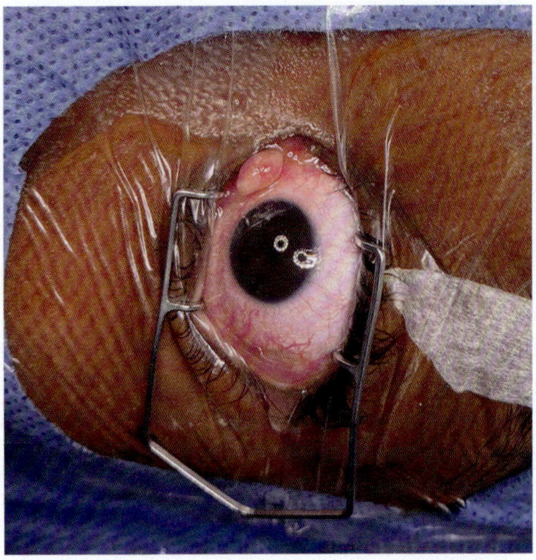

FIGURE 54.4. A postoperative pyogenic granuloma in an 11-year-old child after uncomplicated fornix surgery. This lesion did not respond to topical beta-blocker therapy and was surgically removed. (Courtesy of Laura B. Enyedi, MD.)

- Management:
  - Topical timolol 0.5% twice daily has been shown to result in resolution of these lesions.[24]
  - Use of topical steroids is a common practice, although efficacy is unproven since they may resolve spontaneously. Treatment takes around 30 days, on average.[22]
  - If topical treatment is not successful, remove surgically by excising the lesion at the base of the stalk.[22]
  - They do not tend to recur once treated or excised.[22]

Tenon Capsule Exposure

- Cause—Prolapse of Tenon capsule through the conjunctival incision (Fig. 54.5).
- Signs and Symptoms—White tissue can be seen along the incision line.[18]
- Risk factors—Young age due to increased prominence of Tenon capsule.[20]
- Management
  - May retract back into the conjunctiva without treatment.[18]
  - If a large prolapse fails to resolve, the Tenon capsule will need to be trimmed flush with the conjunctiva.[18]
- Prevention—Careful conjunctival closure with trimming of excess or prolapsed Tenon capsule at the time of surgery.[3,18]

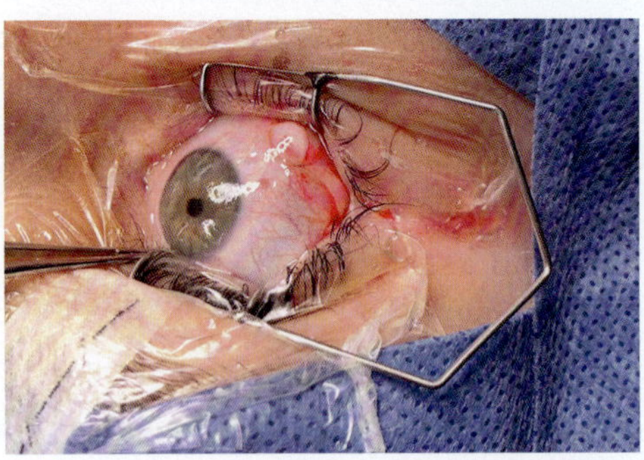

FIGURE 54.5. Tenon capsule is seen as a white tissue prolapsing through the incision site at the completion of strabismus surgery. The prolapsed tissue should be reposited and/or trimmed, and an additional suture placed if necessary. (Courtesy of Laura B. Enyedi, MD.)

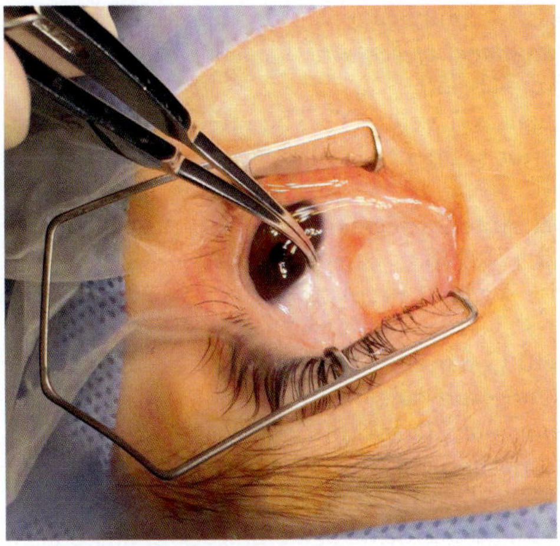

FIGURE 54.6. A large conjunctival epithelial inclusion cyst overlies the medial rectus muscle following previous medial rectus recession. The patient presented with a large consecutive exotropia. This cyst was surgically removed. (Courtesy of Laura B. Enyedi, MD.)

Conjunctival Epithelial Inclusion Cyst (Fig. 54.6)

- Cause—Deposition of conjunctival epithelial cells into the substantia propria or sclera which form a nest that proliferates and creates a central fluid-filled cavity.[20]
- Signs and symptoms—Subconjunctival transilluminating cystic structure occurring anywhere in the operative field that develops days to years postoperatively.[25] These cysts typically arise at the anterior edge of the muscle and the site to which the muscle was sutured during surgery.
- Sequelae—Large cysts may affect ocular motility or alignment or may cause astigmatism with subsequent amblyopia in children.[25]
- Evaluation—If very large, consider obtaining imaging to look for orbital extension and involvement of underlying structures prior to surgical removal.[25]
- Management:
  - Can be observed if small and not cosmetically bothersome.[8,18]
  - Possible treatments include aspiration, injection with alcohol with aspiration of the alcohol,[3,26] thermal cautery,[27] marsupialization with cautery,[26] or removal of the anterior capsule with suturing of the cut edges to the conjunctiva.[25]
  - Complete surgical excision is typically curative.[25] For complete excision, a limbal incision may give better exposure and control of the eye, since the extraocular muscle can be hooked for stability.[3] Dissect very carefully in the area of the reattached muscle, as the cyst may be attached to the muscle or the scleral tracts.[3]

References

1. House RJ, Rotruck JC, Enyedi LB, Wallace DK, Saleh E, Freedman SF. Postoperative infection following strabismus surgery: case series and increased incidence in a single referral center. *J AAPOS*. 2019;23(1):26.e1-26.e7.
2. Bradbury JA, Taylor RH. Severe complications of strabismus surgery. *J AAPOS*. 2013;17(1): 59-63.
3. Olitsky SE, Coats DK. Complications of strabismus surgery. *Middle East Afr J Ophthalmol*. 2015;22(3):271-278.
4. Tsirouki T, Dastiridou AI, Ibanez Flores N, et al. Orbital cellulitis. *Surv Ophthalmol*. 2018;63(4):534-553.
5. Ing MR, Shortell J, Golez J. Extraocular and intraocular infections following strabismus surgery: a review. *J Pediatr Ophthalmol Strabismus*. 2019;56(4):214-221.
6. Koederitz NM, Neely DE, Plager DA, et al. Postoperative povidone-iodine prophylaxis in strabismus surgery. *J AAPOS*. 2008;12(4):396-400.
7. Eustis HS, Rhodes A. Suture contamination in strabismus surgery. *J Pediatr Ophthalmol Strabismus*. 2012;49(4):206-209.

8. Spierer O, Cavuoto KM, McKeown CA. Complications of strabismus surgery. In: Traboulsi E, Miraldi Utz V, eds. *Practical Management of Pediatric Ocular Disorders and Strabismus*. eBook. New York, NY: Springer; 2016:641-650.
9. Oltra EZ, Pineles SL, Demer JL, Quan AV, Velez FG. The effect of rectus muscle recession, resection and plication on anterior segment circulation in humans. *Br J Ophthalmol*. 2015;99(4):556-560.
10. Pineles SL, Chang MY, Oltra EL, et al. Anterior segment ischemia: etiology, assessment, and management. *Eye (Lond)*. 2018;32(2):173-178.
11. Olver JM, Lee JP. Recovery of anterior segment circulation after strabismus surgery in adult patients. *Ophthalmology*. 1992;99(3):305-315.
12. Velez FG, Davila JP, Diaz A, Corradetti G, Sarraf D, Pineles SL. Association of change in iris vessel density in optical coherence tomography angiography with anterior segment ischemia after strabismus surgery. *JAMA Ophthalmol*. 2018;136(9):1041-1045.
13. Saunders RA, Bluestein EC, Wilson ME, Berland JE. Anterior segment ischemia after strabismus surgery. *Surv Ophthalmol*. 1994;38(5):456-466.
14. Ritchie AE, Ali N. The incidence and clinical outcome of complications in 4,000 consecutive strabismus operations. *J AAPOS*. 2019;23(3):140.e1-140.e6.
15. Park K, Hong S, Chung W, et al. Inadvertent scleral perforation after strabismus surgery: incidence and association with refractive error. *Can J Ophthalmol*. 2008;43(6):669-672.
16. Wright K, Hong P. Strabismus surgery. In: Wright K, Strube YN, eds. *Pediatric Ophthalmology and Strabismus*. 3rd ed. New York, NY: Oxford University Press; 2012:368-387.
17. Jordan DR, Stoica B, Dutton JJ. Localizing the lost rectus muscle using the connective tissue framework: revisiting the tunnel technique. *Ophthalmic Plast Reconstr Surg*. 2017;33(6): 477-481.
18. Buckley EG, Freedman S, Shields MB. *Atlas of Ophthalmic Surgery Volume III: Strabismus and Glaucoma*. St Louis, MO: Mosby; 1995.
19. Leoson Y, Ogard C, Mortzos P. Conjunctival autograft as treatment for anterior displacement and scarring of the plica semilunaris after strabismus surgery. *J AAPOS*. 2013;17(5): 528-529.
20. Dos Santos Martins TG, de Azevedo Costa ALF, Centelhas AC, Dos Santos Martins DG. Use of biodegradable collagen-glycosaminoglycan copolymer matrix implant to reduce postoperative fibrosis in strabismus surgery. *Taiwan J Ophthalmol*. 2017;7(4):227-229.
21. Naxer S, Horn M, Schittkowski M. Processed amniotic membrane for conjunctival reconstruction in complex strabismus surgery. *Strabismus*. 2018;1-7.
22. Espinoza GM, Lueder GT. Conjunctival pyogenic granulomas after strabismus surgery. *Ophthalmology*. 2005;112(7):1283-1286.
23. Bradbury JA, Pilling RF. Strabismus surgery complications and how to avoid them. In: Lambert SR, Lyons CJ, eds. *Taylor and Hoyt's Pediatric Ophthalmology and Strabismus*. 5th ed. eBook. Philadelphia, PA: Elsevier Health Sciences; 2016:913-920.
24. Oke I, Alkharashi M, Petersen RA, Ashenberg A, Shah AS. Treatment of ocular pyogenic granuloma with topical timolol. *JAMA Ophthalmol*. 2017;135(4):383-385.
25. Song JJ, Finger PT, Kurli M, Wisnicki HJ, Iacob CE. Giant secondary conjunctival inclusion cysts: a late complication of strabismus surgery. *Ophthalmology*. 2006;113(6):1049.e1-2.
26. Simon JW. Complications of strabismus surgery. *Curr Opin Ophthalmol*. 2010;21(5): 361-366.
27. Hawkins AS, Hamming NA. Thermal cautery as a treatment for conjunctival inclusion cyst after strabismus surgery. *J AAPOS*. 2001;5(1):48-49.

CHAPTER 55

Pharmacologic Management of Strabismus

Jeffrey S. Hunter, MD

Pharmacologic treatments may offer nonsurgical alternatives to surgery for pediatric and adult strabismus/motility disorders.[1]

MIOTICS / PARASYMPATHOMIMETICS (ECHOTHIOPHATE IODIDE [0.125%])

These drugs have traditionally been used for glaucoma treatment but also have been used to treat esotropia since the 1940s. These agents uncouple the mechanism that facilitates the accommodative convergence response, thus allowing the eyes to focus without stimulating convergence. Miotics work best in patients with some fusional potential and small angle deviations (<20 prism diopters [PD]). They may work particularly well in patients with high accommodative convergence to accommodation (AC/A) ratios.[2]

> **Echothiophate iodide has a shelf life of 3-4 weeks and may lose efficacy at the end of that time. It is currently only manufactured by Pfizer, Inc. as phospholine iodide and requires special order to the pharmacy as a "drop shipment."**

- Mechanism of action:
  - Binds cholinesterase in the erythrocytes and plasma irreversibly, causing acetylcholine levels to increase, which potentiates accommodation.
  - Increases uveal outflow.
- Indications:
  - Treating accommodative esotropia (both high and normal AC/A ratio types):
    - As an alternative to single vision glasses for a child who will not wear spectacles.
    - As an alternative to bifocal in a child with high AC/A ratio.
  - Treating postoperative esotropia:
    - Consecutive esotropia after exodeviation surgery.
    - Residual esotropia after eso-surgery (small angle <15-20 prism diopters).
    - Accommodative component esotropia after surgery for infantile esotropia
  - Testing for accommodative component in esotropia—useful in distinguishing accommodative from nonaccommodative esotropia, especially in infants who resist wearing spectacles.

- Dosage—Start with 1 drop of echothiophate 0.125% bilaterally every morning. If effective, the dosage can be reduced to every other day, or even every 3rd day. The dose can be titrated up or down depending on clinical response and side effect profile.[1] The drug may be more effective for controlling esotropia when dosed in the morning, but dosing in the evening may reduce side effects.

If no response is measurable in 2-3 weeks, increase dosing to twice a day. Cease treatment if there is no improvement after a few more weeks at this dosage.

- Side effects:
  - Iris cysts—occurs in 20%-50% of children, usually within 2-40 weeks. Clinicians should monitor for iris cysts at the slit lamp or in the retinoscopy streak at each follow-up appointment when children are using echothiophate. The cysts are not typically visually significant and usually resolve with discontinuation of the echothiophate. The addition of phenylephrine 2.5% daily reduces the incidence of iris cysts.
  - Brow ache—usually subsides after a few days or if dosed at bedtime.
  - Lens opacities.
  - Angle closure glaucoma (very rare).
  - Impaired dark adaptation.
  - Induced myopia.
  - Gastrointestinal hypermotility symptoms.
- Contraindications—uveitis.

Echothiophate iodide depletes cholinesterase from the blood, increasing the patient's susceptibility to the effects of depolarizing muscle relaxants, such as succinylcholine. Advise anesthesia team of usage, consider non-depolarizing agents or discontinue echothiophate 6 weeks prior to general anesthesia.

CYCLOPLEGICS (ATROPINE SULFATE [0.5-1%] AND HOMATROPINE [5%])

These medications can be used to treat accommodative spasm (spasm of the near synkinetic reflex). The diagnosis of accommodative spasm/induced overconvergence is usually made clinically. Signs of accommodative spasm include acute esotropia with or without diplopia, accompanied by miosis of the pupils, and a myopic shift in refractive error.

The two most common etiologies of accommodative spasm are functional, often in association with anxiety and emotional distress, or organic, with underlying head trauma or neurologic disease.

- Mechanism of action—Atropine and homatropine are anticholinergic/antimuscarinic agents that block the effects of acetylcholine leading to relaxation of the ciliary muscle (accommodation), and inhibition of the pupillary sphincter fibers (mydriasis).
- Indications:
  - Blocking or relaxing accommodation in treating accommodative spasm.
  - Inhibiting accommodation (cycloplegia) to allow accurate measurement of refractive error or for amblyopia treatment.

Recently, low dose atropine (0.01% or 0.05%) has been used off-label in children from 6-12 years of age whose myopia is increasing more than 1.0D a year to prevent myopic progression.[3,4]

- Dosage:
  - Accommodative spasm—Instill 1 drop of atropine 1% to both eyes twice a day (with plus lenses) until symptoms resolve.
  - Atropine refraction—Instill 1 drop of atropine 1% to both eyes twice daily for 3 days before and on the day of refraction.
- Side effects:
  - Eyelid edema or dermatitis.
  - Blurred vision.
  - Prolonged mydriasis/photophobia.
  - Confusion/delirium.
  - Dry mouth.
  - Tachycardia and ventricular or supraventricular fibrillation—rare.
  - Anaphylaxis—rare.

If a severe adverse reaction is encountered, use physostigmine (0.02 mg/kg IM or IV).

ONABOTULINUM TOXIN A (BOTOX/BTX)

In the early 1980's, Alan Scott, MD, isolated, purified, and demonstrated effective, safe usage of botulinum toxin A (Botox) to treat strabismus.[5,6]

- Mechanism of action—Botulinum toxin acts by binding presynaptically to high-affinity sites on the cholinergic nerve terminals, blocking the release of acetylcholine, causing a neuromuscular blocking effect that causes a weakening of the muscle.

Botox has a temporary effect that usually lasts 3-4 months. It takes 24-48 hours to see clinically evident paresis. Half of the patients treated with Botox for strabismus will require repeat injections.[6-8]

- Indications:
  - Paralytic strabismus (most commonly CN VI palsy).
  - Infantile esotropia (usually bilateral).[9]
  - Comitant strabismus (exotropia, late-onset esotropia).
  - Thyroid eye disease/endocrine myopathies.
  - Postoperative overcorrections or undercorrections.
  - Acquired nystagmus/oscillopsia.
  - Post-retinal detachment strabismus (scleral buckle).
- Contraindications:
  - Not usually useful in chronic or complete palsies.
  - Not for exceedingly tight or inelastic/fibrotic conditions.
  - Relative contraindication to inferior oblique injection due to spread to the inferior rectus.
- Dosage for EOM injection:
  - Initial dosing starts at 1.25-2.5 units per muscle, escalating to 5.0-10.0 units per muscle (depending on clinical response).
  - No more than 25 units per muscle is recommended.
  - Dilution of the 100 units vial with 4.0 mL of NaCl (0.9%) results in 2.5 units/0.1 cc of Botox. The mixture should be gently swirled, not shaken, and should be used within a few hours of reconstitution.

VIDEO

- Procedure for muscle injection using electromyography (EMG) guidance (Videos 55.1 and 55.2).
    - Anesthetize the eye with a local anesthetic drop then place a cotton swab soaked in lidocaine 4% over the muscle to be injected.
    - Place a drop of betadine and phenylephrine 2.5% in the eye.
    - Connect the patient to the EMG device with a central forehead (glabellar) electrode.
    - Insert eyelid speculum.
    - Connect the EMG adapted needle to a 1- or 3-cc syringe containing the solution at the desired concentration (see above for dosages).
    - Instruct the patient to look away from the injection site.
    - Hold the syringe such that the plunger is easily accessible for injection.
    - Pass the needle, transconjunctivally, in a flat, tangential direction posteriorly over the equatorial region of the desired muscle with the bevel directed down, then redirect the needle in a retrobulbar direction and slowly advance the tip into the muscle belly.
    - Direct the patient to look slowly toward the needle to stimulate the muscle in its field of action in order to elicit a waveform or a static-type noise from the EMG device. If no response is detected, reposition the needle more acutely or advance more posteriorly.
    - Once the proper location is determined, gently depress the plunger to deliver the Botox.
    - Carefully remove the needle straight outward and apply mild pressure if needed.

Some clinicians keep the needle tip in place for 20-30 seconds to minimize the spread of drug to surrounding tissues.

- Procedure for muscle injection in OR without EMG guidance:
    - Use desired anesthesia (general, peribulbar, retrobulbar, or topical) (see Chapter 42).
    - Insert eyelid speculum and place a drop of phenylephrine 2.5% in the eye.
    - Optional: Make a conjunctival incision and expose the muscle (see Chapter 43).
    - Grasp the muscle belly with conjunctival or Mendonca forceps posterior to the insertion and rotate the eye to expose the muscle being injected.
    - Pass the 27G needle bevel down on an insulin syringe through the grasped tendon and rotate the eye back to the straight position, introducing the needle 5-10 mm in a direction parallel with the orbital wall. Slowly inject the desired dosage of drug. Observe a wheal form within the muscle as the medication is injected. Carefully remove the needle. Rinse the area with BSS to prevent inadvertent spread of the medication.

The absence of ballooning of the conjunctiva or Tenon's signifies drug entry into the muscle belly.

    - Optional: Sit the patient up or elevate the head immediately to reduce potential spread into the upper lid.
- Side effects:
    - Ptosis (16%).
    - Induced vertical strabismus (16.5%).
    - Transient diplopia.
    - Overcorrections or undercorrections—common.

  - Retrobulbar hemorrhage—rare.
  - Globe perforation—rare.
- Special considerations:
  - Oscillopsia/intractable nystagmus can be treated with a retrobulbar BTX injection. Usually 15-20 units are injected in 1 cc. A unilateral approach is recommended to reduce risk and to judge the effects. Expect ptosis.
  - Botox can be used to induce a complete ptosis intentionally by injecting 5-10 units in the levator muscle if diplopia is intractable or corneal exposure is threatening the globe (see Chapter 35).
  - Botox can be used simultaneously with bupivacaine (BPX) as an adjuvant to strabismus treatment (see below).

BUPIVACAINE (BPX)

When BPX is injected into the muscle body, it causes a myotoxic degeneration within the myofibrils, followed by regeneration and hypertrophy. This results in a reduction in muscle length and strengthening of the muscle. BPX injection causes an initial paralytic strabismus that turns into a restrictive strabismus (causing a "reversing hypertropia") when an extraocular muscle is inadvertently injected during peribulbar or retrobulbar anesthesia administration. BPX can also be intentionally injected into a muscle to strengthen the muscle and treat strabismus. This effect has been reported to last up to 3-5 years.[10,11]

- Mechanism of action:
  - Initial short-acting paralytic effect secondary to myotoxicity.
  - A sarcomere remodeling process occurs within 2-4 weeks that leads to hypertrophy and shortening of the muscle.
  - Expect 10-20 PD of correction.
- Indications:
  - Comitant, horizontal, strabismus (<20 PD).
  - Nonparalytic strabismus where surgery is contraindicated.
  - Convergence insufficiency exotropia.[12]
- Dosage:
  - 2-4 cc of BPX 0.75-3.0% is injected into the body of the muscle, preferably under EMG guidance. Nonstandard concentrations can be obtained through compounding pharmacies.
  - BPX is most effective when injected into the most posterior one-third of the muscle.
  - The effect is dose and volume related. BPX can be repeated, at graduated concentrations or increased volumes to augment the effects.
  - BPX can be mixed with epinephrine to enhance the effect.
  - BPX can be used in conjunction with BTX to the antagonist muscle.[13]
- Procedure: Same as procedure for injecting Botox under EMG guidance (see above) (Videos 55.1 and 55.3).
- Side effects:
  - Subconjunctival hemorrhage.
  - Spread to other muscles causing strabismus and/or ptosis.
  - Failure to place BPX in the muscle body.
  - Retrobulbar hemorrhage—rare.
  - Globe perforation—rare.
  - Oculocardiac reflex (bradycardia)—rare.

SYSTEMIC TREATMENTS

Medications such as clonazepam, gabapentin, memantine, baclofen, and others have shown inhibitory effects in controlling certain types of nystagmus. However, it is recommended that usage of these drugs to treat nystagmus be done in consultation with a neurologist, or other health care professionals familiar with the disease process, as well medication dosages and side effects.

References

1. Lueder GT, ed. *Basic and Clinical Science Course. Section 6: Pediatric Ophthalmology and Strabismus*. Italy, ITA: American Academy of Ophthalmology; 2014.
2. Von Noorden GK, Campos E. *Binocular Vision and Ocular Motility: Theory and Management of Strabismus*. 6th ed. St. Louis, MO: Mosby; 2005.
3. Chua W-H, Balakrishnan V, Chan Y-H, Tong L, Ling Y, Quah B-L, Tan D. Atropine for the Treatment of Childhood Myopia. *Ophthalmology*. 2006;113:2285-2291.
4. Chia A, Chua W-H, Wen L, Fong A, Goon YY, Tan D. Atropine for the Treatment of Childhood Myopia: 0.01%, 0.1% and 0.5%. *Am J Ophthalmol*. 2014:157:451-457.
5. Scott AB. Botulinum toxin injection into extra ocular muscles as an alternative to strabismus surgery. *J Pediatr Ophthalmol Strabismus*. 1980;17:21-25.
6. Scott AB. Botulinum toxin injection of eye muscles to correct strabismus. *Trans Am Ophthalmol Soc*. 1981;79:734-770.
7. Coats DK, Olitsky SE. Chapter 16. The use of botulinum neurotoxin in the treatment of strabismus. In: *Strabismus Surgery and its Complications*. Berlin, Heidelberg: Springer; 2007.
8. Lionel K, Wong E, Yahalom C. Botulinum toxin in the treatment of strabismus. A review of its use and effects. *Disabil Rehabil*. 2007;29(23):1823-1831.
9. de Alba Campomanes AG, Binenbaum G, Eguiarte GC. Comparison of botulinum toxin with surgery as primary treatment for infantile esotropia. *J AAPOS*. 2010;14(2):111-116.
10. Miller JM, Scott AB, Dahn KK, et al. Bupivacaine injection remodels extraocular muscles and corrects comitant strabismus. *Ophthalmology*. 2013;120(12):2733-2740.
11. Scott AB, Miller JM, Shieh KR. Bupivacaine injection of the lateral rectus muscle to treat esotropia. *J AAPOS*. 2009;13(2):119-122.
12. Josephson M, Mathias SA. Treatment of intermittent exotropia of the convergence insufficiency type with bupivacaine 0.75%: 5-year experience and outcomes. *J Binocul Vis Ocul Motil*. 2019;69(1):3-7.
13. Scott AB, Miller JM, Shieh KR. Treating strabismus by injecting the agonist muscle with bupivacaine and the antagonist with botulinum toxin. *Trans Am Ophthalmol Soc*. 2009;107:104-9.

CHAPTER 56

Sensorimotor Considerations for Strabismus Surgery

Namita Kashyap, CO

PRE- AND POSTOPERATIVE SENSORIMOTOR MANAGEMENT

Ocular misalignment, diplopia, and/or visual confusion can occur for many reasons pre- and postoperatively and need to be addressed accordingly. The management of sensorimotor misalignment depends on the degree of symptoms and the extent of the ocular deviation. Diplopia following eye muscle surgery usually resolves without intervention within 1-6 weeks, and no treatment is required. However, if it persists beyond 4-6 weeks, or is particularly troubling to the patient treatment is typically recommended.

Optical Manipulation—Pediatric

For overcorrection or undercorrection of deviation after strabismus surgery, lenses can be prescribed to manipulate the angle of deviation (Table 56.1).

TABLE 56.1. Optical manipulations for postsurgical strabismus in pediatric patients

Preoperative deviation	Postoperative deviation	Optical manipulation
	Overcorrections	
Esotropia	Exotropia	Cut plus or add minus
Exotropia	Esotropia	Increase plus or reduce minus[a]
	Undercorrections	
Esotropia	Esotropia	Increase plus or reduce minus[a]
Exotropia	Exotropia	Cut plus or add minus

[a]For esotropia at near with a high accommodative convergence to accommodation ratio, consider a bifocal. Bifocal power should be the minimal amount necessary to control the ocular misalignment and promote fusion and binocularity.

Optical Manipulation—Adult

- Monovision can be attempted for older adults with diplopia. This can be particularly helpful in cases of strabismus where there is inability to fuse centrally or peripherally (eg, epiretinal membrane (ERM), retinal detachment (RD), or macular hole causing central vision disruption).
- Trial lenses in clinic are useful to decide which eye is best for distance/near and to determine which lens will blur enough to eliminate diplopia.
- Prism can be combined with monovision to produce the best results.

Fresnel Prisms

Postoperative over- or undercorrections—Fresnel press-on prisms (Fresnel Prism & Lens Co., Bloomington, MN) are useful in instances of over- or undercorrection to eliminate diplopia and encourage binocularity. These temporary "stick-ons" are preferable to ground in prism, especially postoperatively, due to the ease of changing prism amounts as needed during the healing process.

- Apply Fresnel prism to the inside of the glasses/sunglasses (Fig. 56.1). Plano lenses can be used if prescription glasses are not available and/or needed. The lines on the press on-prism will be oriented 90 degrees away from the base (ie, vertical lines for horizontal prism and vice versa).
- Aim to wean down the power of prism slowly. Initially, try the least amount of prism that will eliminate diplopia and provide comfort. Allow time for development of fusional amplitudes.
- Monitor and measure alignment at subsequent visits and adjust the Fresnel prism power as needed. Prism can be ground into spectacle lenses once stability of deviation has been established, and further reduction of power is not possible.

Press-on prisms can be used preoperatively to alleviate diplopia and can be worn up until day of surgery.

The prism adaptation test (PAT) is a diagnostic tool used preoperatively to determine the potential for fusion/stereopsis as well as to elicit the maximum angle of deviation.[1] PAT is done preoperatively by measuring the angle of deviation and correcting it with the corresponding prism. Prism adaptation can be done in office, or the patient can be sent home with a Fresnel prism mounted on glasses, for remeasurement in 1-2 weeks. This is repeated until the maximum angle of deviation is elicited. PAT is particularly useful for cases of acquired esotropia.

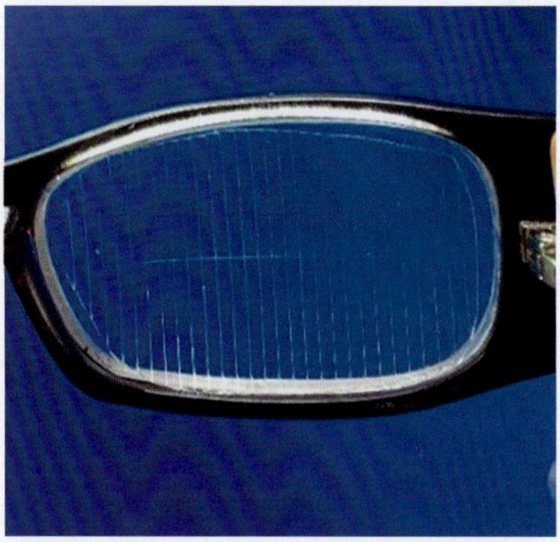

FIGURE 56.1. Horizontal Fresnel prism. The prism/foil should be cut 1 mm inside the edge of the lens and applied with 1-2 drops of rubbing alcohol. Squeeze out any trapped air bubbles. Trapped air/lint can cause significant blur, glare, and discomfort for the patient.

Fresnel prisms cause optical blur (increased power = increased blur).[2] They are best applied to the non-dominant eye. Test in office by holding prism in front of either eye to determine which is least blurry.

Retinal pathology—Fresnel prisms are also useful tools to eliminate diplopia for central image distortion in one eye. Diplopia caused by retina pathology (RD, ERM, macular hole/dragging), often presents with a small angle deviation (or no deviation) and an inability to fuse centrally. The Fresnel prism's purpose, in this case, is twofold: aligning the deviation and causing optical blur to create central suppression in one eye.[2]

- Apply the Fresnel prism over lens of the eye with retinal pathology and/or distorted vision.
- Do not grind in prism as the blurring effect will be lost, and the diplopia will return.

Ground-in Prism

Diplopia caused by a high degree of anisometropia (eg, following cataract surgery) induces prismatic effect between the eyes leading to diplopia when reading. This is usually vertical diplopia and may be correctable with "slab-off" prism (a small base down prism is added to the reading segment of the lens). Prism is added to the more minus or less plus lens with a line bifocal. Slab-off prism cannot be added to progressive add lenses.

Patients with a nervous system disorder that affects movement (eg, Parkinson disease, multiple sclerosis) often have different angles of deviation at distance and near; hence, separate readers and distance glasses with ground in prism are recommended. Try a Fresnel prism first to establish stability before grinding prism into glasses. Computer glasses may not work well for these patients as trying to adjust for the correct viewing distance is difficult due to their limited mobility.

The greatest amount of prism that can be comfortably ground in spectacles is about 10-12 prism diopters.

Blurring Options

- Blurring options may be required when prisms and optical manipulation do not correct diplopia.[3]
- Bangerter occlusion foils (Fresnel Prism & Lens Co., Bloomington, MN) are useful in cases of diplopia caused by ERM, macular hole, and/or fixation switch diplopia (Fig. 56.2). If a foil is not available, Scotch "magic" tape (Scotch brand by 3M, United States) works well for occlusion. Foils eliminate diplopia caused by central vision distortion (ERM or macular hole) or inability to fuse for any reason, by blurring visual acuity and encouraging suppression.

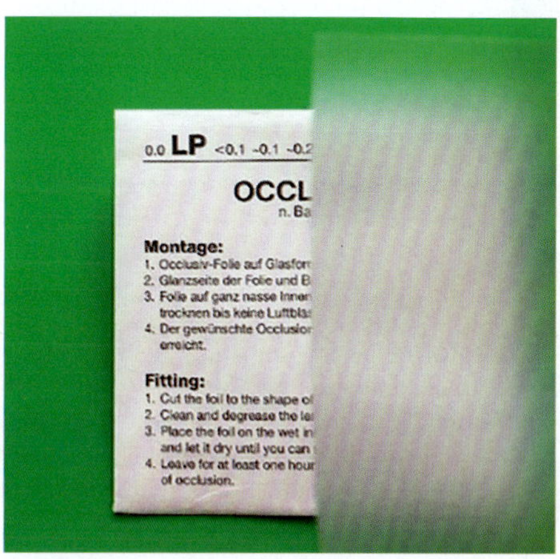

FIGURE 56.2. Light perception Bangerter foil. Bangerter foils are a series of graded vinyl sheets that can be cut to fit the inside of lenses and come in different blurring options ranging from total occlusion to 20/20.

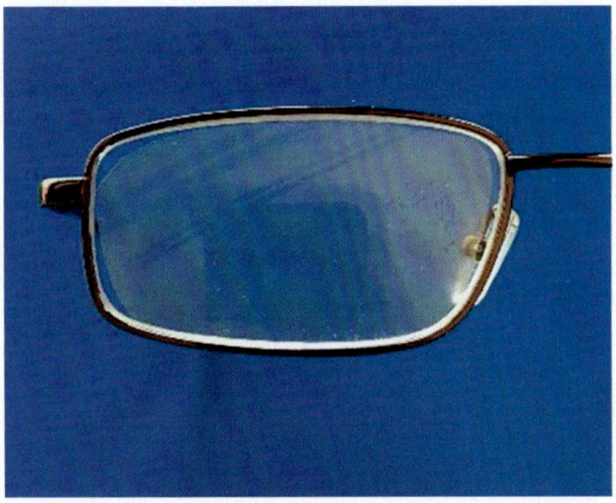

FIGURE 56.3. Bangerter foil mounted on entire lens.

- Different grades of foils can be selected depending on the amount of blur required.
- Foils can be mounted on the entire lens or cut to fit the distance or the reading segment (Fig. 56.3).
- A central occlusion foil (aka "Hoxie" spot) is a small piece of Bangerter foil cut and mounted to a specific position on the lens in order to create central suppression of one eye (Fig. 56.4).
- A "Hoxie" spot is usually placed in front of the eye with the vision distortion and should be positioned carefully on the lens to block the distorted central vision of the affected eye (Fig. 56.4).
- Fixation switch diplopia occurs when the nondominant eye has better vision in the presence of strabismus; this is essentially treated by occluding one eye—use the least "fogging" foil to provide comfort and eliminate diplopia.
- In some instances, prism correction in addition to a Bangerter foil is needed.[4] See also optical manipulation and Fresnel prism above for alternate blurring options.
- Further strabismus surgery may be required in some cases, especially if there is a large residual or consecutive angle of deviation, significant torsion, or if the prism is too large to grind into spectacles.

Computer Orthoptic Exercises

Computer orthoptic exercises can be implemented for small angle deviations that would benefit from improving fusional amplitudes. Binocular function is necessary for this form of treatment. The program can be purchased online and performed at home.

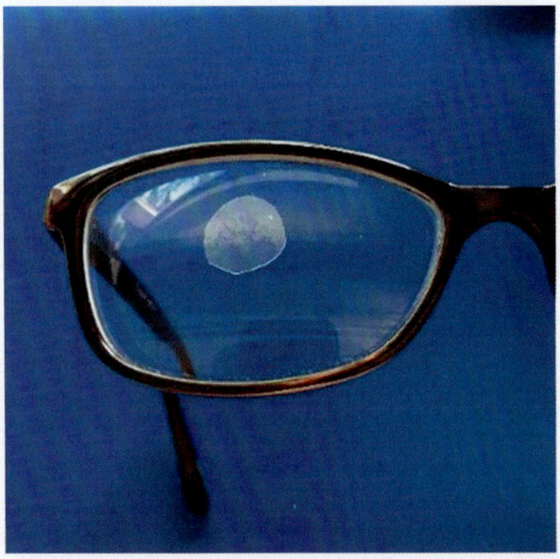

FIGURE 56.4. Central occlusion foil "Hoxie" spot. Cut out a Bangerter occlusion foil (slightly smaller than a dime size) and apply centrally to lens. The Hoxie spot needs to be positioned carefully in order to occlude central vision only. It can be positioned for distance or on the reading segment.

References

1. Velez FG, Rosenbaum AL. Preoperative prism adaptation for acquired esotropia: long-term results. *J AAPOS*. 2002;6(3):168-173.
2. Véronneau-Troutman S. Fresnel prisms and their effects on visual acuity and binocularity. *Trans Am Ophthalmol Soc*. 1978;76:610-653.
3. Kushner BJ. Intractable diplopia after strabismus surgery in adults. *Arch Ophthalmol*. 2002;120(11):1498-1504.
4. Iacobucci IL, Furr BA, Archer SM. Management of binocular diplopia due to maculopathy with combined bangerter filter and fresnel prism. *Am Orthoptic J*. 2009;59(1):93-97.

CHAPTER 57

Imaging in Strabismus

Mays A. El-Dairi, MD

DIAGNOSTIC CONSIDERATIONS

Strabismus is a common presentation for intracranial pathology. Before deciding on surgery in strabismus, it is important to rule out an active neurological cause and manage it. Below is an overview of the indications and type of neuroimaging to consider before strabismus surgery. Additionally, imaging modalities such as UBM, AS-OCT, and MRI may also play a role in identifying the location of extraocular muscle insertions and the presence of a slipped muscle in reoperations.

INDICATIONS FOR IMAGING

Apparent Congenital Strabismus

- **Esotropia:** Neuroimaging is indicated in patients with the following findings:
  - Abduction deficit.
  - Facial palsy (rule out Moebius syndrome or brainstem abnormality)
  - Optic neuropathy.

A mild duction lag in an infant is very difficult to see on simple duction testing. Check duction lag monocularly using a patch and doll's head maneuver, and/or check saccades with an OKN drum.

Bilateral partial facial palsies are difficult to see in an infant. Check for decreased facial expressions. If an infant's facial expressions are less animated than the parents, consider hypotonia or facial palsy.

- **Exotropia:** The presence of a vertical component, ptosis, or anisocoria should alert the examiner to the possibility of a third cranial nerve palsy. A mild third nerve palsy in a child can present with intermittent fusion giving the false diagnosis of intermittent exotropia. Children with a homonymous visual field defect will frequently develop an intermittent or constant exotropia that enlarges their functional field. Pediatric patients with exotropia should have careful visual acuity and visual field testing (Fig. 57.1). Consider formal visual fields testing and OCT if visual acuity is not normal. The presence of a visual field deficit or optic neuropathy should warrant neuroimaging.

A

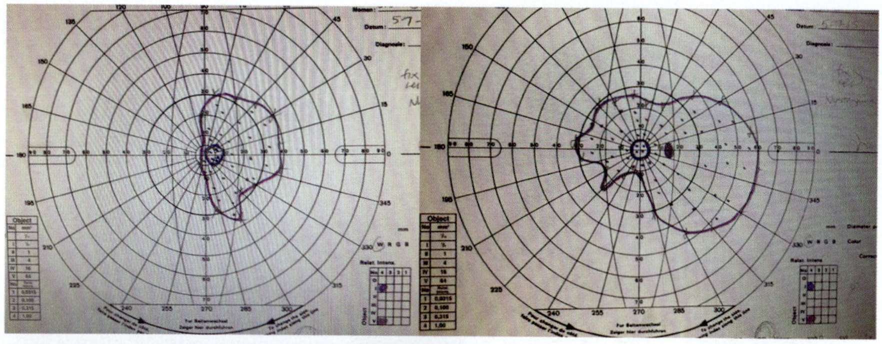

B

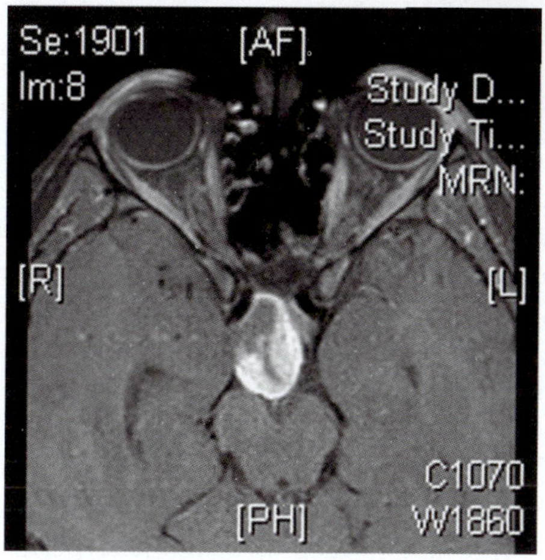

FIGURE 57.1. A, B. A 6-year-old boy with a long-standing history of intermittent exotropia presented with worsening control of his eye alignment. His visual acuity was 20/50 OD and 20/30 OS. Dilated fundus examination was notable for mild bilateral optic nerve pallor. Figure **A** shows a left homonymous hemianopia. Figure **B** is his MRI imaging which revealed a lobulated mass lesion involving the optic chiasm, right greater than left extending along bilateral optic pathways (Courtesy of Tammy Yanovitch, MD MHSc).

> **Check visual fields monocularly in all patients with exotropia, use saccades to check for duction lag, perform prism alternate cover testing in the six cardinal positions of gaze, and look for fundus torsion on examination. A bilateral fourth nerve palsy may look like a V-pattern esotropia (see below).**

- **Fourth nerve palsy:** Imaging is indicated if bilateral or associated with other findings. In the case of a bilateral fourth nerve palsy (V-pattern esotropia with alternating hypertropia and bilateral fundus excyclotorsion), pay special attention to the fourth ventricle. Fourth nerve palsy with a contralateral Horner syndrome is suggestive of a central fourth nerve palsy (see below). A typical isolated fourth nerve palsy with a large vertical fusional amplitude, inferior oblique overaction, and facial asymmetry does not warrant imaging even if noted later in life as these findings indicate that the etiology is likely congenital.
- **Apparent congenital nystagmus:** Poor vision could be from retina pathology (consider OCT and/or ERG). Neuroimaging is indicated if there is an optic neuropathy, or vision is poor and decreased visual acuity cannot be explained by eye examination findings and/or ERG and OCT results.

Acquired Strabismus

- **Trauma:** Image if suspect orbital or intracranial pathology that requires intervention (orbital fracture, hemorrhage, or entrapment). Strabismus surgery should be delayed until full possible recovery (at least 6 months) unless there is entrapment of an extraocular muscle.

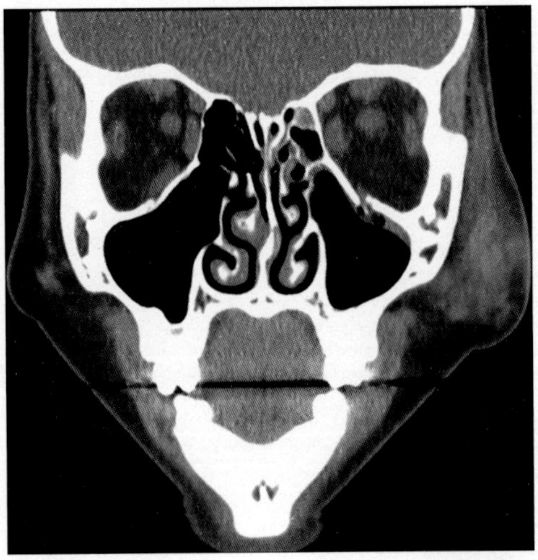

FIGURE 57.2. CT scan of the orbits, coronal view. Soft tissue window. There is a minimally displaced "trap-door" or "greenstick" fracture of the left orbital floor. The left inferior rectus is only minimally visualized in this image, as it is caught within the bony fracture and likely compressed at this level. Comparison can be made to the right orbit with the inferior rectus muscle running above the orbital floor (Courtesy of Jason Liss, MD).

Children are at particular risk of muscle entrapment with inferior orbital wall fractures because their orbital floor is more apt to greenstick and then bounce back ("trap-door fracture"), entrapping the inferior rectus muscle (Fig. 57.2). They may present with a "white-eyed blow-out fracture" (history of trauma with little evidence of soft tissue injury). Nausea and vomiting are common with this type of fracture, and their association with limitation to elevation should make one very suspicious of muscle entrapment.

- **Acute peripheral cranial mononeuropathy (isolated):** An isolated cranial neuropathy in a patient with vasculopathic risk factors such as systemic hypertension, diabetes mellitus, cigarette smoking, hyperlipidemia, and radiation injury is probably ischemic and does not require neuroimaging *acutely* (reminder: ask giant cell arteritis [GCA] symptoms and check erythrocyte sedimentation rate [ESR], C-reactive protein [CRP] if GCA is suspected). However, the patient should be seen again in 3-4 weeks, and imaged if no improvement of motility examination and duction lag.

In a patient with an acute isolated mononeuropathy, neuroimaging studies should be performed if the patient is younger than 50, has a history of any type of cancer, or has evidence of multiple cranial neuropathies or additional neurologic dysfunction.

- **Third nerve palsy:**
  - An ischemic third nerve palsy is usually complete (eyelid, supraduction, adduction, and infraduction are involved) and pupillary sparing. Given that a third nerve palsy can be caused by a life-threatening aneurysm, some physicians would order vascular neuroimaging acutely regardless of the pattern of involvement. If no vascular neuroimaging is performed, the patient should be examined weekly until improvement is seen.
  - If third nerve palsy is incomplete and/or pupillary involving, the cause is compressive until proven otherwise. Vascular neuroimaging (CTA) is recommended STAT to rule out aneurysm. If CTA is normal, obtain MRI/MRA brain and orbits with contrast.
- **Brainstem patterns:** If the motility pattern localizes to a nucleus rather than peripheral nerve, imaging of brainstem is recommended STAT. Specific patterns include:
  - Central third nerve palsy: Inferior division CN III palsy with contralateral supraduction lag, with or without ptosis is suggestive of a nuclear third nerve palsy. Neuroimaging is indicated with special attention to midbrain.

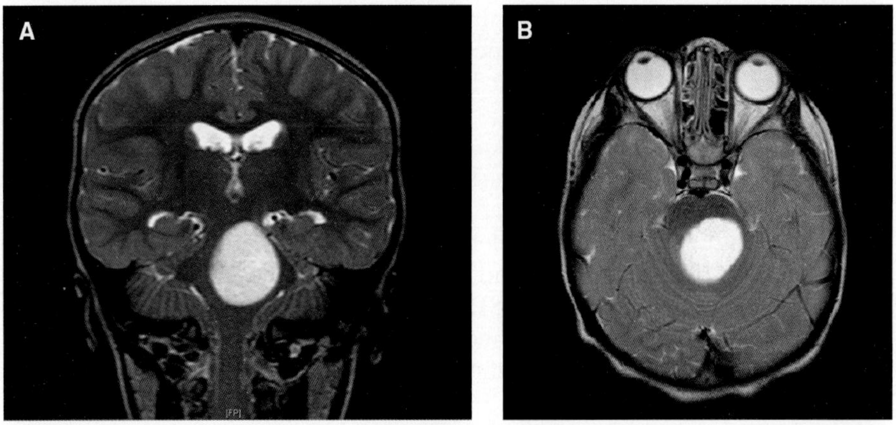

FIGURE 57.3. A, B. A 2½-year-old boy presented with a 1-year history of eye crossing and anomalous head posture. Examination revealed 25 prism diopters of left esotropia worse in left gaze with an anomalous head turn to the right. He had a –2 abduction deficit of the left eye. MRI imaging showed a well-defined mildly lobulated mass arising from the posterior aspect of the pons, slightly more toward the left and compressing the fourth ventricle (Courtesy of Tammy Yanovitch, MD MHSc).

  - **Central fourth nerve palsy:** An acute fourth nerve palsy associated with a contralateral Horner syndrome is suggestive of a central fourth nerve palsy, and brainstem (midbrain/pons) imaging is recommended.
  - **Central sixth nerve palsy:** Pattern consistent with gaze palsy rather than the isolated abduction deficit seen in peripheral sixth nerve palsy. May be associated with facial palsy. Neuroimaging is indicated with special attention to pons (Fig. 57.3A and B).
  - **Skew deviation:** Acquired vertical deviation that can be comitant or incomitant and may be associated with torsional problems including "ocular tilt reaction" (binocular torsion, torticollis, and a tilt in the subjective visual vertical). In skew deviations, the eye torts in same direction as head tilt rather than in the normal compensatory direction away from head tilt. In skew deviations, the deviation improves significantly in the supine position (upright-supine test). Torsion and upright-supine test help distinguish a skew deviation from a fourth nerve palsy. Skew deviations may have pseudoptosis of the hypertropic eye and can be mistaken for partial third nerve palsy. Normal levator function and normal vertical saccades distinguish a skew from a partial third nerve palsy. Patients with skew deviation almost always have diplopia and other signs of brainstem and cerebellar dysfunction. Neuroimaging is indicated with special attention to brainstem.
  - **Internuclear ophthalmoplegia:** Adduction deficit with abducting nystagmus in the contralateral eye. Usually associated with a skew deviation. Also can be mistaken for partial third nerve palsy (check levator function and vertical saccades). Neuroimaging is indicated with special attention to brainstem.
- **Acute comitant esotropia:** Although the most common cause is accommodative, an acute comitant esotropia that cannot be explained or treated with refraction requires neuroimaging to rule out a thalamic or brainstem tumor.
- **Multiple cranial neuropathies:** Location could be brainstem, cavernous sinus, orbital apex, or orbit. All require neuroimaging.

Chronic Strabismus in an Older Child or Adult

- **Bilateral external ophthalmoplegia:** Saccades will be normal in a restrictive process (thyroid eye disease: make sure you rule out a compressive optic neuropathy). If saccades are decreased, neuroimaging is indicated to rule out a bilateral orbital or cavernous sinus pathology. Chronic progressive external ophthalmoplegia will be associated with diffuse thinning of the extraocular muscles (EOM) on MRI. Chronic myasthenia gravis is also associated with thin EOM on MRI. Other diagnoses to consider if acute include Miller Fisher (Guillain Barré) syndrome, botulinum toxicity, and Whipple disease.

- **Divergence insufficiency:** An esotropia that is worse for distance than near needs neuroimaging to rule out a bilateral sixth nerve palsy. Lumbar puncture can be considered if there are other signs of elevated intracranial pressure (ICP). A small comitant esotropia in an elderly (>75 years) is not uncommon and can be observed carefully for a few weeks and treated with prisms or surgery if stable.
- **Heavy eye syndrome (HES):** Usually adults older than 50 years old. High axial myopia. Pattern: Esotropia and limited abduction due to superotemporal globe shift relative to the extraocular muscles. Orbital imaging shows the displacement of the EOM.
- **Sagging eye syndrome (SES):** Older patients (>50 years) myopic or nonmyopic. Pattern: Distance esotropia and cyclovertical strabismus with limited supraduction due to lateral rectus muscle inferior displacement. Patients typically have bilateral ptosis with high lid creases and deep orbital sulci. Orbital imaging shows the displacement of the EOM.

MRI enables differentiation between HES and SES in myopic patients. HES shows a larger angle between the lateral rectus and superior rectus and also shows superotemporal prolapse of the globe.

- **Silent sinus syndrome:** Hypoglobus and collapse of the orbital floor due to opacification of the maxillary sinus from a chronic maxillary sinusitis. Orbital imaging shows thinning of inferior orbital wall with sagging of the globe.

Variable Strabismus

- Myasthenia gravis is always on the differential diagnosis of any type of strabismus and should be investigated if there is variability during the examination or on follow-up. The blood panel has poor sensitivity (<50%) despite high specificity. Single fiber EMG is more sensitive but cannot be obtained in children so the motility examination is used for diagnosis and treatment monitoring. The aim of treatment in ocular myasthenia is to stabilize the strabismus rather than to completely eliminate it. EOM atrophy can be seen in chronic severe myasthenia that will not respond to medical treatment and would eventually need EOM surgery (strabismus needs to be stable >6 months).
- Thyroid eye disease (TED) is a common cause of variable strabismus (especially incomitant vertical deviations and esotropia) in adults. The diagnosis is usually made clinically, but orbital imaging (CT or MRI) can be particularly helpful in atypical cases (eg, unilateral cases) and to rule out other disorders in the differential diagnosis (eg, orbital inflammatory disease). In TED, the extraocular muscle belly is enlarged with sparing of the tendons (Fig. 57.4A and B). The inferior and medial rectus muscles are most commonly affected, followed by the superior and lateral rectus muscles, and rarely oblique muscles. Involvement is usually bilateral but may be asymmetric.

Strabismus Reoperations

Both wide-field UBM and AS-OCT provide reasonable estimates of EOM insertion distance from the limbus. In addition, MRI can be used to detect slipped muscles, in which case the distance from the limbus to the muscle is significantly increased compared with recessed muscles and recessed muscles with stretched scar.

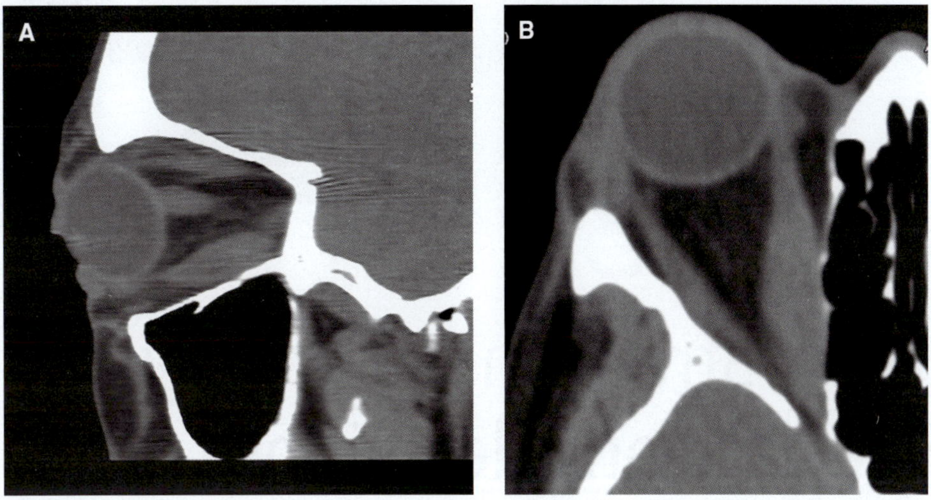

FIGURE 57.4. Note the enlargement of the muscle belly with sparing of the tendon in the inferior **(A)** and medial **(B)** recti of this patient with TED (Courtesy of Michelle Cabrera, MD).

Suggested Readings

Clark RA. Orbital imaging in strabismus. *J Binocul Vis Ocul Motil*. 2018;68(3):87-98.

Sargent J, Miller NR, Newman NJ. *Walsh and Hoyt's Clinical Neuro-Ophthalmology*. 6th ed. Philadelphia, PA: Lippincott Williams & Wilkins; 2005.

Shuan D, Kraft SP, Smith DR, et al. Ultrasound biomicroscopy in strabismus reoperations. *J AAPOS*. 2006;10(3):202-205.

Siakallis LC, Uddin JM, Miszkiel KA. Imaging investigation of thyroid eye disease. *Ophthalmic Plast Reconstr Surg*. 2018;34(4S suppl 1):S41-S51.

Wei LA, Durairaj VD. Pediatric orbital floor fractures. *J AAPOS*. 2011;15(2):173-180.

Wong AM. Understanding skew deviation and a new clinical test to differentiate it from trochlear nerve palsy. *J AAPOS*. 2010;14(1):61-67.

CHAPTER 58

Adult Strabismus Surgery: Special Considerations

Matthew D. Gearinger, MD

PREOPERATIVE CONSIDERATIONS

Adult strabismus patients are more likely to have had prior ocular surgery and experience diplopia than pediatric patients. In addition, many adult patients will have incomitant strabismus as a result of neurologic disease or orbital processes and may have limited improvement with prism.

Patient Expectations

It is important to establish appropriate expectations of outcomes prior to surgery. The following indications may be improved in adults with strabismus:

- Diplopia: An appropriate surgical goal is to create a large area of single binocular vision surrounding primary position and downgaze. Patients should be counseled preoperatively if there is a reasonable expectation of postoperative diplopia in eccentric gaze. A secondary goal is to reduce incomitance and the angle of strabismus to allow use of prism spectacles to create a large field of single binocular vision.
- Anomalous head position: Adults with strabismus or nystagmus may adopt a face turn or head tilt to improve ocular alignment or to utilize a null-point. Strabismus surgery can be performed to improve head position and visual functioning.
- Cosmesis/Reconstruction: Unfortunately, many adult patients with strabismus have been counseled by their primary physicians and eye care providers that strabismus surgery is not possible. These patients can suffer from poor self-esteem, employment bias, and social anxiety. Strabismus surgery can restore physical appearance and improve binocularity.

Latent Hyperopia

Prepresbyopic patients with latent hyperopia may develop asthenopia or manifest strabismus with diplopia similar to accommodative esotropia. A cycloplegic refraction can be useful to determine if the patient has been chronically over-minused or can accept a more hyperopic correction.

Role of Imaging

Adult-onset strabismus may be due to cranial neuropathy or orbital processes, (including myopathy, slipped muscle, mass, or anomalies of the pulleys and intramuscular septum). Direct communication with the radiologist including the likely localization of pathology can improve diagnostic yield. Personal review of the images can help surgical planning (see Chapter 57).

Anomalous Retinal Correspondence

Adults with long-standing strabismus since childhood may have anomalous retinal correspondence (ARC) and experience diplopia postoperatively with good motor alignment. An indication of ARC is if diplopia persists when a prism is used to neutralize the deviation. This test can be augmented by using a red filter over the fixating eye in a darkened room. If ARC is present preoperatively, a trial with a temporary prism that simulates motor alignment can determine if the ARC can be overcome before performing surgery.

Torsion

Patients may be unable to fuse despite the correction of their horizontal and vertical angles. This may be due to torsion, aniseikonia, macular pathology, or central disruption of fusion after head injury. The presence of torsion can be determined by using the double Maddox rod test. A synoptophore can allow torsional correction of images to see if sensory fusion is possible in these cases.

Surgical Planning

In patients who have had prior surgery, it is helpful to review any prior operative notes to determine the current location of the extraocular muscles and any prior complications. When operative notes are not available, the locations of conjunctival scars (sometimes elicited with a cotton-tipped applicator to move the conjunctiva) and the type of strabismus that was present preoperatively can allow a reasonable guess at what prior surgery has been performed.

SURGICAL PROCEDURE

Anesthesia

Anesthesia for adult strabismus surgery can include pure topical anesthesia (at times augmented with subconjunctival or sub-Tenon injections), topical anesthesia with intravenous sedation, retrobulbar block, or general anesthesia. The decision depends on the surgeon's experience and comfort with these methods, the patient's medical comorbidities, the extent of surgery planned, and whether an adjustable suture is used (see Chapter 1).

Location of Incision

Either a limbal or fornix incision can be used (see Chapter 43). A limbal incision (or hemi-limbal "7" incision) may be more stable and offer improved exposure and dissection in adults with prior strabismus surgery. Fornix incisions in the very elderly (with thin conjunctiva and absent Tenon capsule) are at risk of extending to the limbus. Marking the corners of a limbal incision with a marking pen or tagging suture can allow for improved reapproximation during closure.

Managing Scarring

In patients with prior strabismus surgery, there is often scarring of conjunctiva and Tenon capsule to the prior insertion site. Careful blunt and sharp dissection can reestablish tissue planes and maintain conjunctival integrity. In reoperations, it can be difficult to distinguish scleral adhesions from the true muscle insertion. In this situation, it is prudent to secure the scleral adhesion with a suture in the typical fashion prior to disinserting it and exploring posteriorly. There can also be extensive scarring in cases of orbital hardware (glaucoma drainage devices, scleral buckles), or prior scleral incisions, trauma, or sutures.

Adjustable Sutures

Many strabismus surgeons will utilize an adjustable suture technique in adult patients and children with complex strabismus (see Chapter 48).

- Type of knot: Sliding noose, simple loop, or bowtie knots can be used in cases of immediate or delayed adjustment.
- Timing of adjustment:
  - Intraoperative adjustment usually requires topical anesthesia or quick-acting intravenous agents. Advantages include the ability to maintain monitoring in a sterile environment with the same surgical instruments, minimal muscular edema or inflammation, and no loose sutures or patching postoperatively.
  - Adjustment in the recovery room can be done if OR efficiency, anesthetic choice, or patient cooperation precludes intraoperative adjustment.
  - Delayed same-day adjustment is needed if a retrobulbar block is used (often requiring 4-8 hours for recovery of muscle function). Full ocular rotations should be achieved to assure the block is no longer active.
  - Many surgeons utilize a delayed adjustment, checking the patient's alignment daily until stability is demonstrated and adjusting the suture in the office. The muscle position may be adjusted up to 7 days postoperatively.

POSTOPERATIVE CONSIDERATIONS

Postoperative Diplopia

There may be variable alignment in the initial days to weeks following strabismus surgery as a result of edema, hemorrhage, or inflammation. A slipped muscle should be suspected if rotations are significantly limited into its field of action. Management of disabling postoperative diplopia can include patch or temporary prism (see Chapter 56).

Post-op Spectacles

Patients who wear prism glasses preoperatively may have old glasses without prism; a Fresnel prism with the same power but opposite prism orientation can be placed to neutralize the prism; or new glasses with most recent prescription without prism can be prescribed preoperatively.

ACKNOWLEDGMENTS

Supported by an unrestricted grant from Research to Prevent Blindness.

Suggested Readings

Arnoldi K. Factors contributing to the outcome of sensory testing in patients with anomalous binocular correspondence. *Am Orthopt J*. 2011;61:128-136.

Flodin S, Karlsson P, Andersson Grönlund M. Cyclotorsion measured in a patient population using three different methods: a comparative study. *Strabismus*. 2016;24(1):28-36.

Szigiato AA, Caldwell M, Buys YM, Kraft SP, Mireskandari K. Population trends in adult strabismus surgery. *Can J Ophthalmol*. 2019;54(4):501-508.

CHAPTER 59

Complex Strabismus Pearls

Laura B. Enyedi, MD

GENERAL PEARLS FOR COMPLEX STRABISMUS

- If you do not know which surgery to perform, select the one that is easier and/or has fewer complications.
- Always think ahead. Have a plan B (and C!). Consider staging surgery if very complex.
- Think about comitance and matching deficits.
- Patients usually accept undercorrection better than overcorrection.
- Do not "flip the hyper," especially in downgaze (see below discussion in thyroid eye disease [TED]).
- If there is a muscle restriction, do a surgery that relieves the restriction.
  - Recheck forced ductions intraoperatively after a restricted muscle is removed. Sometimes restrictions will remain even after the muscle is completely off the eye because of orbital tissue involvement (ie, TED). This problem is very difficult to correct.
  - If you cannot relieve the restriction, consider matching the deficit on the fellow eye.
- Make sure you understand the patient's goals for surgery (eg, do they want to "look normal" or are they hoping to regain stereopsis or improve vision), and during the preoperative discussion, carefully communicate what is realistically attainable (see Chapter 58).
- Identify if the patient has any special needs for work or hobbies (eg, diplopia in upgaze is a problem for competitive cyclists or skydivers).
- Adjustable sutures (see Chapter 48) can be a great option in unpredictable situations. BUT…:
  - Choose patients for adjustable sutures carefully. A "rehearsal" with q-tips preoperatively can yield valuable information.
  - Be prepared for bradycardia, asystole, fainting, and vomiting during adjustment procedures. If the patient has a vagal response, have the patient lean the head forward between the knees or lay the examination chair flat with the feet elevated. An alcohol wipe directly under the nose can sometimes alleviate nausea. Be wary of vagal responses in family members present during adjustment.
  - If you cannot make things perfect at the end of a muscle adjustment, leave the patient with the easier deviation to correct during the next surgery.

- Operating on the "good eye" is sometimes necessary for the best outcome.
- Consider the "Law of Diminishing Returns," an economic theory that applies to complex reoperations: The more surgery done on a patient, the lower the expectation for a great result.
  - The patient did not respond to the other surgeries as expected.
  - The anatomy is distorted from the previous surgeries making results even less predictable.
- You cannot fix everyone, and some eyes do not want to be straight!
- In the words of Edward G. Buckley, MD, "Once you operate on a patient, their problem becomes your problem."

STRABISMUS IN THYROID EYE DISEASE (TED)

TED is one of the most common and most challenging forms of incomitant restrictive strabismus.

- General guidelines
  - Smoking is a modifiable risk factor for strabismus in TED. Encourage patients to stop or reduce smoking!
  - Patients often need multiple surgeries (orbital, strabismus, lid).
    - Orbital decompression is done first because it can affect strabismus.
    - Strabismus surgery is done next.
      - Can impact lid position.
        - Especially worsened lid retraction with vertical muscle recessions.
        - Warn patients about worsening of dry eye and cosmesis.
    - Eyelid surgery is the last step.
  - Avoid operating on patients in the active phase of disease.
    - Patients are often eager for their surgery and may pressure you to do surgery expediently.
      - TED is often disfiguring, and diplopia can be very disabling for patients.
      - Depression and anxiety are common in patients with TED.

Using a clinical activity score can be helpful in determining if a patient has active disease. Signs of active disease vary and may include conjunctival chemosis and injection, lid swelling, lid retraction, proptosis, strabismus, exposure keratopathy, and optic neuropathy. If a patient has moderate to severe active disease consider treatment with IV pulse steroid administration (commonly used in Europe). In addition, teprotumumab (insulinlike growth factor-1 receptor inhibitory antibody) has shown promising results in clinical trials for reducing proptosis and alleviating diplopia.

Some patients with dysthyroid optic neuropathy do not show signs of active disease. Abnormal color vision, exophthalmometry >20 mm, and visual field defects (arcuate or altitudinal defects, central/paracentral scotomas, or generalized depression) are common. Most of these patients have normal-appearing optic nerves. Apical muscle crowding is usually seen in patients with dysthyroid optic neuropathy. If there is a delay in treatment, patients can develop permanent optic nerve atrophy and irreversible vision loss.

- Strabismus measurements should be stable for 4-6 months pre-op.
  - While awaiting stability, the goal is to help the patient function with diplopia (see Chapter 56).
    - Incomitance limits the use of prisms to correct diplopia.
    - Fresnel prisms are often used because of the size and variability of the deviation.
    - For some patients, the size of the deviation makes suppression or ignoring the second image easier. When the strabismus improves and the images

come closer together, the brain may have more difficulty ignoring the second image. Discuss this with patients preoperatively.
    - Patching or use of occlusive foils can be helpful.
  - Consider oral steroids for a short time (days-week) before and after strabismus surgery if the patient has had a difficult course (very severe, difficult to control, relapses) or still seems inflamed.
- Set realistic goals for surgery with the patient.
  - Focus on achieving orthotropia in primary and reading position.
  - Expand binocular field of single vision.
  - Decrease anomalous head position.
  - Alleviate torsion.
  - Patient may still be able to "find" diplopia.
    - Incomitance is common postoperatively.
    - Patients may need prism postoperatively.
- Consider comitance and torsion:
  - The most important fields for most patients are primary gaze and down gaze.
  - Beware of "flipping the vertical" in downgaze!
    - Patients do NOT tolerate reversing the hypertropia and will usually be more comfortable undercorrected than overcorrected.
    - The amount of prism the patient can tolerate in downgaze helps determine how much inferior rectus (IR) recession can be done without causing reversal of the hypertropia.
  - Consider torsion especially with involvement of vertical muscles.
  - Consider torsion if the patient cannot fuse with prism at the corrected angle.
- The normal strabismus tables (see Chapter 42) are guidelines for surgical amounts but often do not apply well in TED.
  - May need big surgery for small deviations and small surgery for big deviations:
    - Small vertical deviations may require asymmetric bilateral surgery in larger amounts than would be expected for the size of the deviation.
    - Small recessions of very tight muscles may give larger than anticipated effects, especially if antagonist muscles are involved.
  - Results are unpredictable and reoperation rates are high (40%-60%):
    - Some need for postoperative prism is common.
  - Consider the use of adjustable sutures (see Chapter 48):
    - The deviation can change days to weeks after surgery.
    - Late overcorrections are the most common postoperative change.
      - Especially problematic with IR recession to "flip the hyper."
        - In general, patients tolerate undercorrection of hypertropia better than any overcorrection.
      - Leave patients undergoing IR recession undercorrected by several prism diopters, especially if they can fuse with a slight chin up.

Because of the tendency for late overcorrection in these cases possibly due to scar elongation and slippage, there has been debate regarding the use of adjustable verses nonadjustable suture techniques and absorbable verses nonabsorbable suture in TED. It is felt that the use of absorbable and adjustable sutures might impede anchorage of the muscle to the sclera. However, multiple studies have found better success rates with adjustable suture use.

      - If you do overcorrect these patients and reverse the hypertropia:
        - Consider advancing the recessed IR rather than recessing a superior rectus (SR) so that you can get the desired correction in downgaze.
        - Consider posterior fixation suture ("adjustable Faden") on the contralateral eye (see Chapter 49).

- Forced duction testing (FDT) is important to evaluate restrictions and guide the surgical approach and surgical amounts.
- Patients often have dry eye and exposure; keep the cornea well lubricated during strabismus surgery. A small moistened Weck-cell sponge can be placed over the cornea to keep it from drying out during surgery.
- Strabismus is often complex with multiple muscles involved in one or both eyes.
  - Imaging may help guide diagnosis and surgical approach (see Chapter 57).
  - The most common muscles involved are the IR and medial rectus (MR).
  - The SR and lateral rectus (LR), and rarely the oblique muscles may also be involved.
  - Most patients have bilateral but asymmetric involvement.
  - Orbital tissues are also involved and can contribute to the restrictive strabismus. Taking the muscle off the eye may not completely relieve the restriction.
- Consider effects of restriction and strabismus surgery on the secondary and tertiary actions of the muscle as well as the primary action.
  - IR involvement may worsen esotropia.
    - Be cautious with MR recession at same time as IR recession—because of A-pattern exotropia (XT) postoperatively (see below).
- Be particularly cognizant of torsional effects and pattern strabismus.
  - Extorsion is common and often relieved with IR recession.
  - Intorsion is less common and can be difficult to treat.
    - Superior oblique (SO) involvement (uncommon) may cause more intorsion (or less extorsion) than one would expect with tight IR's.
    - SO tenotomies may not have as much torsional effects in TED as one would normally expect because of orbital tissue involvement.
    - DelMonte described inferior oblique (IO) advance and superior transposition (see Chapter 46) as an effective technique for intorsion in TED (Fig. 59.1, VIDEO Video 59.1).
      - Transpose the IO under the LR and suture the IO at the superior edge of the LR and 8-mm posterior to LR insertion.
      - Corrects about 10 degrees intorsion per eye.
      - Can do bilaterally for more torsion effect.
      - Collapses A-pattern.
  - For vertical deviations with small amounts of torsion, consider combining IR recession w/contralateral SR recession (also see below).
    - Balances torsional effects.
    - Reduces the amount of IR recession needed (and potentially avoids overcorrecting the hyper in downgaze).

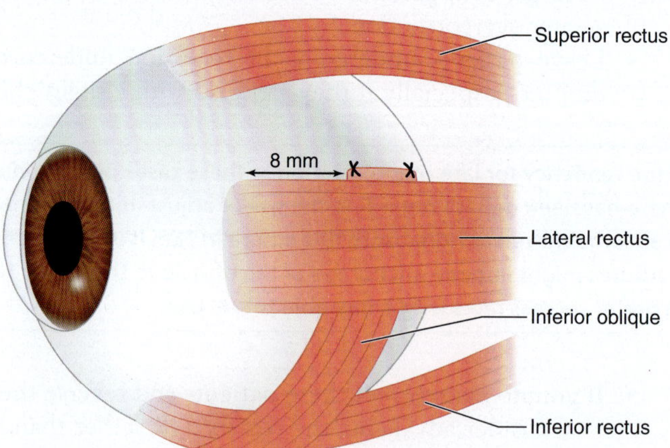

FIGURE 59.1. Inferior oblique advancement under the lateral rectus to treat intorsion in TED.

- Bilateral IR recession can create A-pattern XT in downgaze.
  - To avoid this problem, consider unilateral IR recession if possible.
  - For bilateral IR involvement with hypertropia:
    - Do bilateral asymmetric recessions of IR, and leave patient fusing with a slight chin up position.
  - Consider nasal transposition or nasal collapse of the IR (this may worsen the intorsion).
  - Consider superior transposition of the MR (this may worsen the intorsion).
- Be aware of masked restrictions.
  - SO involvement can be masked by tight IR's.
    - Difficult to assess the SO with FDT in the presence of tight IR's.
    - SO involvement may contribute to postoperative A-pattern following IR recession.
  - LR involvement may give bigger than expected results with MR recession.
  - SR involvement may contribute to large vertical deviations.
    - Consider IR recession w/contralateral SR recession:
      - Will limit torsional effect (balancing extorter and intorter).
      - Will help prevent overcorrection in downgaze.
      - Will help correct esotropia (ET) (weakening 2 adductors).
- Typically avoid resections in TED, BUT sometimes a small resection of an LR or SR is a better option than overrecession of the MR or IR, respectively.
- Remember myasthenia gravis (MG) in TED patients:
  - Patients with TED have a higher than normal incidence of MG.
  - Patients with MG have a higher than normal incidence of TED.
  - Both can cause incomitant, variable strabismus.
  - Be particularly suspicious of MG in patients with TED with ptosis instead of lid retraction.

STRABISMUS SURGERY AFTER SCLERAL BUCKLE (SB)

Strabismus after SB can be challenging and unpredictable.

- Obtain operative report from SB procedure if possible.
- Consider preoperative examination by a retina specialist to ensure that the retina is attached on the buckle and whether or not the buckle can be partially or completely removed.
- If the patient is amenable, surgery on the fellow, non-SB, eye is usually easier and more predictable.
- If there is significant restriction in the eye with the SB, then surgery on the buckled eye may be necessary.
- Results are unpredictable so consider use of adjustable sutures (see chapter 48).
- Be prepared for anatomic challenges:
  - Conjunctival scarring makes access and closing challenging.
  - Expect adhesions between muscles and between the muscle and the buckle.
  - The buckle may be located where the muscle should attach.

The muscle and buckle can be thoroughly exposed and cleaned, and sutures and the muscle can be passed underneath the buckle and be permanently attached or left for adjustment. If using this technique on an adjustable suture, be sure that the muscle slides well under the buckle (Fig. 59.2).

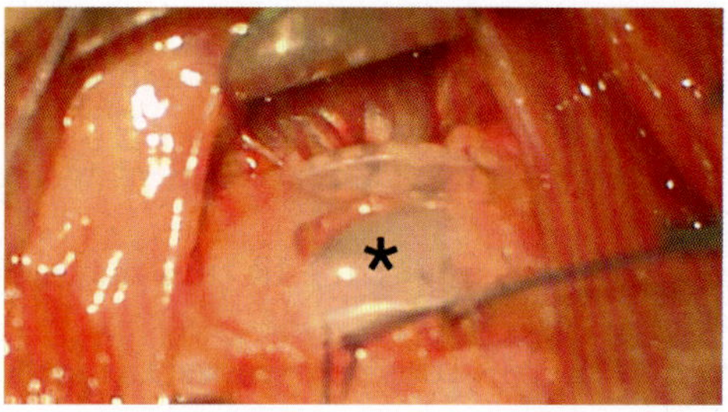

FIGURE 59.2. The buckle (*asterisk*) has been dissected free, and the rectus muscle has been disinserted and the sutures secured at the original insertion (anterior to the buckle). Both the sutures and the muscle slide under the buckle. This technique can be used for adjustable sutures with either recession or resection. (Courtesy of Federico Velez, MD.)

- The muscle tissue overlying the buckle may be friable, increasing the risk of muscle damage or slippage (see Chapter 54).
- The sclera around the implant may be thin, impacting where and how deep scleral passes are made:
  - Increased risk of muscle slippage (see Chapter 54).
  - Increased risk of scleral perforation (see Chapter 54).

If the muscle is being attached posterior to the buckle, the sutures can be passed under the buckle and secured to more anterior sclera or through the buckle itself and the muscle allowed to hang back.

- Sensory challenges (see Chapter 56):
  - Fusion may be disrupted.
  - The patient may have torsion.

STRABISMUS SURGERY WITH GLAUCOMA DRAINAGE DEVICE (GDD)

Patients often have large incomitant restrictive strabismus making prisms unhelpful. If the restriction is mild, then consider operating on the fellow eye without the GDD. Patients often have significant vision loss and may be reluctant to undergo surgery on the fellow "good eye." Visual field restriction and vision loss can also cause sensory difficulties. Finally, these surgeries are technically challenging and carry significant risks not usually associated with strabismus surgery.

- Etiology of strabismus:
  - Trauma to extraocular muscle.
  - Muscle stretching or distortion by the bleb.
  - Fibrous capsule formation.
  - Fat adherence.
  - Scarring of extraocular muscles to the GDD, capsule, and/or sclera.
- Pre-op:
  - Review operative notes and determine location, type, and size of GDD.
  - Consult glaucoma specialist about surgical plan and consider joint surgery:
    - The strabismus surgery could jeopardize the function of the GDD.
    - The GDD may need to be altered or removed.
      - Resection of the plate.
      - Repositioning of the plate.
      - Ligature of the tube.
    - The patient is at risk for hypotony and/or IOP spikes.

SURGICAL PROCEDURE: STRABISMUS SURGERY WITH GDD (VIDEO 59.2)

- Perform FDT to identify restrictions, repeat intraoperatively to confirm release of restrictions.
- Use an operating microscope.
- Be aware that the patient is at risk of abrupt hypotony and collapse of the anterior chamber if the GDD capsule is perforated:
  - Consider creating a limbal paracentesis prior to dissection in case the anterior chamber needs to be reformed.
  - Inject viscoelastic or filtered air to reform the chamber; viscoelastic may need to be removed at the end of the case to prevent a large IOP spike.
  - Consider suturing a small capsule rupture using an 8-0 or 9-0 Vicryl on a BV (round) needle.
  - If extensive capsule resection planned, consider tube ligation.
  - If valved GDD, ligation may not be necessary.
- Use a fornix incision on the side of the muscle away from the GDD.

If the capsule is very large and/or a decision has been made preoperatively to dissect the capsule or alter the GDD, then a limbal incision or fornix incision over the GDD may give better exposure. This should be carefully planned with the glaucoma specialist as these approaches are very likely to disrupt the capsule.

- Hook the muscle using a thin hook (eg, Katena).
- Use the hook to gently dissect the muscle away from the fibrous capsule.

It is usually better to split the muscle leaving a bit of the muscle attached to the capsule rather than to enter the capsule.

- Once the muscle is dissected free and disinserted, recheck FDT. If the restriction is not significantly improved, consider more dissection (but be ready for hypotony as discussed above).
- Consider a hang-back recession if scarring and/or small incision size make exposure difficult.
- Risks (in addition to typical risks of strabismus surgery):
  - Jeopardization of functioning GDD.
  - Cataract.
  - Dislocation of IOL.
  - Hypotony.
  - Difficulty closing conjunctiva.
  - Endophthalmitis.
  - Intraocular pressure spikes postoperatively.

SLIPPED, LOST, SEVERED, TRAUMATIZED MUSCLES (SEE ALSO CHAPTER 54)

Muscles can retract or "slip" within their capsule or the muscle and surrounding tissues can retract into the orbit and become "lost." These situations may be recognized intraoperatively or postoperatively. Muscles can spontaneously rupture intraoperatively (see pulled-in-two syndrome (PITS) below) or the muscle can be contused, torn or severed from trauma (eg, orbital fracture, penetrating orbital injury, sinus surgery).

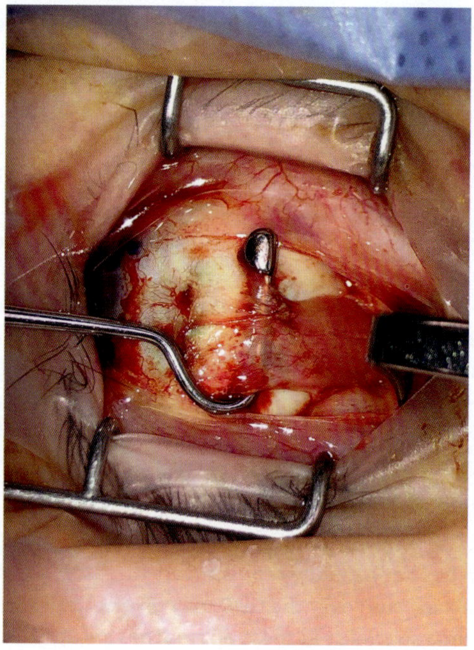

FIGURE 59.3. Stretched scar on recessed MR. Note the whiter fibrotic tissue closer to the muscle hook and the more normal MR tendon slanting more posteriorly. The patient had undergone bilateral MR recessions as a child and presented with long-standing large alternating XT with mildly reduced adduction in both eyes. Both MR had a similar appearance. The scar was resected and the muscle advanced OU with good results.

Slipped and Lost Muscles

- Clinical signs:
  - Incomitant deviation with either over- or undercorrection.
  - Duction lag in the field of action of the affected muscle.
  - Slight proptosis.
  - Lid fissure widening in the field of action of the affected muscle (eg, lid fissure widening on adduction with a slipped MR).
- Differential diagnosis:
  - Over recession of the muscle: treat by advancing muscle.
  - Stretched scar (Fig. 59.3): treat by resecting the stretched scar and reattaching the muscle.

In some cases, it may be difficult to distinguish a slipped muscle from stretched scar because areas of thin translucent tissue and areas of thick white scar may occur within the same attachment. Regardless, there is abnormal rectus muscle attachment, and the treatment requires excision of the anomalous connective tissue and reattachment of the muscle fiber firmly to the sclera. Secure any questionable tissue with suture before disinserting to avoid transecting and losing muscle.

- Surgical Diagnosis and Treatment:
  - Consider preoperative orbital MRI to assist in locating muscles (see Chapter 57).
  - In the case of trauma, consider waiting a few weeks for hemorrhage and edema to subside before exploration and repair. One potential downside to waiting is contracture of the antagonist muscles, so some surgeons advocate early repair in the case of trauma.
  - In the case of postoperative slipped/lost muscles, consider early intervention as the muscle sutures can aid in finding the muscle.
  - Avoid aggressive FDT as the remaining attachments could be disrupted.
  - The MR is the most likely muscle to be "lost" because of its angle of attachment and lack of surrounding muscles to keep it from retracting into the orbit.
    - Consider working with an orbital surgeon as exploration will be along the medial orbital wall (not usually along the globe).

- Do NOT abduct the eye in an attempt to find the MR; this will only allow the muscle to retract back more.
- Use a retractor to push the globe against the lateral orbital wall and retroplace it to expose the area of Tenon capsule where the muscle is most likely to be found.
- The oculocardiac reflex can help identify muscle tissue. Discuss the need for an intact oculocardiac reflex with the anesthesia team and ask them to help identify slowing of the heart rate.

Pulled-in-two Syndrome (PITS)

- Most common muscles: MR and IR.
- Can occur anywhere along length of muscle, but often at junction of tendon and muscle belly, about 10 mm posterior to insertion.
- Risk factors:
  - Cranial nerve palsy.
  - Advanced age.
  - Previous surgery (strabismus or SB).
  - Abnormal muscle (TED, metastases to the muscle, radiation, congenital fibrosis of the extraocular muscles).
  - Excessive traction on the muscle.
- Prevention:
  - Consider using a grooved hook if the muscle is very tight.
  - Use the Wescott scissors with the tips down if the muscle is very tight. Alternatively, a no. 15 Bard Parker Blade may be used to disinsert the muscle.
- Treatment:
  - Try to find and the severed end of the muscle (see lost muscles above).
    - The muscle can be reanastomosed to the stump that is attached to sclera.
    - The muscle stump can be disinserted, and the severed muscle belly can be reattached to the sclera (usually recessed). Expect this to give an effect similar to an "adjustable Faden" (see Chapter 49).
    - If you cannot find or reattach the muscle at the time of surgery, there are several options.
      - A portion of Tenon or muscle capsule can be attached to the globe with variable results.
      - A transposition procedure can be performed (see Chapter 50). Consider ½ tendon width (TW) transposition or Nishida-type procedure to reduce risk of anterior segment ischemia (ASI).
      - Consider waiting to see the resulting deviation and intervening later if needed.
    - Consider using nonabsorbable sutures when reapproximating torn muscle.
    - Be wary of ASI (see chapter 54) with further surgical intervention.

> **Particularly with the IR, the deviation and duction lag may not be as bad as one would think even if the severed muscle is not recovered. The torn muscle attaches to the globe or surrounding tissues during healing, and many of the orbital pulleys remain operational even after the muscle is disinserted.**

Extraocular Muscle Trauma

- **Contusions with blunt trauma:**
  - Hematomas and edema of the muscle can cause restrictions and/or weakening of muscle action.
  - Suspect in blunt trauma with no perforation.
  - The IR is most commonly involved because of the Bell phenomenon.
  - Commonly resolve spontaneously, but complete recovery may take weeks to months.

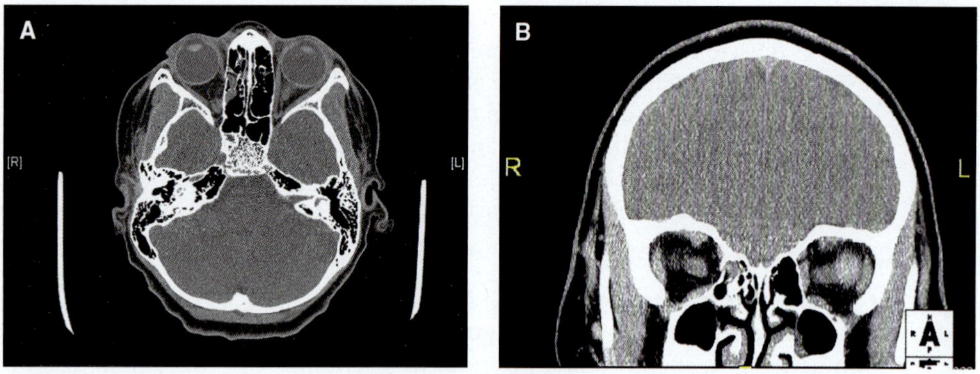

FIGURE 59.4. Axial **(A)** and coronal **(B)** CT images of an 8-year-old child who sustained blunt trauma with right medial wall fracture and entrapment of the MR muscle. The child was exotropic for 2 months after fracture repair, but eventually regained orthotropia with no strabismus surgery. (Courtesy of Jason Liss, MD.)

- **Orbital fractures with extraocular muscle involvement:**
  - Inferior and medial wall fractures most common with blunt trauma (Fig. 59.4A and B).
  - Entrapment of muscles.
    - IR, IO, MR, and SO more common; SR and LR less common.
    - Entrapment of multiple muscles possible, especially if both the medial wall and orbital floor fractured.
    - Inferior fractures:
      - Usually present with incomitant hypotropia:
        - Positive FDT with restriction to upgaze.
        - Positive force generation (ie, the muscle functions).
      - May present with incomitant hypertropia:
        - Forced duction test shows restriction to downgaze.
        - Forced duction may show restriction to upgaze also.
        - Posterior fracture with entrapment.
        - Flap tear of IR with adhesions.

The bigger the fracture, the less likely that the muscle will be incarcerated and compromised. Large blow-out fractures present with periorbital edema and enophthalmos, but little motility disturbance. Small trapdoor fractures carry a high risk of muscle incarceration and significant motility disruption.

- **Special considerations in children:**
  - Children are at higher risk for roof fractures than adults.
  - Children and young adults are at risk for trapdoor fractures:
    - Linear, minimally displaced fracture that "greensticks" open and then bounces back, incarcerating muscle and/or surrounding soft tissues.
    - Significant motility disturbance, especially restriction to upgaze.
    - Early surgery may be indicated to prevent ischemia and necrosis of muscle.
    - "White eye blow-out fracture" more common in children:
      - History of trauma (sports or assault usually) with little evidence of soft tissue injury.
      - Vasovagal symptoms such as nausea, vomiting, and bradycardia are common:
        - High positive predictive value for a trapdoor fracture.
        - Indicate need for urgent intervention.

- **Flap tears of muscle:**
  - Shearing of the outer orbital layer of muscle away from the inner global layer of muscle.
  - Can occur with blunt or penetrating trauma.
  - Usually produces limitation toward the affected muscle (muscle weakening).
  - May also have restrictive component away from affected muscle (eg, restriction to upgaze with IR flap tear).
- **Direct muscle injury:**
  - IR and MR most common, but any muscle at risk.
  - Initially negative FDT (which may become positive later with scarring and restrictions) and reduced force generation.
  - Imaging may be helpful to identify the location and extent of injury.
  - Reapproximation of lacerated muscles should be attempted.
    - If the laceration is posterior, consider an orbitotomy approach with the assistance of an orbital surgeon (see above discussion of slipped and lost muscles).
    - Consider waiting a few weeks for hemorrhage and edema to subside before exploration and repair. One potential downside to waiting is contracture of the antagonist muscles, so some advocate early repair in the case of trauma.
    - Use nonabsorbable sutures to reattach the ends of the muscle if recovered.
    - If the muscle cannot be found or there is significant tissue loss:
      - Transposition procedures (see above and Chapter 50).
      - Tethering procedures (see below).
      - Additional surgeries are often postponed to allow healing and make a more informed surgical plan.
      - Beware of risk of ASI (see Chapter 54).

OCULOMOTOR NERVE (CN III) PALSY

Lesions at different sites along the path of the oculomotor nerve can result in a variety of imbalances of elevation, depression, and adduction as well as effects on levator function, pupillary constriction, and accommodation. Surgical procedures are chosen with a goal of centering and widening the field of single binocular vision. The surgical plan depends on the severity of palsy, muscles involved, presence of secondary contractures, and effects of aberrant regeneration. Large angle XT secondary to complete oculomotor palsy can be very difficult to treat, and the surgical goal for these patients is alignment in primary position. Even this outcome is not always achievable, and patients may not regain binocularity.

Correctly diagnosing and localizing the lesion in CN III palsies is critical prior to surgical intervention. In adults, complete pupil-involving CN III palsy (ptosis, dilated pupil, eye down and out with limited elevation, depression, and adduction) is aneurysm (internal carotid, posterior communicating, posterior cerebral arteries, or cavernous sinus) until proven otherwise and requires urgent imaging. An incomplete CN III palsy also requires MRI/MRA to rule out possible aneurysm. Isolated muscle involvement is more typical of neoplastic masses in the cavernous sinus or orbit and require imaging. Complete pupil-sparing CN III palsies (severe ptosis, eye down and out with limited elevation, depression, and adduction, normal pupil and no other CN palsy or neurologic signs/symptoms) in adults is typically secondary to ischemia, but other causes such as trauma, giant cell arteritis, neoplasm, and rarely aneurysm should be considered. Isolated ischemic CN III palsies should resolve in 6-8 weeks. Further evaluation is required with involvement of other CN's (IV, V, and VI need to be carefully evaluated), other neurologic signs/symptoms, failure to resolve, young age, history of cancer, absence of cardiovascular risk factors, or development of aberrant regeneration (which does not typically occur in ischemic palsies). In children, CN III palsies are rare and usually congenital or secondary to trauma, but children should also be imaged to rule out other etiologies (neoplasms, vascular anomalies). (See also Chapter 57.)

In a patient with acquired ptosis and unusual strabismus, consider MG in the differential diagnosis.

General Considerations

- Ischemic CN III palsies often resolve and typically do not need surgery.
- CN III palsies associated with closed head trauma rarely get spontaneous recovery of binocular single vision.
- Patients need thorough preoperative motility assessment of which muscles are involved and the severity of involvement.
- Carefully evaluate for associated CN IV palsy, which will impact workup and surgical planning.
- There are often restrictions of antagonist muscles in long-standing palsies, and these are addressed with weakening procedures.
- Results may be unpredictable:
  - Consider adjustable sutures (see Chapter 48).
  - Make sure that goals of surgery are clear to the patient and that expectations are reasonable.
- Patients may need multiple procedures:
  - Consider pros/cons of staging strabismus procedures.
  - Ptosis surgery usually follows strabismus surgery.
    - Congenital CN III palsy with amblyogenic ptosis may need earlier ptosis surgery.
    - A ptotic lid blocks diplopia.
    - Make sure the patient will be able to fuse, suppress, or tolerate diplopia prior to lid surgery.
    - A frontalis sling will likely be necessary (see Chapter 38).
    - Consider a conservative approach with impaired Bell phenomenon.
- Children with congenital CN III palsy need aggressive and long-term amblyopia therapy.
- With large MR resections (see below), the medial conjunctiva and plica semilunaris tend to get advanced toward the limbus:
  - Consider tacking the conjunctiva down anterior to the plica with a double-armed 8-0 Vicryl passed through the sclera or muscle belly to keep the plica in place.
  - Consider tacking the conjunctiva down with fibrin glue.
  - Securing the conjunctiva not only makes the appearance better but may also help tether the eye medially.
- Aberrant innervation (synkinesis that occurs from persistent partial oculomotor nerve dysfunction after failure to completely recover):
  - Traumatic CN III palsies almost always develop synkinesis syndromes.
  - If there is elevation of the lid on attempted adduction and an XT.
    - A large LR recess/MR resect of the affected eye may help with ptosis as well as the XT.
    - An LR recess/MR resect of the contralateral eye may work at least as well for the XT and ptosis.
      - Hold up base in prism in front of contralateral (sound) eye, which causes abduction of that eye and synergistic contraction of the palsied MR and contraction of the levator on the affected side (because of the aberrant innervation).
      - Removing the action of the aberrantly innervated muscle may be necessary if it is not helpful to the strabismus.

Surgical Plans for Isolated Muscle Involvement in CN III Palsy

- **Medial rectus:**
  - Mild involvement:
    - Large recession of yoke LR.
    - +/− MR resection.
  - Moderate involvement:
    - Large MR resection.
    - Very large recession of ipsilateral LR.
  - Severe involvement:
    - Large MR resection (>10 mm), very large recession of ipsilateral LR, recession of yoke LR:
      - In general, the patient needs to be esotropic at the end of the procedure or probably not enough surgery has been done.
      - Consider staging recession of yoke LR.
      - Consider adjustable suture on yoke LR.
      - Consider posterior fixation or adjustable faden on yoke LR (see Chapter 49).
    - Consider IR and SR transpositions (see Chapter 50):
      - Transpositions to the MR do not work as well transpositions to the LR (especially in complete palsy affecting the SR and IR function).
      - Large resections of the IR and SR will improve the effect.
      - The transposition will tether the eye medially, NOT provide significant adduction.
      - Partial TW transposition if LR recession planned to avoid ASI.
- **Vertical Rectus Muscles (SR or IR):**
  - Mild involvement:
    - Resection of involved muscle.
    - Weakening of yoke oblique (contralateral IO for SR, contralateral SO for IR).
  - Moderate involvement:
    - Resection of involved muscle with recession of ipsilateral antagonist (ie, vertical recess/resect of involved eye).
  - Severe involvement:
    - Vertical transposition of horizontal rectus muscles.
    - +/− weakening of contralateral eye to match deviation.
      - SR: recess contralateral SR.
      - IR: recess/faden contralateral IR.
- **Inferior oblique:**
  - Mild involvement:
    - Recession of yoke (contralateral) SR.
  - Moderate-severe involvement:
    - Weakening ipsilateral SO.
    - Recession of yoke (contralateral) SR.

Surgical Plans for Multiple Muscle Involvement

- Tailor surgery individually.
- Refer to guidelines for isolated muscle involvement for guidance:
  - Resect involved muscle or transposition to paralytic muscle.
  - Weakening of antagonist.
  - Weakening of contralateral yoke.
- Avoid ASI.
- Small vertical deviations in association with MR weakness:
  - Imbalances of the SR and IR function (hyper- or hypotropia).
  - Intact SO function (hypotropia).

- May be addressed with vertical displacement of the horizontal rectus muscles in conjunction with the horizontal recess/resect to treat XT (eg, shift the MR and LR superiorly ½ TW to correct up to 5 PD of hypotropia).

Surgical Plans for Complete (or Near Complete CN III Palsy)

- Difficult to treat because four of six rectus muscles involved.
- Leave eye slightly adducted with resistance to abduction at the end of surgery.
- **Crippling of the LR:**
  - Adequately weakening the LR is difficult.
  - Very large LR recession (10-14 mm behind insertion).
  - Resection of up to 20 mm and then release of LR.
  - Tethering of LR to the lateral orbital periosteum:
    - Challenging, but often best way to ensure LR will not reattach to globe.
    - Clean the LR very far back (~15 mm posterior to insertion).
    - Use a nonabsorbable polyester suture such as 5-0 or 6-0 Prolene or Mersilene on a curved cutting needle to imbricate the muscle, then disinsert the muscle.
    - Expose the adjacent periosteum ~5 mm posterior to the orbital rim and use two periosteal bites to attach the LR to the lateral orbital wall.
      - Exposure can be difficult.
      - Consider working with an orbital surgeon.
    - Close the cut edges of the intermuscular septum over the sclera to help prevent reattachment of the LR to the globe.
    - Close the conjunctiva, recessing if tight.
  - The eye should be free to adduct after LR crippling. If not, consider that the SO tendon may also be tight and may also need to be weakened (which may result in hypertropia).
- **Globe tethering procedures:**
  - Goal is to tether eye in primary position; eye will have little movement.
  - MR resection (10-14 mm).
  - Medial globe tethering to orbital periosteum (Fig. 59.5) with nonabsorbable suture (5-0 or 6-0 Prolene or Mersilene) from the MR insertion to the medial periosteum.
    - This can be especially useful if the MR cannot be resected or if the globe is not in adduction after maximal MR resection and LR recession.
    - Be careful to avoid injury to nasolacrimal sac and medial canthal tendon.
    - Consider working with an orbital surgeon.
  - Attach the SO tendon to the superior border of the MR.
  - Y Split and transpose the LR to the MR insertion (Fig. 59.6):
    - Technically challenging.
    - The upper half of the LR is transposed to the superior border of the MR insertion, and the lower half of the LR is transposed to the inferior border of the MR insertion.
    - Split the LR as far posteriorly as possible and imbricate each half on a nonabsorbable suture.
    - Pass the superior ½ of the LR behind the SO insertion under the SR and SO complex. Attach adjacent to the superior edge of the MR insertion.
    - Pass the inferior ½ of the LR between the IR and sclera. Attach adjacent to the inferior edge of the MR.
    - Tighten the two halves simultaneously, rather than doing one at a time because the globe may be too tight after tying the first ½ of LR down to transpose the other half.
    - If the muscle is tight, may need to symmetrically hangback the two halves.
    - Consider adding a posterior fixation suture to each 1/2 of the LR (Fig. 59.6).
    - Complications include transitory serous retinal detachment.

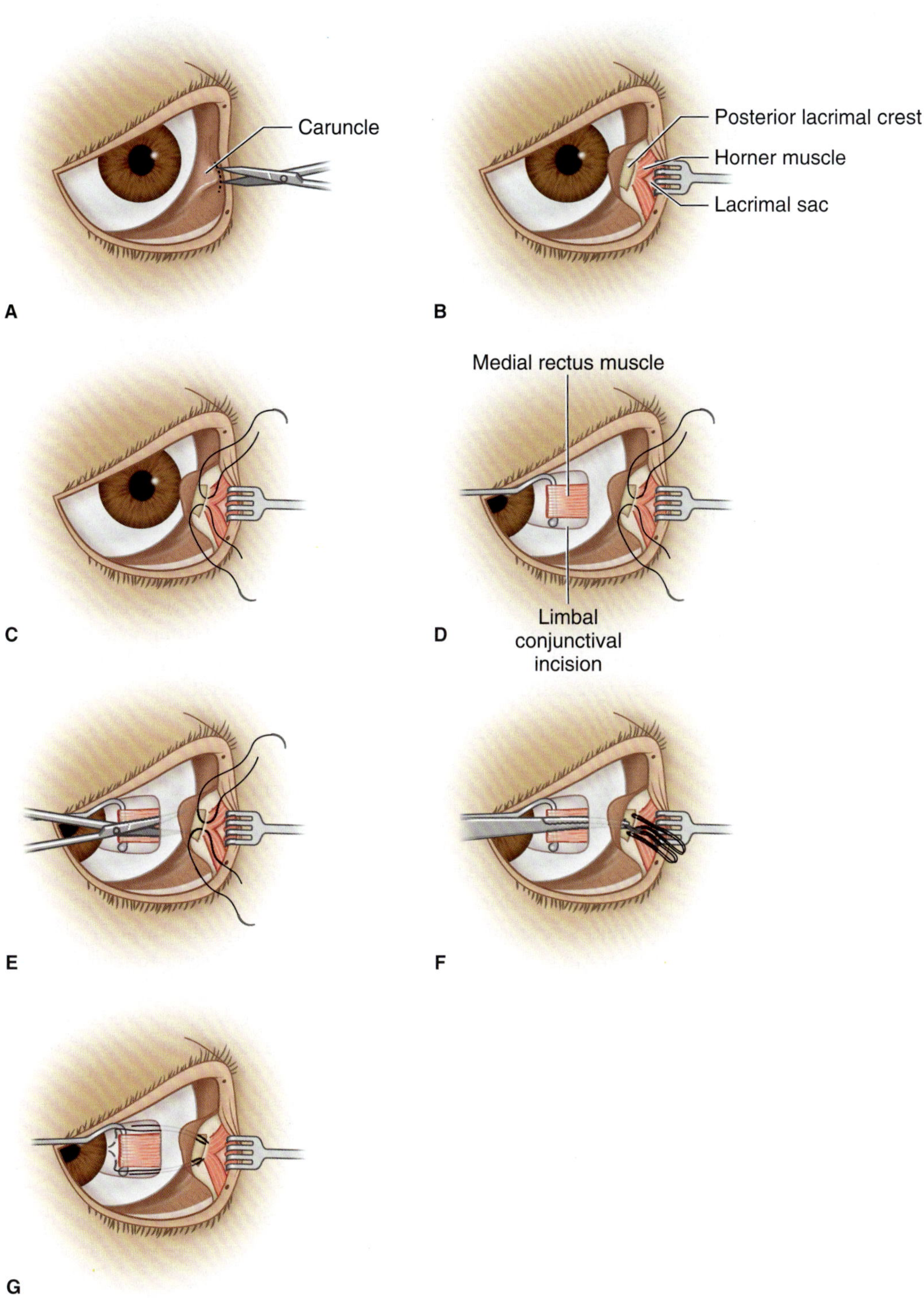

FIGURE 59.5. Schematic diagram showing medial periosteal fixation of the right globe. **(A)** Incision at precaruncular area, **(B)** exposure of posterior lacrimal crest, **(C)** passing of nonabsorbable sutures through posterior lacrimal crest, **(D)** exposure of medial rectus muscle through limbal conjunctival incision, **(E)** creating a sub-Tenons tunnel with the Wescott scissors, **(F)** The nonabsorbable suture are passed towards the limbus through the conjunctival tunnel with a hemostat or blunt forceps. **(G)** Secure the sutures just anterior to the medial rectus insertion with partial-thickness scleral bites and tie down to pull the globe medially.

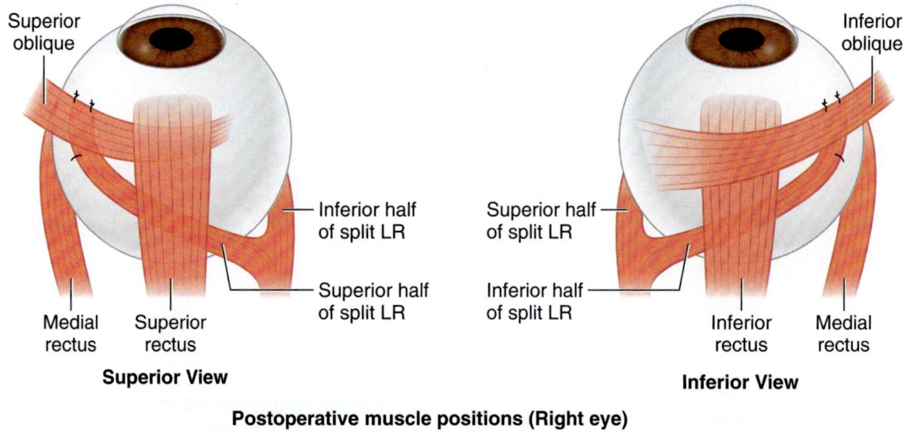

FIGURE 59.6. Y split and transposition of lateral rectus (LR) to medial rectus. (Modified from Saxena R, Sharma M, Singh D, et al. Medial transposition of split lateral rectus augmented with fixation sutures in cases of complete third nerve palsy. *Br J Ophthalmol*. 2016;100:585-587.)

SURGICAL ERRORS AND MIX-UPS

The nature of strabismus surgery makes surgical errors and confusion common. It is easy and relatively common to do the wrong strabismus procedure (eg, resect a muscle that should be recessed) and/or the wrong muscle and/or the wrong eye. In addition, globe torsion and anatomical difficulties can be disorienting and contribute to surgery on the wrong muscle, especially with fornix surgery and reoperations.

- Reducing human error in strabismus surgery:
  - Preoperatively:
    - If your preoperative measurements are confusing, unstable, or difficult to obtain or interpret, consider another appointment and/or examination by another person (eg, orthoptist, partner).
    - Make and document a specific surgical plan preoperatively (eg, plan: BMR recession for ET 20), preferably when you are examining the patient.
    - Have the patient's strabismus measurements and specific surgical plan available in the operating room (eg, taped to the wall) and refer to it prior to each incision.
      - "Recess" and "Resect" look very similar, especially when viewed from across the room; consider using terminology like "Strengthen" and "Weaken" when writing up the surgical plan that you will refer to intraoperatively.
    - Perform a surgical time-out to include correct patient, deviation, specific muscles, and intended procedure (eg, this is Jane Doe who will have right medial recess and right lateral plication for esotropia).
  - Intraoperatively:
    - Beware of possible sources of error and clues for identifying the correct muscle:
      - Significant bleeding.
      - Muscle not in anticipated location.
      - Muscle fibers not oriented in the expected direction.
      - The insertion appears too wide or narrow.
    - If in doubt, pause; recheck position of globe; hook adjacent muscles if necessary, to confirm orientation.
    - If you are not sure of the identity of tissue (muscle vs connective tissue), put a suture in the tissue to tag it before removing the tissue from the globe.
    - Be particularly alert to the possibility of error when there are multiple distractions or other unusual events occurring.

- In the event of an error:
  - Try to correct the problem as soon as possible.
  - Call risk management.
    - Document as advised.
    - Discuss billing with risk management.
      - Make sure that the patient is not charged for any surgery needed to correct the problem.
      - Risk management may or may not advise waiving charges for the original procedure.
  - Disclosure:
    - Explain to the patient what happened and how you will remedy the situation as well as any plans to prevent similar problems in the future.
    - Apologize. It will make you feel better and has been shown to reduce litigation.
    - File a safety report in the hopes that "system changes" can occur to help prevent similar errors in the future.
    - Make yourself available to the patient and family postoperatively for questions or concerns, even if you refer the patient to another specialist. The patient and family will need your support as they navigate the postoperative period. Try to show empathy, concern, and patience. Make sure to listen carefully to what the patient has to say.

The patient you most want to avoid is often the one you need to spend the most time with, and these patients can take a lot of time.

    - Assist the patient in finding another qualified surgeon if they do not want to continue your relationship. Offer to arrange a second opinion if you feel it would help the patient.
      - Consider contacting the new doctor by phone to explain what happened and give him or her a "heads-up" about the upcoming consultation.
      - Make sure records are accurate and available to the new physician.
  - Take care of yourself:
    - Seek support from trusted colleagues, mentors, and friends, while maintaining confidentiality. If you are concerned about medicolegal risk, speak in theoreticals and abstractions (eg, tell your partner about a "friend" who did the wrong surgery on a patient and feels awful about it).
    - Expect to feel shame, anxiety, loss of confidence, sadness, frustration, regret, and anger (at yourself, the patient, others involved in the case). You may experience insomnia and depression.
    - Consider seeking professional help if symptoms are severe or long-lasting.

Suggested Readings

Cherfan CG, Traboulsi EI. Slipped, severed, torn, and lost extraocular muscles. *Can J Ophthalmol.* 2011:46:501-509.

Del Monte MA, Richard G. Scobee Memorial Lecture. 2001—An ocular odyssey: Lessons learned from 25 years of surgical treatment for Graves' eye disease. *Am Orthoptic J.* 2002;52:40-57.

Del Monte MA. Management of direct extraocular muscle trauma. *Am Orthoptic J.* 2014;54:32-44.

Ellis EM, Kinori M, Robbins SL, Granet DB. Pulled-in-two syndrome: a multicenter survey of risk factors, management and outcomes. *J AAPOS.* 2016;20:387-391.

Gokyigit B, Akar S, Satana B, Demirok A, Yilmaz OF. Medial transposition of a split lateral rectus muscle for complete oculomotor nerve palsy. *J AAPOS.* 2013;17:402-410.

Kim A, Nejad M, Pineles S, Chang M, Velez F. A modified technique for strabismus surgery in the presence of a scleral buckle. *J AAPOS.* 2016;20(4):376-378.

Lee AR, Talsania SD, Go M, Freedman SF. Strabismus surgery in the setting of glaucoma drainage devices in the pediatric population. *J AAPOS*. 2019;23:83.e1-83.e8.

Molinari AD. Strabismus following extraocular muscle trauma. https://www.aao.org/disease-review/strabismus-following-extraocular-muscle-trauma

Morad Y, Kowal L, Scott AB. Lateral rectus muscle disinsertion and reattachment to the lateral orbital wall. *Br J Ophthalmol*. 2005;89(8):983-985.

Shen E, Porco T, Rutar T. Errors in strabismus surgery. *JAMA Ophthalmol*. 2013;131(1): 75-79.

Wang Y, Patel A, Douglas RS. Thyroid eye disease: how a novel therapy may change the treatment paradigm. *Ther Clin Risk Manag*. 2019;15:1305-1318. doi: 10.2147/TCRM.S193018. PMID: 31814726; PMCID: PMC6858302.

Yanovitch T, Buckley E. Diagnosis and management of third nerve palsy. *Curr Opin Ophthalmol*. 2007;18:373-378.

Index

Note: Figures and tables are indicated with "*f*" and "*t*," respectively.

H

R

T

U